THE MATTER OF THE HEART

THE MATTER OF THE HEART

A History of the Heart in Eleven Operations

THOMAS MORRIS

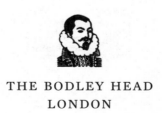

THE BODLEY HEAD
LONDON

1 3 5 7 9 10 8 6 4 2

The Bodley Head, an imprint of Vintage Publishing,
20 Vauxhall Bridge Road,
London SW1V 2SA

The Bodley Head is part of the Penguin Random House group of companies
whose addresses can be found at global.penguinrandomhouse.com.

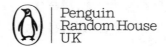

Penguin
Random House
UK

First published by The Bodley Head in 2017

www.penguin.co.uk/vintage

A CIP catalogue record for this book is available from the British Library

Hardback ISBN 9781847923912
Trade Paperback ISBN 9781847923929

Typeset in India by Integra Software Services Pvt. Ltd, Pondicherry

Printed and bound by Clays Ltd, St Ives plc

Penguin Random House is committed to a sustainable future for
our business, our readers and our planet. This book is made
from Forest Stewardship Council® certified paper.

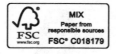

MIX
Paper from
responsible sources
FSC
www.fsc.org FSC® C018179

CONTENTS

The heart and its blood vessels

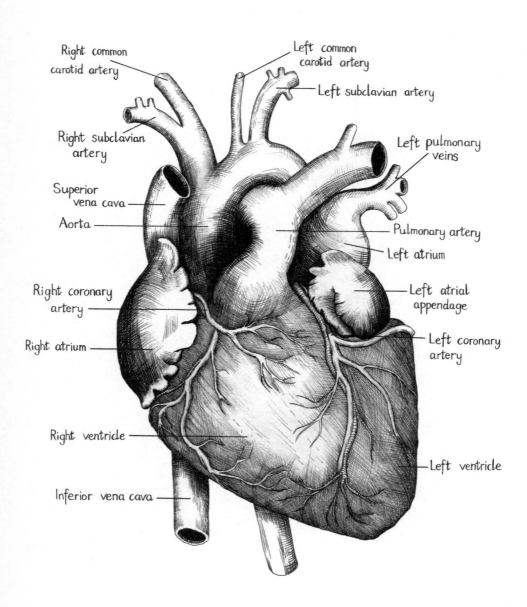

Right common carotid artery

Left common carotid artery

Left subclavian artery

Right subclavian artery

Left pulmonary veins

Superior vena cava

Aorta

Pulmonary artery

Left atrium

Right coronary artery

Left atrial appendage

Right atrium

Left coronary artery

Right ventricle

Left ventricle

Inferior vena cava

Interior structures of the heart

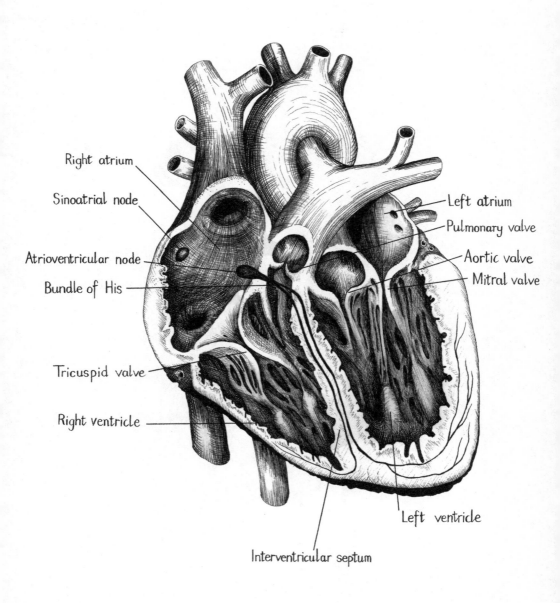

Right atrium

Sinoatrial node

Atrioventricular node

Bundle of His

Tricuspid valve

Right ventricle

Left atrium

Pulmonary valve

Aortic valve

Mitral valve

Left ventricle

Interventricular septum

INTRODUCTION

A few months ago I was walking through a large teaching hospital with one of the consultants, a surgeon of some eminence, when he turned to me and asked: 'Why do you want to write a book about heart surgeons? We're all psychopaths.'

Although tempted to reply, 'Precisely *because* you're all psychopaths,' I just laughed; while this affable man had an impressive ability to monopolise any conversation, I was pretty sure he was no psychopath. And after spending many hours in the company of cardiac surgeons, both in their operating theatres and in more unguarded moments, the one thing that struck me about them was how difficult they were to pigeonhole. True, I'd met one or two who spoke fluently and with a startling lack of modesty about their own achievements, deftly sidestepping any questions that threatened to take us into neutral territory. But others were diffident almost to a fault, more comfortable talking about their mentors and patients than about themselves. Then there were those who were simply fascinated by the minutiae of their craft, happily explaining techniques and procedures to me at length until an exasperated secretary put a head round the door to shoo them off to a more important engagement. Most seemed to be normal and well adjusted – more blessed with self-confidence than most of the population, perhaps, but also friendly and compassionate, and manifestly devoted to helping their patients get better.

So at first I dismissed the surgeon/psychopath association as a self-deprecating joke. But why had he said 'psychopaths'? 'Egotists' or 'narcissists' would have been just as funny, and probably more accurate, I thought. And then I stumbled across a study in the *Bulletin of the Royal College of Surgeons of England* which asked simply: 'Are surgeons psychopaths?'[1] The authors assessed 172 doctors for the traits typical of psychopathy, including 'Machiavellian egocentricity', 'social potency' and 'cold-heartedness'. Surgeons scored particularly highly on this scale, exceeded only by paediatricians in their psychopathic tendencies.* The most commonly identified personality traits in surgeons were stress immunity and fearlessness – qualities which, the researchers noted, are 'beneficial or even essential' when providing care in difficult situations.

Not long afterwards I spent a day in the operating theatre of Marjan Jahangiri, a charismatic surgeon based at St George's Hospital in Tooting. Standing next to the anaesthetist at the head of the table, I had the best possible view as Professor Jahangiri prepared to replace a diseased heart valve. The first part of the procedure had already been completed, the patient's chest lay open and I could clearly see his motionless and empty heart, temporarily relieved of its work by the heart-lung machine a few feet away, which was now oxygenating his blood and circulating it through his body. Professor Jahangiri picked up a pair of scissors and in one smooth motion severed the aorta, the artery that normally carries oxygenated blood from the heart to the rest of the body. Involuntarily I took a large gulp of air: I was taken aback by the insouciance with which she had cut the heart loose from its moorings, somehow transforming it from an integral part of the human machine into a distinct and isolated viscus.

Why was this moment so shocking? It was only later, as I watched her replace the man's diseased aortic valve and then reconstruct his aorta with a tubular graft of synthetic fabric, that I understood. It was the point at which there could be no turning back, when the patient became entirely reliant on the skill of an experienced surgeon

---

* As the authors of the study point out, the test they used 'only confers an actual diagnosis of psychopathic personality when an individual scores highly across *all* of the subdivisions'. Displaying a few traits typical of a psychopath is a long way from actually being one.

to ensure that he left the operating theatre alive and with his heart beating once more. Only somebody with absolute confidence in their abilities could pick up those scissors and be happy to continue. This, I realised, was the fearlessness that all cardiac surgeons need in order to do their job.

Every contemporary heart surgeon has lost a patient, and all need to confront the sobering fact that a single mistake may be all that separates life and death. But the truth is that cardiac surgery today is safer than it has ever been: there is a wide repertoire of operations which have become routine, and so safe that the vast majority of patients make an excellent recovery. Many surgeons walk into theatre expecting every patient to pull through; it is the rarity of death that makes it all the more shocking. So what must it have been like to be a member of the profession in the early years, when death was not merely an occasional visitor but the cardiac surgeon's constant companion?

Surgeons were so convinced of the unique fragility of the heart that they scarcely dared touch it until the last years of the nineteenth century. The first successful operation on the beating heart took place in 1896, but for almost forty years the only interventions possible would remain simple suture repairs for stab or bullet wounds. Specialists were sure that the scalpel would one day provide relief from many other cardiac conditions – and they were right – but achieving that progress took many decades and entailed a shocking loss of life. The only way of establishing the efficacy of a new procedure was to test it on a patient, and the few plausible candidates for such experimental surgery would usually be so sick that their death was likely whatever happened. For some new operations, therefore, surgeons were braced for the possibility that few, if any, of their patients would make any sort of recovery. And it was not just human lives at stake: virtually every major cardiac procedure was first tested on rabbits, dogs, apes, calves or pigs, many thousands of them – indeed, far more experimental animals died during the twentieth century than did patients.

Pioneers in such a brutal field required perseverance and an extraordinary degree of emotional resilience. Unsurprisingly, many of those attracted to this unforgiving occupation were powerful characters, with strong opinions and unshakeable faith in their own abilities. This was a true medical elite: it is easily forgotten that fifty years ago heart surgeons were the most glamorous and best paid professionals in the world, celebrities who were photographed for the cover of *Time* magazine and became the friends of royalty and film stars. Some made colossal fortunes which they spent on property empires or fleets of luxury cars; others donated their considerable surgical income to the hospitals for which they worked. Many were tyrants, impossible men who worked seven days a week and expected the same of their juniors, and bitter rivalries were commonplace. And they were usually men: for years this was an almost exclusively male club, a bastion of inequality which did not begin to admit women in significant numbers until the turn of the millennium.

Much else has changed. If cardiac surgeons were quasi-deities in the 1960s, it was partly because there were so few of them, a select number willing and able to tamper with an organ traditionally seen as the repository of the soul. Today there are close to fifty centres of cardiac surgery in the UK alone, and every developed nation has hundreds or even thousands of highly trained surgeons. There is no longer such mystique surrounding the profession, and (with few exceptions) the surgeon has willingly stepped down from his pedestal. In some hospital departments, treatment is now overseen by a multi-disciplinary 'heart team', in which anaesthetists, surgeons, cardiologists and medical-imaging specialists all play an equal role, and discussion of a case may only take place if the patient is present.[2] The dictator has become a member of a democratic assembly.

Though the body count in this story is high, it is also full of unexpected recoveries, exhilarating moments of discovery, and celebrations of human ingenuity. Its heroes and heroines are not just those who held the surgical instruments, but also the armies of nurses, physiologists, engineers, biochemists and inventors who made their work possible; and of course the many patients, and their families, who willingly allowed their bodies to be used as glorified laboratory specimens. This is not a comprehensive history of the subject, and I have had to be highly selective in which operations and individuals to include; many other important contributions were made which, with regret, I was unable to acknowledge. At times progress was driven by competitive individuals, at others it was a team effort; but what they achieved was miraculous, and I hope readers will share my admiration for these brave pioneers.

1. BULLET TO THE HEART

Stowell Park, Gloucestershire,
19 February 1945

A few minutes' drive south of the pretty market town of Northleach, in the heart of the Cotswolds, is a pub called the Inn at Fossebridge. If you park here, as I did one blustery spring afternoon, and climb a steep hill, you'll soon come to a small wood that lies beside a Roman road, the Fosse Way. It's a peaceful spot filled with birdsong, and as you tramp through the undergrowth it seems scarcely possible that this was the scene of one of the great feats of modern medicine. But seventy years ago this unremarkable little wood was the birthplace of modern heart surgery.

The trees, although tall, were planted only a few decades ago, and beneath them some relics of what used to be here are still visible. Dozens of low brick structures protrude through a light covering of moss and dead branches: these are the bases of long-demolished Quonset huts,* and just off the footpath I found one still intact, preserved – or so I hoped – as a reminder of what happened here in wartime.

In late 1944 you would have seen lines of these huts, hundreds of them, covering several acres of the Stowell Park estate. This was a

---

* A prefabricated structure of American design, based on the British Nissen hut.

huge military hospital, with its own airstrip, constructed in haste to cope with the flood of casualties expected to follow an Allied invasion of continental Europe. In April that year it became the headquarters of the 160th General Hospital of the US military, a unit specialising in chest injuries which at its peak had 500 patients under treatment[1] – and in an improvised operating theatre in one of these huts, a young Iowan surgeon called Dwight Harken removed bullets and shell fragments from the chests of 134 soldiers without experiencing a single fatality.[2] This was impressive in itself, but what makes his unblemished record all the more remarkable is that he extracted many of these pieces of twisted metal from inside a beating heart.

A metal hut is not the ideal environment for heart surgery. Sixteen feet wide by twelve high, Harken's ramshackle operating theatre had a roof of corrugated iron and was poorly insulated: the summer sun turned it into a stifling furnace, while in winter it was heated by a small stove. But the cold was the least of his concerns as he prepared for surgery on 19 February 1945. He already knew his patient well: Leroy Rohrbach, an infantry sergeant who had been involved in the Normandy landings the previous summer, a tricky case who had been in Harken's care for some time. A month after D-Day he had been caught up in the fierce fighting which obliterated the town of Saint-Lô, and an exploding shell had sent a piece of shrapnel through the lower part of his chest.

He was evacuated to England, where an X-ray showed a small piece of metal lodged inside his heart. On the fluorescent screen it could be seen pulsating gently with the throb of his heartbeat, indicating that it had passed through the outer wall of the organ and was now inside one of the cardiac chambers. On 15 August Harken operated and came desperately close to removing it: after making a small incision in the heart he managed to grasp the metal fragment with a pair of forceps, but it was jerked from his grasp as the organ contracted, and slipped back into the bloodstream. He made frantic attempts to find it, but it had vanished from view and could not be felt through the heart's thick walls. Three months later he tried once more. Again he found it; and again it defied him, slipping from his forceps just as success seemed assured.

Yet despite these failures his patient continued to improve. This was not unheard of: soldiers with similar injuries might never need an operation, living quite happily with pieces of shrapnel – or even bullets – inside them as permanent reminders of their military service. The sergeant showed no signs of infection, and electrocardiograms revealed that his heart rhythm, which had been disturbed by the injury, was slowly returning to normal. Given that his patient had already endured two major and fruitless operations, Harken was reluctant to risk a third: it would be dangerous and possibly unnecessary.

But there was another consideration. Although many soldiers lived active lives after such injuries, others developed crippling anxiety about the alien shard of metal lodged deep inside their chests. They became depressed, fretful, and lived in perpetual fear of sudden death, terrified that a single careless movement could be enough to dislodge the shrapnel and kill them. This phenomenon was well known by 1945, and had been given a name: cardiac neurosis. Indeed, Harken's patient had become increasingly nervous about the inch-long shell fragment inside his body and begged the surgeon to persevere. Appreciating that such distress constituted a significant clinical consideration, Harken agreed to make a final attempt.

At thirty-four, Dwight Harken was already one of the most highly regarded surgeons in the US medical corps. A tall and muscular redhead, he had been born into medicine, delivered by his father, a doctor who ran the small Harken Hospital in Osceola, Iowa, and had grown up in a basement flat in the building. During his childhood the antiseptic smell of the wards had never been far away, and his father's hope was that he would eventually take over the family business; but small-town life had little appeal, and he left to study at Harvard. A few years later he moved to Britain to work with the country's leading chest surgeon, Arthur Tudor Edwards, at the Brompton Hospital in London.[3] During the war Tudor Edwards had an immense impact on military medicine, training surgeons and developing new techniques in his treatment of air-raid casualties. Given this pedigree, and despite his youth, Harken was a natural choice to run the new specialist thoracic unit in Gloucestershire.

Although Harken's operating theatre was little more than a shack, he was otherwise in a fortunate position. By February 1945 he had state-of-the-art equipment and drugs, including the new antibiotic penicillin, and a close team of surgical colleagues who had assisted him in over a hundred operations. Charles Burstein, the anaesthetist, had been with him since the beginning;[4] he now put the patient to sleep, administering a mixture of ether and air through a facemask. Today the hut was more than usually cramped. Word had got around about this remarkable young American doing wondrous things in a field in Gloucestershire, and a delegation of eminent British surgeons, including Tudor Edwards, had come to watch Harken at work. Above the operating table a cameraman was lying on a scaffold, ready to film proceedings for the benefit of medics in America.[5]

The sergeant's body bore obvious scars from the first two operations, one a snaking line across his back from shoulder blade to hip, the other a smaller curve around his left nipple. Harken chose to renew his attack through the chest, using a scalpel to reopen his earlier incision. With a pair of Tudor Edwards retractors, an instrument named after his mentor, he separated the patient's ribs and exposed the heart by cutting through the pericardium, the tough sac around it. He could see the scar in the cardiac wall left by his first operation, and elsewhere the tissue appeared flabby and discoloured, evidence of trauma. By gently squeezing the beating heart he was able to locate the foreign body, a small area of hardness in the right ventricle, near the organ's base.

Now the shell fragment had been found, the delicate task of removing it could begin. Harken held it in place with a finger placed firmly on the outside of the heart, while inserting two rows of catgut sutures on either side, an otherwise straightforward procedure rendered more difficult by the constant contraction and relaxation of the muscle. In the event of catastrophic bleeding these could be pulled together, a simple but effective way of staunching the flow of blood. As Burstein watched the electrocardiogram nervously, looking for signs that this manipulation was disturbing the heart's rhythm, Harken's assistant picked up the loose ends of the catgut and waited for a signal. This was the critical moment.

Working as quickly as he could, Harken now made a small incision in the heart wall and inserted a pair of forceps to widen the opening. Through this aperture he introduced a clamp and fastened it around the elusive piece of metal. For a moment all was quiet. And then, as he related in a letter to his wife, 'suddenly, with a pop as if a champagne cork had been drawn, the fragment jumped out of the ventricle, forced by the pressure within the chamber. Blood poured out in a torrent.'[6] His assistant pulled the control sutures taut, but the wound continued to bleed. Harken put a finger over it, and picking up a needle started to sew it shut. The opening was closed, but when he tried to remove his finger he discovered that he had sewn his glove to the wall of the heart. Finally his assistant cut him loose, and the job was done. Opening the heart, removing the shell fragment and repairing the incision had taken three minutes. His distinguished guests were deeply impressed: this was surgery of a sophistication and audacity which none had seen before.

Some of Harken's operations were still more dramatic. Sometimes when he cut into the heart the resulting jet of blood entirely obscured his view, and he was forced to fish around blindly for the metallic fragment in a churning scarlet sea. The degree of haemorrhage was often so severe that patients had to be given rapid transfusions. Today, blood comes pre-packed in plastic bags which are hooked on a drip stand, and enters the body under atmospheric pressure; in 1945 the blood bag had yet to be invented, and so it was instead poured into a bottle into which air was then pumped to create the high pressure necessary to force it into the patient's veins. Most of the time this worked without any problems, but every so often the bottle would explode, showering the entire operating theatre and its staff with blood and shards of glass.[7]

On another occasion Harken tried a novel method of removing foreign objects. During the First World War several surgeons had realised that since many bullets were made of iron it should be possible to remove them magnetically. Harken took up this idea, ordering a huge mains-powered electromagnet which was mounted above the operating table. After the patient's chest had been opened it was turned on. The bullet remained stubbornly in place, but every surgical instrument in the room flew lethally through the air and landed on the surface of the electromagnet with an alarming metallic clink.[8]

In an age when open-heart surgery takes place in thousands of hospitals all over the world every day, it is difficult to appreciate quite what a momentous achievement Harken's work was. He was not the first to remove bullets from the heart, but never before had a surgeon operated on so many patients without a single death, or made a terrifying procedure look almost routine. The magnitude of the accomplishment is noted in the official account of British surgery in the Second World War: 'His outstanding success, his daring interventions, and his brilliant results underline one of the most striking chapters of surgical achievement in any war, and in a symposium of this type all British surgeons will unite in offering their tribute to him.'[9]

Such hyperbole is easier to understand if you consider that less than half a century earlier heart surgery was widely regarded as impossible. In 1896 the author of the most widely read British textbook on chest surgery, Stephen Paget, wrote, 'Surgery of the heart has probably reached the limits set by Nature to all surgery: no new method, and no new discovery, can overcome the natural difficulties that attend a wound of the heart.'[10] One of his contemporaries, the American Benjamin Merrill Ricketts, observed gloomily that 'there is probably no organ or disease about which so much has been said and written, with so little accomplished, as the heart with its diseases.'[11]

By the end of the nineteenth century surgery had made great strides, thanks to two recent discoveries: anaesthesia and antisepsis. The first anaesthetic agents, ether and chloroform, were discovered in the 1840s and made it possible to undertake quite radical procedures without inflicting excruciating pain. Twenty years later Joseph Lister showed that if instruments and dressings were sterilised, infections could be prevented, and the age of modern surgery had begun. It was now possible to operate at leisure on an unconscious patient, and to be reasonably confident that they would not then succumb to gangrene.

Progress was rapid. Within a few decades surgeons were operating on virtually every part of the human body. By 1890 detailed surgical textbooks were available for the skeleton and its muscles,[12] the mouth and jaw,[13] the ear,[14] the eye,[15] the kidney,[16] the reproductive organs,[17] the urinary system,[18] the intestines[19] and the rectum.[20] Not even the brain was out of bounds: in 1884 Rickman Godlee successfully removed a tumour from inside the skull of a twenty-five-year-old man in an operation in London, prompting editorials in national newspapers.[21]

So why was the heart, alone among the major organs, still taboo? There were certainly practical difficulties: its position beneath the ribcage made it inaccessible, and operating inside the chest could cause the lungs to collapse as air entered the space around them, causing catastrophic respiratory failure. And then there was the fact that if the patient were to remain alive the heart had to keep pumping: how could you possibly operate on an organ that wouldn't stay still?

But there was something else, too: a reverence for the heart rooted in centuries of tradition. It was not merely another organ, but an object far more mysterious and freighted with significance. This was eloquently expressed in the sixteenth century by the French surgeon Ambroise Paré, who described the heart as 'the chief mansion of the Soul, the organ of the vitall faculty, the beginning of life, the fountain of the vitall spirits'.[22] This attitude is even apparent in the oldest surviving medical texts, those from ancient Egypt. The heart was then believed to be the seat of the intelligence, the emotions and the soul, and was preserved after death: admission to the afterlife could only be granted when it had been weighed by the god Anubis. Later, Greek scholars agreed on the fundamental importance of the heart. In the fourth century BC Aristotle pointed out that it was the first organ to form, and the last to die; it occupied a central position; it moved; and it communicated with all other parts of the body. He also saw the heart as the source of the 'animal heat', the life force inherent to all organisms.[23]

Given the fundamental importance assigned to the heart by early thinkers, it was natural to assume that injuries to it must necessarily be fatal. In his great 37-volume encyclopaedia *Natural History*, compiled in the first century AD, Pliny described the heart as 'the primary source and origin of life'. He claimed that it 'is the only one among the viscera that is not affected by maladies, nor is it subject to the ordinary penalties of human life; but when injured, it produces instant death'.[24] A century later the most celebrated surgeon of the ancient world, Galen, was able to describe the effect of cardiac injuries at first hand. For a few years he was the official doctor to the gladiators of his hometown of Pergamon, and witnessed many die from the effects of a stab wound to the heart. He noted that such a death was often instantaneous, but that the length of survival depended on the location of the wound:

> When a wound pierces the ventricle of the heart, they die immediately with great flow of blood, and especially so if the ventricle of the left part has been wounded; but if it does not reach the ventricle, but the wound stops in the substance of the heart, some of those affected can survive not only the day on which they were wounded but as long as the following night.[25]

Galen's writings remained the foundation of medical education until superseded by Renaissance scholarship almost 1,500 years later, so it is unsurprising that his conclusions went undisputed for centuries. In a wince-inducing treatise on the treatment of wounds, the seventh-century Byzantine physician Paul of Aegina gave a vivid description of a cardiac injury and its fatal consequences: 'When the heart is wounded, the weapon appears at the left breast, and feels not as if in a cavity, but as fixed in another body, and sometimes there is a throbbing motion; there is a discharge of black blood if it can find vent, with coldness, sweats ... and death follows in a short time.'[26]

That description was echoed eight hundred years later by Paré, the greatest surgeon of the Renaissance. Like Galen he had seen such injuries for himself, having spent many years as a military surgeon on the battlefields of France: 'If the heart be wounded, much blood gusheth out, a trembling possesseth all the members of the body: the pulse will be small and weak: the colour of the face will become very pale: a cold sweat, and frequent swooning will assault the wounded party: and when the limbs grow cold, death is at the door.'[27] But Paré also pointed out that death was not necessarily instant. He had witnessed a duel in Turin during which one of the combatants had been stabbed through the left breast; he nevertheless continued to fight, chasing his enemy for two hundred paces before falling down dead. When Paré examined the body he found a wound in the heart so large that he could insert his finger into it.[28]

Yet by the end of the sixteenth century surprising discoveries were being made which threatened to challenge the dogma that cardiac wounds were inherently fatal. Barthélémy Cabrol, physician to the French king Henry IV, described conducting an autopsy on two men and finding scars on their hearts. One had 'a lesion the size and width of a myrrh leaf, which penetrated quite deeply; and lest anybody think that these injuries were the cause of death, both men had been hanged: one for thieving, the other for producing counterfeit coin'.[29] Still more perplexing was the discovery of Johann Dolaeus, who wrote of a 'bullet of lead found in the heart of a boar, covered with flesh, that no way endangered his life: for he was a large boar, and when it was taken out with a huntsman's knife, any one might observe that the wound was not made two or three days, but a long time before'.[30]

Though many physicians continued to insist that cardiac wounds spelled death, the body of evidence to the contrary continued to grow. In 1778 Henry Thomas, a marine on board HMS *Foudroyant*, slipped off a gangplank while the ship was in dock at Portsmouth and fell on his bayonet. He removed the blade and declared himself fit to resume his guard duty, before collapsing in a faint. He died nine hours later, and when they opened his body doctors were amazed to find that after impaling his colon and liver the bayonet had passed right through his heart.[31] A few years later a similar injury was seen at the same hospital in Gosport; in this case the soldier survived for two days, but died suddenly while defecating. At a post-mortem the surgeon concluded that a clot had formed in the wound, blocking the escape of blood from the heart, but had been dislodged as the soldier strained to empty his bowels.[32]

Throughout medical history some of the greatest advances in surgical knowledge have been made in the theatre of war. Military surgeons encountered injuries so numerous and terrible that they were tested to the limits of their ingenuity, devising new therapeutic approaches if existing techniques proved unequal to their needs. During the Napoleonic Wars, for instance, the Frenchman Dominique Larrey devised the modern process of triage, prioritising casualties according to the urgency of their condition, and introduced ambulances to the battlefield. His British counterpart George Guthrie, meanwhile, introduced new treatments for gunshot wounds of the legs – in particular, early amputation – that drastically reduced mortality. But one of the most celebrated cases of that conflict was one in which the surgeon did nothing at all.

At the Battle of Corunna in northern Spain in January 1809, a private in the Queen's Royals, Samuel Evens, was shot in the chest. His comrades carried him off the battlefield and he was put on a troopship back to England. It was crowded with wounded and ill soldiers and the only treatment he received was a plaster, but he was still in a fair condition when taken to hospital in Plymouth a few days later. Evens told the Scottish doctor who examined him, John Fuge, that a musket ball was still lodged in his chest, and begged him to remove it, saying that he was sure it was in easy reach. Fuge inserted a probe into the wound, but it was so deep that the entire instrument disappeared into it, and he abandoned the attempt. Three days later Evens died. His body, when Dr Fuge examined it, contained a huge surprise. The musket ball had ripped through the wall of the heart, leaving an inch-long tear, and had lacerated one of the heart valves. This was a catastrophic injury, and yet the soldier had lived for a fortnight after receiving it. Fuge's report of the case, illustrated by an engraving of the preserved heart in a jar, was widely circulated in Europe and America – graphic evidence of the resilience of an organ hitherto believed to be uniquely fragile.[33]

Several similar cases came to light over the next few years, and doctors were now confronted with the question of how to treat them. From a twenty-first-century perspective, the emergency care received by Victor Janson in 1828 leaves a lot to be desired. Aged sixteen, he had been messing around with a friend in the cellar of his parents' house, and while play-fighting had stabbed himself with a knife. He felt no pain and assumed he had only cut his waistcoat, but ten minutes later noticed his clothes were covered in blood. He was taken to hospital, where doctors bandaged the wound, put him on his back and bled him. For the next three days they repeated this bleeding at regular intervals. The results were evidently unsatisfactory, because a few days later the therapy was intensified and twenty leeches were applied to his anus. Apparently intent on killing his patient, the doctor then inserted a probe into the wound, whereupon 'the blood sprung to the height of several feet'. Unsurprisingly, the boy soon died.[34]

Venesection, bleeding a patient by opening a vein, is one of the oldest therapies known to medicine. It was widely practised in the ancient world, when physicians believed that disease was caused by an imbalance of the four fundamental fluids or 'humours' of the human body: blood, phlegm, yellow bile and black bile. According to the humoral system, removing blood was a simple way of restoring the natural balance between the four fluids. By the nineteenth century most physicians had abandoned this antiquated notion, yet many retained an evangelical belief in the powers of bloodletting. It was often used in cases where the heart seemed to be under strain: doctors reasoned that reducing the amount of blood in the body was a simple way to reduce its workload.

Baron Guillaume Dupuytren, who was appointed chief surgeon of the hospital of Hôtel-Dieu in Paris in 1815, was a passionate advocate of venesection, and had no doubt that heart wounds could be survived. He advised treating patients as if the organ had not been injured: doctors should dress the wound, bleed the patient regularly and keep them cold.[35] Some took this last measure to extremes, packing the patient in bags of ice and cooling the room to sub-zero temperatures, while in summer they might resort to using a cellar.[36] This was intended to depress the circulation and reduce the strain on the heart; but others believed that stimulation was the key to survival. Rather than chilling their patients, they enveloped them in warm blankets and piled hot water bottles all over them.[37] There was also little agreement about what they should be given to eat or drink. Baron Dupuytren suggested acidulated drinks,[38] while hot brandy and water,[39] barley water,[40] and water-gruel and strawberries[41] were also tried. The patient in the last of these cases was a student who survived for six weeks after being stabbed in the heart; his attending physician, a Dr Lavender, concluded that the strawberries had contributed to his demise.

The first indication that more positive surgical intervention was possible came in 1872, when a thirty-one-year-old pewterer became involved in a pub brawl in London. After the tussle he noticed that a needle he had been carrying in his coat had disappeared, and he wondered whether it had entered his chest. The following day he was in some pain, and went to St Bartholomew's Hospital. The doctors could find no evidence of injury, so he went back to work; but nine days later he returned, still in pain and troubled by palpitations. He was examined by a surgeon called George Callender, who noticed a tiny bump between two of the ribs. He decided to investigate further, and after the patient had been given chloroform made a small incision into the pectoral muscle. To his surprise this revealed a small metallic object which vibrated with every heartbeat. With great delicacy he pulled at it with a pair of forceps, and a needle almost two inches long emerged from the man's chest, having apparently been lodged inside the cardiac muscle. The patient made a good recovery, and when the details of the procedure were made public it quickly became the talk of medical London. It even earned the surgeon the rare distinction of becoming an eponym: 'Callender's operation' was notable as the first occasion on which a patient had recovered after surgery to remove an object from the heart.[42]

While a few early textbooks refer to Callender's operation as the first heart surgery, he had not actually needed to expose the organ or make an incision into its surface. The first person to do this deliberately – albeit not on a human patient – was Dr Block, a surgeon from Danzig. At a meeting of the German Surgical Society in 1882 he began a presentation of his work by brandishing a rabbit's heart. Some weeks earlier, he explained, he had cut open the animal's ribcage and created an artificial wound in the surface of the organ. He had then repaired the damage with three stitches, and a few days later the rabbit had completely recovered. To make sure this outcome was not a one-off he repeated the experiment, on the same animal and others.[43]

What particularly surprised Block was the organ's resilience. In order to insert sutures into the rabbit's heart he had to lift it out of the ribcage. He noticed that when he did this it stopped beating, and all breathing ceased. But as soon as it was released into its normal position all function resumed. Surgeons had long been terrified of touching the heart, fearing that even gentle manipulation might be enough to disturb its rhythm and cause instant death. But a much earlier writer, working in the seventeenth century, had already shown that it was quite a robust organ which would easily withstand careful handling.

The seventeenth-century English physician William Harvey contributed more than anybody to our understanding of what the heart is and what it does. He devoted years to his study of the movement of blood around the body, experimenting on an extraordinary range of creatures including dogs, rabbits, toads, lizards and crabs. Cold-blooded animals proved particularly useful, because they had a slow metabolism and therefore a slow heartbeat, allowing him to see more clearly what was going on. When Harvey began his work, most authorities still subscribed to Galen's version of the action of the blood, a rather convoluted theory according to which arterial blood was manufactured in the heart and cooled by the lungs, while the liver produced the blood found in the veins. So great was Galen's reputation in the seventeenth century that dissent from his views amounted to medical heresy; it says much for Harvey's dedication to scientific truth that he was prepared to brave the consequences. His great discovery, laid out in his 1628 book *De Motu Cordis* ('On the Movement of the Heart'), was that blood travelled around the body in a closed circuit, propelled by the heart.

For over a decade Harvey was physician to Charles I, who took an interest in his work, allowing him to conduct dissections on deer in the royal parks. In the 1640s Harvey met a young nobleman, the son of Viscount Montgomery, who had suffered a serious accident in child-hood. This left him with a cavernous wound in his side which had failed to heal. When Harvey examined the opening, he found a large open space in the thorax, into which he could easily fit three of his fingers. Looking more closely, he noticed 'a protuberant fleshy part' which, he realised with astonishment, was the young man's heart. He knew that his employer would be fascinated:

> I carried the young man himself to the king, that his majesty
> might with his own eyes behold this wonderful case: that,
> in a man alive and well, he might, without detriment to the
> individual, observe the movement of the heart, and with his
> proper hand even touch the ventricles as they contracted.

Charles inserted the royal fingers into the gaping chasm in the youth's flank and held the heart for himself, noting that this caused no pain or visible disturbance.[44] Here was clear evidence that the organ could be handled without danger; yet strangely this knowledge had already faded from view two centuries later.

Block was not the only researcher of the 1880s to suggest that it might eventually be feasible to stitch a human heart. An American surgeon, John Roberts, raised the possibility in 1881, although the main subject of his article was the pericardium, the fibrous sac that surrounds it. Sometimes when the heart is injured this natural envelope fills with blood, preventing the organ from beating effectively. This condition, known as cardiac tamponade, is potentially fatal, and at least two surgeons of the early nineteenth century are believed to have treated it by inserting a sharp probe to puncture the sac, allowing the blood to drain away. Roberts suggested that it might even be safe to open the pericardium to retrieve foreign objects, or to enable minor repairs of the heart muscle: 'The time may possibly come when wounds of the heart itself will be treated by pericardial incision, to allow extraction of clots, and perhaps to suture the cardiac muscle.'[45]

It was a decade before this prediction was proved correct. On 6 September 1891, a young man in St Louis, Missouri, was stabbed in a fight. He was taken to the city hospital, where his wound was dressed, but ten hours later his condition had deteriorated and he was taken into the operating theatre. No anaesthetic was used, presumably because time was of the essence – a decade later one prominent surgeon still thought anaesthesia 'improper' for such a procedure,[46] and it would not be routinely used for such major surgery until after the First World War.[47] When the dressings were removed, blood and air gushed from the wound. Henry Dalton, the surgeon in charge, opened the patient's chest and turned him on his side in order to drain the blood. The incision revealed a two-inch wound in the pericardium which he managed to repair, after many attempts and with great difficulty: 'I had no precedent to guide me, no authority to uphold me in attempting to sew up this wound over a heart that was beating at the rate of 140 per minute.'[48]

At several points in the operation the patient appeared close to death, but on each occasion he was injected with a cocktail of strychnine and whiskey, which improved his condition. Strychnine is a highly toxic compound which was once used as rat poison, but at this date it was believed to be a useful stimulant which in small doses would elevate the heart rate. Whiskey also enjoyed something of a vogue in American operating theatres at the turn of the century: in 1900 John DaCosta recommended enemas of hot coffee and whiskey when treating heart injuries,[49] while the post-operative medication of a stab victim in Georgetown nine years later included three pints of whiskey administered in a single day.[50] European surgeons preferred Old World drinks: during an operation in the 1890s, Charles Ballance injected his patient with a mixture of brandy and saline, which had so dramatic an effect that by the end of the procedure, 'he no longer seemed dead, but was so drunk and obstreperous that five men were required to hold him down'.[51]

Dalton's patient made a rapid and uninterrupted recovery; an impressive success, but he had not interfered with the heart itself. That remained a threshold that few were willing to cross. From a modern perspective it can be difficult to understand what it was that deterred surgeons from taking the decisive final step, when they had already come so close. Writing a few years later, the American surgeon Charles Elsberg explained why he and his colleagues were so petrified of touching the beating heart:

> We must remember that we have to deal with an organ of first importance which is in constant motion, and which, more-over, was believed to be very sensitive to the smallest mechanical insult or injury. It was feared that during the slightest manipulation the heart might suddenly stop, that the mere passage of a needle might be followed by the direst results.[52]

What changed their minds? A flamboyant piece of theatre staged by the Italian researcher Simplicio Del Vecchio in 1894 may have been the catalyst. At a conference of surgeons in Rome he appeared on stage with a dog on a lead and proceeded to tell his colleagues that he had operated on this animal forty days earlier, puncturing its heart and repairing the wound by stitching. Two days later it was killed, and members of the audience were able to see for themselves that the wound had healed perfectly, leaving only a small scar. Del Vecchio

was cautious about the prospects for human heart surgery, acknowledging that there were still important questions to be answered, such
as whether it would be possible to administer an anaesthetic. But, he
concluded, 'I am confident that in the not too distant future surgery
will answer all these questions, and that with the protection afforded
by asepsis it will surmount still more serious obstacles.'[53]

He did not have long to wait, for within a matter of months a surgeon in Norway had the courage not only to open the pericardium,
but to attempt an operation on the structure of the heart itself – and
even to insert a needle through its pulsating muscle. In the early hours
of 4 September, a young man was rushed to the National Hospital in
Oslo in a taxi, having been found at home lying in a pool of blood. He
had been stabbed in the chest. When the thirty-seven-year-old duty
surgeon, Axel Cappelen, examined him he found his unconscious
patient 'pale as a corpse'. The man briefly stopped breathing, and an
hour later his pulse was barely detectable. Cappelen decided to operate. Once the patient had been put to sleep with chloroform and his
chest opened, Cappelen found massive internal bleeding. There was
a wound about three-quarters of an inch long in the left ventricle of
the heart, which he sutured with catgut, timing each stitch to avoid
the violent leaps of the organ as it contracted. This delicate job was
eventually completed, and when the patient awoke the next day he
said he felt much better. But his recovery was only temporary: he died
on the morning of 7 September, having succumbed to blood loss from
an undetected arterial wound.[54]

Cappelen felt that his patient had been unlucky: the position of
the wound concealed the fact that the heart had been injured in two
places. If this had been spotted, and the operation had begun more
promptly, he might have been successful. A second attempt to repair a
cardiac wound took place in Rome in March 1896 when Guido Farina
placed three silk sutures in the heart of a man who had been stabbed
with a stiletto; his patient died two days later from an infection.[55] But
there was something encouraging even in these failures, a hint of
greater deeds to come, and the mood began to change. The *Journal*

of the American Medical Association declared bullishly: 'The opinion seems warranted, that "the citadel of life" itself will no longer be exempt from the incursions of the surgeons.'[56]

Indeed, disaster would soon be followed by triumph. Six months after Farina's disappointment, a surgeon from Frankfurt, Ludwig Rehn, achieved lasting fame and the adulation of his colleagues when he conducted the first successful operation on a human heart. On the last day of August 1896 a twenty-two-year-old gardener was discharged from the army – ironically, as it turned out, because he had been diagnosed with a heart problem. A week later he was stabbed and collapsed, unconscious. He was taken to hospital in the early hours, drenched in blood. When Rehn saw him the following day his initial assessment was that the man was dying. A colleague inspected the wound and concluded the heart was injured, so the decision was taken to operate.

When Rehn reached the chest cavity he could see a small wound in the pericardium. He opened the sac further; blood and clots were being continuously discharged from the area around the heart. He soon noticed a wound half an inch long in the surface of the cardiac muscle. He was able to control the bleeding by putting a finger over this aperture, although every time the heart contracted his finger slipped off and more blood gushed out. Rehn quickly decided to suture the laceration with silk thread, a material which was easy to handle and which – unlike catgut – would not be absorbed by the body. In the pause between heartbeats he passed his needle through both sides of the wound, and was alarmed to find that the heart halted for a moment before resuming its movement. When three stitches had been inserted the bleeding stopped; 'the heart continued to work, and we could breathe freely.'[57]

The worst was over, and all that Rehn now needed to do was wash the remaining blood and clots from the chest cavity and replace a rib which had been sawn through in order to reach the heart. These tasks were completed without alarm, and the patient returned to the ward. His condition remained a cause for concern for some weeks, but his life was out of danger and he eventually made a full recovery. When Rehn described the operation to a meeting of surgical colleagues in Berlin the following April, he concluded his speech by bringing his patient on to the stage to demonstrate that he was in perfect health. This caused a sensation. Within hours telegraph wires were humming with the news, which was reported all over the world. Foreign correspondents were in too much of a hurry to check the spelling of Rehn's name: the front pages of newspapers in America and New Zealand attributed the triumph to a 'Dr Rehe',[58] while British readers were treated to breathless accounts of the operation performed by 'Herr Relin'.[59] Rehn had shown that while operating on the heart was daunting, the hazards were not insurmountable; emboldened by his example, many younger surgeons chose to intervene where once they had stood by impotently.

Most of the earliest attempts to emulate him took place in Europe. When an Italian surgeon reported a second successful operation in 1897, the physician G. S. Brock remarked: 'Happily it is only in Italy that surgeons have many opportunities of practising cardiac surgery – opportunities they owe to the terrible frequency with which the dagger is resorted to in this country in the quarrels of the lower orders.'[60] It was another five years before a surgeon in the US would follow suit, and in conditions far removed from the modern operating theatre. Luther Leonidas Hill's patient was Henry Myrick, a boy from an impoverished black family in Alabama, and the operation took place on their kitchen table, illuminated by kerosene lamps. Hill was assisted by his brother, who held the heart steady while stitches were inserted.[61] The case seized the attention of national newspapers, one of which headlined the story 'Lived with Stabbed Heart'.[62]

All these early cases involved patients with stab wounds; the American surgeon Rudolph Matas was not alone when he stated in 1899 that this was the only type of injury which could be treated: 'As to the gunshot perforations of the heart, they will continue, for obvious reasons, to spare the surgeon even the contemplation of his helplessness to relieve them.'[63] Like many of the pessimistic predictions made by surgeons, this was both emphatic and completely wrong. On 3 March 1902, a twenty-six-year-old man was admitted to hospital in Paris after being shot with a revolver. The surgeon, M. Launay, operated and found that the bullet had passed right through the heart, leaving entry and exit wounds. The first of these was easily sutured, but the second, on the underside of the organ, was less easy for the surgeon's hands to reach and so caused more difficulties. Nevertheless, the operation took only thirty-five minutes and the patient was out of bed ten days later.[64]

Launay's task was simplified by the fact that the bullet had not lodged in the cardiac tissue but passed through it; removing a foreign body from inside the heart represented an altogether more formidable challenge. The evidence suggested that such injuries were always fatal, although there were records of a few fascinating cases where a victim survived for days or even weeks. The first surgeon to accept the challenge – the forerunner of Dwight Harken forty years later – was an Estonian, Werner von Manteuffel. A well-heeled young woman, Marie Plavsona, had fallen in with a bad crowd and been shot during an argument a short distance from his hospital in Dorpat on 12 September 1903.[65] When he uncovered the heart a wound came into view, out of which a fountain of blood half a metre high splashed with every beat. He closed the opening and found the bullet, which was embedded in the wall of the right ventricle, but by lifting the heart he was able to cut out the missile and repair the wound. Plavsona remained in hospital for several months, but survived.[66] For an obscure surgeon working in Estonia's second city this was a remarkable feat, and it was reported widely; von Manteuffel was rewarded with a prestigious position as personal physician to Tsar Nicholas II.

Manteuffel's description of a 'fountain of blood' gives some hint of the gory challenges faced by these brave pioneers. One spoke of being confronted by 'a lake of blood in which were churned bubbles of air',[67] another found himself 'operating in a mass of bloody foam, which is not conducive to equanimity'.[68] 'If it is in plain view', one surgeon remarked sardonically, 'the stream spurting from a ventricle strikes the eyes of the operator with surprising accuracy.'[69] The blood in a contracting heart is at surprisingly high pressure, comparable to that at the bottom of a five-foot-deep swimming pool. Like a hairline fracture in a hot-water tank, even a minor puncture can rapidly produce startling amounts of fluid. The average human body contains around five litres of blood, and the heart pumps that entire volume every minute – making it quite possible for a large stab wound to kill a patient in a matter of seconds. But Charles Ballance, the first eminent British surgeon to venture into such territory, offered bracing encouragement to his colleagues: 'The surgeon having this job in hand will take it all in the day's work, and just as he plunges his hand into the abdomen into a mass of blood in a case of ruptured spleen . . . so he will now plunge his hand into the pericardium and seize the heart.'[70]

The First World War confronted surgeons with new and more horrible sights. The rapid evolution of military technology resulted in wounds more catastrophic than anything seen on the battlefields of the Crimea or the Boer War: machine-gun bullets tore through flesh with unprecedented power, and high-explosive shells riddled bodies with shrapnel or lacerated them with blast wounds. Ballance was one of several surgeons whose new prowess in cardiac surgery was invaluable in these circumstances. The apparently endless flood of casualties prompted a new manual on the treatment of war wounds, written by Henry Gray, a Scottish surgeon who spent most of the war at hospitals in northern France. As well as being an expert in gunshot injuries he was also an innovator who realised that for some procedures it was not always necessary to put the patient to sleep. His use of the newly discovered local anaesthetics meant that serious wounds could be treated quickly while the patient was spared the worst of the pain, saving time and allowing him to get through more operations each day.

While local anaesthetic is not obviously a method applicable to cardiac surgery, in 1915 Gray removed a bullet from the heart of a soldier who remained awake throughout the operation. The patient in question could count himself doubly unlucky, having been shot by a round which passed straight through the man in front of him. After giving him morphine, Gray made a large incision into the man's chest; at this point the patient became anxious and complained that he was breathless, but 'settled down in about one minute, after being reassured by the surgeon'. Gray must have had a wonderfully calming bedside manner: in order to remove the bullet he had to lift the heart out of the man's chest, make an incision and extract the missile with forceps, and then stop the considerable bleeding that ensued. The patient lived another four days, but again died from an infection.[71]

Cardiac surgery was a major undertaking and rarely attempted during the war, but surprisingly successes outnumbered such failures. When the French surgeon Pierre Duval attempted to compile a list of every heart operation undertaken during the conflict he found that 23 of 26 patients had survived[72] – a triumphant result. One reason for this improvement was the increasingly sophisticated use of radiography, which gave surgeons a clear idea of what to expect before they made the first incision. X-rays, a form of high-energy electromagnetic radiation, had been discovered in November 1895 by the German physicist Wilhelm Röntgen, who also found that they could be used to visualise the internal structures of the human body. X-ray radiation is absorbed by bone and other dense materials, but passes through soft tissue virtually unaltered. Röntgen demonstrated this effect by getting his wife to place her left hand on a photographic plate and then exposing it to a burst of X-rays: when the plate was developed it revealed a skeletal image of her fingers and wedding ring. This had such obvious application to medical practice that within only a few months the technique was being used clinically to locate fractures, gallstones and bullets. Twenty years later X-ray machines were commonplace in military hospitals and even as mobile installations on the battlefield – and were often used to do more than simply take a picture.

One new technique was stereoscopic radiography, in which two images were combined to produce a three-dimensional picture. This provided invaluable information when foreign bodies were involved, because it enabled surgeons to work out whether a shrapnel fragment was actually inside the heart or sitting a few inches in front of it. If the patient were placed between the X-ray machine and a fluorescent screen it was also possible to produce moving images, a technique known as fluoroscopy. When objects were lodged inside the heart they pulsated in time with the heartbeat, or danced hypnotically as they were buffeted by the bloodstream. Alphonsus d'Abreu, a British surgeon who served in Africa and Italy during the Second World War, remarked that these swirlings and gyrations were watched 'with the same interest that astronomical observers bestow on minor planets'.[73] A particularly ingenious use of the fluorescent screen was made by a French medic, Petit de la Villéon. Instead of making an eight-inch incision through flesh and bone to remove shrapnel from the heart, he operated through a tiny opening between two ribs, using an X-ray screen to guide a pair of forceps to the site of injury. This was the first keyhole heart operation, but it horrified de la Villéon's colleagues, one of whom stated that 'no matter how satisfactory this method had proved in the lung and in other parts of the body, it had no place in the surgery of the heart.'[74] The remark is revealing, since it shows that the old, quasi-religious belief in the exceptional status of the organ still lingered; it would be many decades before minimally invasive cardiac surgery was contemplated again.

One of the more mystifying experiences for a surgeon was opening up a patient only to find that a bullet clearly visible in X-rays was nowhere to be found. Usually this meant that it had been swept away by the bloodstream and lodged elsewhere. Foreign objects could travel quite surprising distances: in one particularly dramatic example, two British surgeons found themselves in marathon pursuit of a jagged shell fragment as it migrated around the body of a teenage soldier. It had entered a vein in his chest but soon moved ominously towards his heart, where the surgeons managed to seize it briefly; but before it could be extracted it was sucked into the cardiac chambers, eventually coming to rest in an artery behind his bladder, from which it was finally removed.[75]

In 1921 Rudolph Matas, one of the titans of early twentieth-century medicine, described these extractions of foreign bodies from the heart as 'one of the crowning triumphs of surgery'.[76] But there was little need for such expertise in peacetime, and it was not until the Second World War and the feats of Dwight Harken that any surgeon would again regularly experience the exhilaration and terror of rummaging inside a beating heart.

On the evening of 18 February 1945, Harken wrote to his wife Anne from his quarters in Gloucestershire. The following morning he would operate on Leroy Rohrbach, and he was anxious: 'If I kill this man, I shall be regarded as foolhardy rather than bold, and heart surgery could be set back by decades. If I succeed, heart surgery may well be on its way.'[77] Why such trepidation? Removing a bullet from the heart was, after all, nothing new, and Harken had himself done it many times before. But this time was different: word had got around about the young American who made cardiac surgery so safe that it was almost routine, and the pick of London's surgeons would be watching intently to find out if the rumours were true. This was not just another case, but one by which he and the future of his specialism would be judged. As it turned out, it was a triumph: two years later in America a hall full of Harken's colleagues would watch awestruck as the drama of his operation unfolded on a cinema screen in front of them. Many of them would be inspired to follow his example.

Harken's tour de force in a hut in the Cotswolds was the culmination of half a century's progress, in the course of which surgeons had overcome ancient fears about the heart and learned to treat it as one of the ordinary tissues of the body. They now knew that it could be held, manipulated and even repaired without fatal result. But heart injuries are rare, even in wartime; what of the millions living with faulty heart valves or blocked arteries, or the thousands of babies born every year with congenital cardiac deformities? These were challenges crying out for a surgical revolution. As it happened, that revolution had already begun a few months earlier, in an operating theatre on the other side of the Atlantic; and Dwight Harken would continue to play a leading role.

2. BLUE BABIES

Baltimore, 29 November 1944

One afternoon in November 1944 the chief of surgery at Johns Hopkins Hospital in Baltimore, Alfred Blalock, sat in his office deep in thought. As usual he had a cigarette on the go: even after losing two years of his early career to tuberculosis, he had never quite managed to give up his forty-a-day habit. With his neatly combed hair, immaculate chalk-stripe suit and donnish glasses, he might easily have been mistaken for a prosperous lawyer, but at the age of forty-five he was already known as one of America's foremost clinical researchers. A few years earlier he had revolutionised the treatment of circulatory shock, a life-threatening condition in which blood loss makes it difficult for the heart to pump enough fluid to the body. Shock was one of the biggest killers in wartime, frequently the consequence of injury by shrapnel or explosives. Blalock's experiments led to the routine use of blood-plasma transfusions to treat those with severe wounds, a measure which saved the lives of thousands of servicemen in the Second World War.[1]

This achievement alone was enough to ensure Blalock's place in the medical pantheon, but this afternoon he felt only frustration. When his senior resident surgeon, William Longmire, walked into the room he found his boss sitting disconsolately behind a pile of books. In recent weeks Blalock had attempted a series of ambitious and difficult procedures on patients seriously ill with abdominal disorders:

none had been successful, and most of the patients had died. 'Bill, I am discouraged,' he said to Longmire. 'Nothing I do works.'[2] Blalock was desperate to make an original contribution to surgical history, and to silence colleagues who complained that he was a competent researcher but a mediocre clinician. Recently he had been concentrating his efforts on developing new methods to treat problems with the pancreas and intestines. But only a few days later he would perform a novel and entirely different kind of operation, one that would catapult him to fame and make Johns Hopkins a place of pilgrimage for patients and surgeons from all over the world.

Shortly after their conversation Longmire was summoned to the third floor of the clinic, where Blalock took him to a cot containing one of the hospital's youngest patients. Her name was Eileen Saxon, and she had been born at Johns Hopkins the previous year. Now fifteen months old, she was desperately ill and being kept alive in an oxygen tent. Longmire was shocked by her condition. She was unusually small for her age, but the first thing he noticed was her colour. Her skin had a deathly pallor, and her lips and fingernails were a dark, inky blue. Eileen was suffering from a congenital condition called tetralogy of Fallot; children unlucky enough to be born with it were known as 'Blue Babies', and there was little that could be done for them. The blue tinge to Eileen's skin was cyanosis, the result of blood bypassing the lungs and circulating through the body unoxygenated. Half of all children in her position would die before the age of three, and fewer than a quarter would make it to the age of ten.[3] Those who survived for any length of time endured a miserable existence. Many physicians believed that the smallest degree of excitement would be fatal, and everyday pursuits – school, outdoor play, the cinema, even travel by motor vehicle – were often prohibited.[4] Eileen's future looked bleak.

When Blalock told his junior that he intended to try a new type of operation on her, Longmire was horrified: given her state, he could not believe that she would survive an anaesthetic, let alone a procedure that had never before been attempted.[5] The chief anaesthetist, Austin Lamont, concurred. When he heard of Blalock's plans he flatly refused to take part in proceedings, and the operation was cancelled.[6] But one of Lamont's colleagues, Merel Harmel, was prepared to take the risk, and it was rescheduled for the following day.

Early on the morning of Wednesday 29 November little Eileen was taken into room 706, an operating theatre on the seventh floor of the building that in later years would be known simply as 'the heart room'. Two large windows provided most of the light; in the summer these were usually thrown open in a futile attempt to gain some respite from the fierce Maryland heat. There was a small observation gallery overlooking the operating table, and several hospital staff were leaning over its rail, having heard rumours that something unusual was about to take place. As Blalock scanned the faces of the spectators he caught sight of his laboratory assistant, and called out to him: 'Vivien, you'd better come down here.'

In his early thirties, Vivien Thomas was a talented surgical technician with a sophisticated grasp of anatomy and physiology – and almost entirely self-taught. Thomas had planned to become a doctor, but his chances of going to university evaporated after the bank holding his savings collapsed in the aftermath of the Wall Street crash. Instead he found a job working in Blalock's laboratory in Nashville, where the authorities paid him a pittance and categorised him as a janitor because he was black.[7] He soon became so essential to Blalock's work that when the surgeon moved to Baltimore he insisted that Johns Hopkins employ Thomas too. Since he had no medical qualifications, Thomas usually had no contact with patients. His role was in the animal laboratory, where he performed physiological experiments and helped to develop new surgical procedures. He had perfected the operation Blalock was about to perform, practising it hundreds of times on dogs and refining every detail.

But the idea to operate on these desperately ill children had come from one of the other people standing expectantly in the operating theatre. Helen Taussig was the paediatric cardiologist looking after Eileen Saxon; like Thomas, she had faced prejudice and personal setbacks in her early career. As a student she had been rejected by

Harvard Medical School on the grounds that she was a woman, but had nevertheless managed to become the world's leading expert on congenital heart conditions. Profoundly deaf since her thirties, she had taught herself to diagnose rare conditions using her hands as a stethoscope.[8]

Thomas and Taussig would play no active part in proceedings, but Blalock leaned heavily on them for advice. The surgical team assisting him was young and formidable; it included William Longmire and William Muller, two outstanding protégés who would soon be appointed to major professorships. Standing at the foot of the table, ready to administer intravenous fluids to the patient, was a twenty-four-year-old intern whose career would outshine even theirs: his name was Denton Cooley, and he was destined to become one of the most celebrated surgeons in the world, and the first to implant an artificial heart.

The mood was far from optimistic. Longmire was convinced the girl would die, and Cooley's considered opinion was that the operation would be 'a big disaster'.[9] Merel Harmel put a mask over Eileen's face and dripped ether on to it. This was a primitive way of putting a patient to sleep, used since the dawn of anaesthesia in the 1840s; it was also dangerous, as it was difficult to control how deeply or for how long the patient would remain unconscious. As Eileen succumbed to the ether, Blalock and his colleagues – eight in total – gathered around her tiny body. Vivien Thomas remarked that she was so small that it was difficult to believe that there was a patient underneath the sterile drapes.[10]

Blalock made the first incision on the left side of her chest, starting at her breastbone and extending it to her armpit. As he cut through her muscle in order to gain access to the heart, blood welled up from a number of small arteries. The surgeons were taken aback by its appearance: rather than the free-flowing, bright red fluid they were used to seeing, this was a glutinous blue-black. Longmire described it as 'like purple molasses'; had he been in charge, the operation would have been abandoned there and then.[11]

The alarming colour of Eileen's blood was the cause of her infir-
mity. Although people often refer to 'the circulation' when talking
about the movement of blood, there are really two: the pulmonary circulation and the systemic. When the blood has completed its journey
around the body and arrives back at the heart it has given up most of
its oxygen to the organs and tissues; in this state, it has a blueish tint.
The right side of the heart then pumps it to the lungs, where it passes
through tiny vessels that allow freshly inhaled oxygen to pass into the
red blood cells. At the same time, carbon dioxide – a waste product of
processes inside the body's cells – moves in the opposite direction and
is then exhaled. The freshly oxygenated blood, now bright red, travels
back to the left side of the heart, ready to be pumped through the rest
of the body. Blood therefore passes through the heart twice: first as
part of the pulmonary circulation through the lungs, and then as part
of the systemic circulation that nourishes all our major organs.

In tetralogy of Fallot this neat arrangement is hopelessly compromised. Those with the condition have four separate cardiac deformities, of which two are responsible for the characteristic skin pallor.
Whereas the left and right sides of a normal heart are separated by a
wall of tissue, in tetralogy there is a large aperture between the two,
known as a septal defect. As a result, oxygenated blood from the lungs
mixes freely with blue, deoxygenated blood from the rest of the body.
In addition, the pulmonary artery, the vessel through which blood is
pumped to the lungs, is drastically narrowed so that its flow is greatly
reduced. When the heart of a tetralogy patient contracts, only a small
proportion of the deoxygenated blood in the right ventricle is able to
escape through the narrowed pulmonary artery towards the lungs;
most of it instead passes through the septal defect and into the systemic circulation. Because so little of their blood has travelled through
the lungs, Blue Babies have extremely low blood oxygen levels, causing
breathlessness, stunted growth and the unhealthy coloration which
typifies the condition.

Blalock could not entirely correct this malformation, but by some
ingenious plumbing he hoped to improve Eileen's condition. Having

exposed her heart and its major vessels, his plan was to redirect one of her arteries so that instead of delivering blood to her left arm it would instead send it back towards her lungs, increasing her overall oxygen levels. In surgical parlance this type of procedure, in which blood is redirected to where it is most needed, is called a 'shunt'; within a few years Blalock's operation would be universally known as the 'Blalock–Taussig shunt'.*

The first challenge was identifying the correct blood vessels. Unless you have seen the inside of the human body at first hand, it's difficult to appreciate how little it resembles the neat arrangement of nerves and vessels depicted in a textbook. Every patient is different: arteries vary greatly in size or trace entirely unexpected paths; blood vessels sit so close together that they become almost impossible to differentiate. And they lie snugly embedded in tissue, requiring meticulous dissection in order to lay eyes on them in the first place. It took Blalock some time to be sure he had found the two arteries he was looking for.

The first of these was the left pulmonary artery, which takes blood from the heart to the left lung. The procedure would involve shutting off this vessel for as much as half an hour, with the result that Eileen would be breathing through a single lung. This was a huge risk in an already oxygen-deprived patient, and so Blalock temporarily clamped the vessel to see how she would tolerate it. To everybody's alarm her skin became an even more icy blue, as if her life was ebbing away before their eyes. Harmel attempted to put a tube into the girl's windpipe in order to deliver oxygen straight to her one functioning lung, but without success: endotracheal tubes for such small children had not yet been manufactured, and the only implement available – a urinary catheter – was hopelessly unsuited to the job.[12]

---

* It has since been argued, with some justification, that given the importance of Vivien Thomas's contribution the operation should instead be known as the Blalock–Taussig–Thomas shunt.

There was an anxious wait as the surgeons decided what to do. To their relief, Eileen's colour improved slightly without further interference; they could continue. With infinite care, Blalock freed a second artery from its surrounding tissue. This was new territory for him: although he had watched Vivien Thomas carry out the procedure on dogs, he had never attempted it himself. He had installed Thomas – the expert, with 200 trial runs under his belt – on a stool behind him, a vantage point from which he could observe and make suggestions. Periodically Blalock would turn to his assistant and ask for advice: is this artery long enough? Is this the right part of the vessel to clamp?

Eileen's blood vessels were even smaller than those of the dogs Thomas had operated on: the one Blalock needed was no bigger than a matchstick.[13] This was the vessel taking blood to her left arm, the left subclavian artery. After isolating a section of the vessel with clamps to ensure no blood was flowing through it, he cut through the artery with a scalpel. He made a small incision in the side of the pulmonary artery and began the most challenging part of the procedure. A fine needle threaded with silk was used to attach the tiny subclavian artery to the pulmonary artery. Placing the sutures required almost inhuman accuracy, and the instruments at Blalock's disposal were ill-suited to such delicate work. Nothing of this kind had been attempted before on the miniature vessels of a child: the needle and forceps Blalock was using were designed for adult surgery and felt unpleasantly cumbersome, as if he were trying to repair a Swiss watch using a plumber's wrench.

After what seemed like an eternity, the two vessels were united.[14] In theory, a proportion of the blood leaving the heart would be pumped into the subclavian artery and then be redirected back into Eileen's left lung, increasing its oxygenation. But the vessel was so small that Blalock was unsure if the operation would have much effect. He released the clamps, allowing blood to pass through the new junction for the first time. After checking carefully for signs of bleeding, he closed the chest and stitched the external wound. The operation had lasted a little over an hour and a half; although there was no obvious improvement in Eileen's condition, she had survived.* Complications followed, however, and for two weeks the little girl's life hung in the balance. Thereafter she began to make good progress, and on 25 January, almost two months after the operation, she was well enough to go home. Helen Taussig was pleasantly surprised to find that she had started to gain weight, and her episodes of cyanosis became less pronounced. Her parents were delighted: previously too ill to go outside, she was now learning to walk and could join them on outings to their local park.[15] The operation had been a modest but definite success.†

This outcome seemed to justify further attempts, and on 3 February Blalock operated on a second patient, this time a nine-year-old girl. On her arrival in hospital she was only able to walk thirty feet, stooping and panting; a month after surgery she could walk upright for twice that distance, without any sign of discomfort.[16] This was an encouraging development – but better was to come. On 7 February 1945 a desperately ill six-year-old boy was admitted to Johns Hopkins. He was extremely undernourished and could manage only a few paces without losing his breath. Taussig examined him and noted that he was severely cyanosed, recording in her notes that the insides of his cheeks were a deep mulberry colour.[17] His parents were adamant that they would take any chance to save their son, and three days later Blalock operated.

This time he used the innominate artery, a vessel supplying blood to the arm, head and neck. First he severed it just before the point at

* In their accounts of the operation both Cooley and William H. Muller state that Eileen's colour improved markedly within a few minutes. Blalock and Taussig's journal article, based on notes made on the day of the procedure, suggests otherwise. It seems likely that Cooley and Muller confused the first operation with the third, in which a dramatic colour change *was* observed.
† Despite this initial improvement, Eileen Saxon lived only a few months longer: her symptoms returned and a second operation was unsuccessful. It later became clear that children under the age of three gained only temporary benefit from the procedure.

which it split into the two branches supplying the head and left arm. After suturing its upper extremity closed, he attached the lower part of the vessel, the end nearer the heart, to the right pulmonary artery. This new circuit would redirect some of the boy's blueish systemic blood back into the lungs for an additional dose of oxygen. When he released the clamps, a stream of blood gushed out of an undetected hole between the sutures; he quickly reapplied the clamps to cut this off and repaired the opening with an extra stitch. This time the join was perfect, and when the circulation was allowed to flow again it did so without any problems.

As the patient's right lung received its first blood in over an hour, something extraordinary happened. Merel Harmel, the anaesthetist, suddenly cried, 'He's a *lovely* colour now! Take a look!' Blalock and Taussig moved to the head of the table, and were astonished to see a pink-faced little boy with healthy red lips. Within a few minutes he was awake and asking to get out of bed.[18] Elation filled the room. A young medical student who had been observing the operation, Mary Allen Engle, was so moved that she decided then and there to become a cardiologist; she would go on to be one of the field's leading authorities.[19] For the next few days, nurses accustomed to tending critically ill children found themselves dealing with a patient who was desperate to run around and play. The transformation was miraculous: in her case notes, Helen Taussig recorded that 'his disposition has changed from that of a miserable whining child to a happy smiling boy.'[20]

That dramatic colour change – from sickly blue to healthy pink – was a proof of success that both medics and the public could readily understand. Blalock and Taussig wrote a report of their three cases for the *Journal of the American Medical Association*. Before the article had even been printed a journalist from the Associated Press somehow got hold of a copy, realised its significance, and published a story. Editors leapt upon it: at a time when newspapers were full of harrowing details of American deaths in the war in Europe, this was a rare morsel of good news: a happy story of terminally ill children being magically restored to life.[21]

The effect was electrifying, and the medical world was utterly unprepared for it. Tetralogy of Fallot is one of the more common congenital heart conditions, affecting one in every 2,400 newborns.[22] There were thousands of children in the US alone who might be saved by the new operation, invalids presumed to be beyond medical help. Family doctors who knew nothing about Blalock's breakthrough suddenly received visits from parents demanding a referral to the hospital in Baltimore. Children began to arrive at Johns Hopkins from across the country and then from abroad, and before long a trickle had become a flood. Not all parents could afford the operation, and some small-town newspapers launched public appeals to fund them. Such patients often turned up with a local journalist in tow, and surgeons found themselves constantly answering questions from uninvited members of the press.[23]

Within a few months the paediatric beds of Johns Hopkins were full, with tetralogy patients (known to the staff as 'tets') spilling out into the adult wards. This was an exhausting period for Blalock's team, who were constantly operating during the day and often called to the wards at night; they barely took a day off. Regular delegations of surgeons arrived from abroad to observe the operation and find out what equipment they would need in order to do it themselves.[24]

A still more rapturous reception awaited Blalock in Europe. He was invited to spend a month at Guy's Hospital in London, and on 22 August 1947 Blalock and his wife Mary sailed for England on the *Mauretania*. He had spent the day before his departure frantically trying to procure a month's supply of Viceroy cigarettes, which were unobtainable in Britain.[25] During his short residency at Guy's, Blalock operated successfully on ten Blue Babies. His visit was widely reported: one woman from Sevenoaks in Kent, a Mrs Gallard, read about the celebrated American heart surgeon and promptly jumped on a London train to ask him to operate on her eight-year-old son Roger, who was confined to a wheelchair. Four months later a local newspaper reported that he was now able to run around and play with his friends. His mother explained to the journalist, not entirely accurately, that the surgeon had 'removed Roger's heart, and while it lay pulsating in his hands, he remodelled it'.[26] Displaying a similarly hazy grasp of surgical minutiae, a *Daily Mail* article the following month claimed that during the procedure another patient's heart was 'removed and massaged'.[27]

Towards the end of his stay, Blalock shared the stage with Helen Taussig for a joint lecture to a packed hall at the British Medical Association. Their presentation ended in spectacular fashion when a spotlight beam suddenly pierced the darkened hall to pick out a nurse sitting on a chair with an angelic and healthy two-year-old on her lap; Blalock had operated on the little girl a week earlier. The leading British surgeon of the day, Russell Brock, described it as 'a Madonna-like tableau, a perfect climax to an impressive lecture on an epoch-making contribution'.[28]

Blalock's tour (his 'royal progress', as one of his juniors described it) continued with visits to hospitals in Sweden and France. He left behind an important legacy in Europe: a 'Blue Baby clinic' was set up at Guy's,[29] and within a few months the operation was being successfully performed in many other centres across the continent. As they boarded their plane back to America, Blalock remarked to his wife that they had been treated like gods; now they must come down to earth again.[30] This was no exaggeration: a massive backlog of cases awaited him in Baltimore. By 1948 there was a three-year waiting list for the operation,[31] and two years later a photographic portrait of Blalock was commissioned to commemorate the 1,000th case.[32]

Despite the hundreds of lives it saved, the work of Blalock, Taussig and Thomas was also fiercely criticised. Antivivisection campaigners were outraged at the number of animal experiments taking place in the Johns Hopkins laboratories, and fought tirelessly to put a stop to them. Experimental surgery on animals had long been standard practice in developing new operations; dogs, whose hearts and major vessels were similar in size to those of humans, were easily available, since most cities had large numbers of unwanted strays. But some of these experiments were of dubious value and inflicted unnecessary suffering. In 1901 one of the pioneers of cardiac surgery, Benjamin Merrill Ricketts, performed experiments on forty-five dogs at his laboratory in Cincinnati, deliberately injuring their hearts and surrounding tissues. 'The object was to induce as many complications as possible,' he explained, and in this he was certainly successful: the vast majority of the animals died shortly afterwards.[33]

By the 1940s researchers had a more enlightened attitude, and Vivien Thomas's surgical trials on dogs were all conducted with full anaesthesia; those that developed complications were humanely killed. Nevertheless, there were repeated attempts to shut down his research, with campaigners harassing laboratory staff and the suppliers of animals. A national animal-rights movement had emerged in the 1880s, and later succeeded in presenting to Congress a bill to ban animal experimentation.[34] It was defeated, but vigorous local campaigns continued in many states. In February 1946, as Congress considered new antivivisection legislation, Blalock gave evidence before a House committee with three of his young patients, explaining that without animal experimentation none of them would have survived.[35] He made a powerful case, and the bill was voted down.

Local activists in Baltimore were more tenacious, and succeeded in preventing medical researchers from using unclaimed stray dogs for their experiments. Without a ready supply of animals, hospitals took to buying them in from neighbouring states, and when this practice was also deemed unlawful matters came to a head.[36] Baltimore City Council announced a public vote – popularly known as the 'dog referendum' – to decide whether the use of animals for medical research should be prohibited. The pro-vivisection camp indulged in some emotive tactics in its attempt to win the public over. When Helen Taussig spoke at an open meeting she was accompanied by a brigade of her patients: healthy, smiling children, many of whom had brought their pet dogs.[37] The star of the campaign was a playful and photogenic mongrel called Anna, an early survivor of Vivien Thomas's surgical trials. She appeared in an educational film and was photographed for *Life* magazine with one of the children who had been saved by the operation.[38] The result of the dog referendum was decisive: the anti-vivisection faction was resoundingly defeated by a margin of more than four to one.[39] To commemorate the win, Blalock commissioned a portrait of Anna, which remains on display at the hospital today.[40]

Blalock and his first Blue Baby success of 1944 captured the public attention as no operation had before. Most modern surgeons would agree with Russell Brock's assessment that it represented the starting point of modern heart surgery, although Blalock had not operated on the organ itself, but on the blood vessels around it. Nor had he cured his patients: the operation was palliative, improving their quality of life rather than correcting the underlying condition. It was not until a decade later that another surgeon, C. Walton Lillehei, succeeded in curing a cyanotic infant.[41]

Tetralogy of Fallot is only one of a vast array of cardiac malformations, many of which at the time offered a still gloomier outlook for patients, with no hope of cure. The battle against congenital disease was only just beginning, but Blalock had made an effective assault on its ramparts. To give a sense of quite how significant a shift this represented, here is what the Scottish cardiologist James Mackenzie had to say about therapy for congenital conditions in his influential textbook *Diseases of the Heart*, published in 1908: 'If the heart maintains the circulation well, no treatment is required. In more serious cases, beyond attending to the child's comfort and nourishment, special treatment for the heart is of little benefit.'[42] In a work of several hundred pages Mackenzie devotes only a couple to congenital heart disease, and two meagre sentences to its treatment. Other experts had little else to offer: parents were advised to keep their children warm and, if possible, move to a balmy climate. In a lecture delivered at Great Ormond Street Hospital in 1906, Frederick Poynton recommended fattening them up like a Christmas turkey: 'No overcoat fits so well and acts so effectually as an undercoat of adipose tissue.'[43]

The fact that so little could be done for congenital heart disease at the turn of the twentieth century made it a deeply unfashionable area of research, and knowledge of individual disorders was virtually non-existent. Doctors could generally offer a diagnosis no more specific than 'malformation of the heart'. This is in some ways strange, since giant strides had already been made in the understanding of other types of heart disease, and congenital conditions had been among the first to be identified. Indeed, a Babylonian tablet once held by the Library at Nineveh, now in the collection of the British Museum, refers to a probable cardiac malformation from more than 2,500 years ago: 'When a woman gives birth to an infant that has the heart open and has no skin, the country will suffer from calamities.'[44] This appears to be a description of ectopia cordis, a rare condition in which the heart is formed outside the ribcage and protrudes through the chest, exposed to the air and beating in plain sight. In ancient civilisations such horrible deformities were often seen as an evil portent, making them worthy of record.

Early modern science also had a fascination with the grotesque. In 1665 the inaugural issue of the first scientific journal, the Royal Society's *Philosophical Transactions*, contained an article by Robert Boyle entitled 'An Account of a very odd monstrous calf'.[45] Prodigies and monsters were a common feature of the journal in its early years, and malformations seen in stillborn infants were a particular source of fascination. One such description, entitled 'A Monstrous Human Foetus, Having Neither Head, Heart, Lungs, Stomach, Spleen, Pancreas, Liver, nor Kidneys', was reproduced as a pamphlet and widely circulated. It was in an article of this kind that tetralogy of Fallot was first described.

The seventeenth-century Danish scientist Nicolas Steno enjoyed a varied career during which he made important contributions to anatomy and geology, and later became a bishop. His most celebrated achievement was to prove that heart tissue was muscular. In 1673 he published an account of an autopsy he had carried out on a stillborn infant, sensationally entitled 'Monstrous Embryo Dissected Near Paris'. The child exhibited a number of deformities, including a cleft lip and palate and webbed fingers on one hand; many of the organs had passed through a hole in the abdomen and were visible externally.

When questioned by Steno and his colleagues, the mother suggested that these anomalies had been caused by her fondness for rabbit stew.[46] This was not what interested them most, however: 'The unusual form of the arteries arising from the heart attracted the chief attention and called for admiration.' Steno was struck by the form of the pulmonary artery, which was much narrower than normal. Intrigued, he then dissected the heart and found that there was a septal defect – a hole in the tissue between the left and right ventricles. In addition the aorta, the main artery supplying blood to the rest of the body, did not arise from the left ventricle as it should, but communicated with both the left and right ventricles.[47]

These cardiac deformities – a narrowed pulmonary artery (known as pulmonary stenosis), a ventricular septal defect and an overriding aorta – are three of the four characteristic defects of tetralogy of Fallot. The fourth, not mentioned by Steno, is a thickening of the wall of the right ventricle: its clinical name is right ventricular hypertrophy, and it is caused by the difficulty the heart encounters in pumping blood through the narrowed pulmonary artery.* Steno was flummoxed by the discovery, concluding with the observation, 'As to the cause of this phenomenon, I have nothing to say.'[48]

By the late nineteenth century at least seven investigators had described this combination of cardiac malformations and the symptoms it caused. So it may seem strange that the condition is now named after an obscure French medic whose research took place a full two centuries after Steno's. In 1888, Étienne-Louis Arthur Fallot published a long article based on his observations of three cyanotic young men he had encountered at his hospital in Marseille. The first two patients died, and at a post-mortem he found the four characteristic deformities in their hearts. When the third patient was admitted with identical symptoms not long afterwards, Fallot diagnosed him with the same congenital disease, and predicted the cardiac malformations

---

* Heart muscle becomes stronger and more bulky if extra work is required of it, just as a bodybuilder's biceps are bulked up by weight training.

that would be found at autopsy. The man died shortly afterwards, and Fallot was shown to be correct. He then made a careful study of all the documented examples he could find of cyanotic disease, which he called 'la maladie bleue'. Earlier writers had often been confused about what caused the blue colour of their patients, attributing it to a single cardiac deformity or to a secondary feature which was absent in other cases. Fallot asserted that he had identified four separate features of this disease which were always present: pulmonary stenosis; a ventricular septal defect; right ventricular hypertrophy; and an overriding aorta. 'The constancy with which this group is reproduced is no less remarkable than its coexistence with the clinical syndrome of blue disease,' he wrote.[49] He called this group of four features a 'tetralogy', a misnomer that has pained classically educated medics ever since.[*]

The year after Fallot's paper appeared, a young Canadian called Maude Abbott applied to study medicine at McGill University in Montreal. Despite a vigorous campaign which was endorsed by several of the city's grandees, the faculty refused to admit her to a department which had hitherto been exclusively male. Rebuffed, Abbott instead went to Bishop's University, where as part of its first intake of female medical students she won numerous prizes.[50] For most of the twentieth century the field of heart surgery would be dominated by men; it was not until the 1960s that the first woman, Nina Starr Braunwald, would make inroads into this very male world.[51] It is therefore notable that the two people who added most to our knowledge of congenital heart disease – Abbott and Taussig – were both women who had to fight even to be admitted to the medical profession.

Abbott was later appointed to what might have been a dreary job as assistant curator of the medical museum of McGill, the university that had rejected her as a student. Browsing its collections she became intrigued by one specimen in a glass jar, a heart with a strange

---

[*] A 'tetralogy' is a set of four linked works of art, such as Ford Madox Ford's *Parade's End* or the *Lethal Weapon* franchise. Fallot's group of related heart lesions should strictly be known as a 'tetrad'.

deformity. She sought the advice of Sir William Osler, Canada's most eminent clinician and one of the founding professors of Johns Hopkins medical school. He encouraged her to make congenital heart conditions the subject of her research, commissioning her to write a chapter on the topic for his textbook *The Principles and Practice of Medicine*.

Abbott tracked down and examined 412 separate cases of cardiac malformations. She became so immersed in the subject that she continued to amass examples long after the publication of Osler's book, and by the 1920s had studied over 1,000 hearts with abnormalities.[52] This was an undertaking unprecedented in its scope, and by 1936, when she published an illustrated book based on her findings, the *Atlas of Congenital Cardiac Disease*, she was the world's acknowledged expert. When Helen Taussig, then a young paediatrician, first became interested in congenital heart conditions she went on a pilgrimage to McGill to tap this vast reservoir of knowledge; Abbott was enormously helpful, showing Taussig specimens from her collection, and comparing them with X-ray images of the same defect.[53] Maude Abbott died in 1940, four years before Taussig's astonishing Blue Baby triumph. But she did live long enough to see a surgeon from Boston, Robert Gross, achieve the first outright cure of a congenital abnormality.

In the first century AD the Roman surgeon Galen made a startlingly accurate observation whose true significance would not be appreciated until a millennium and a half later. In book XV of his study of human anatomy, *De Usu Partium*, he wrote: 'The ductus joining the aorta to the pulmonary artery not only ceases to grow after birth, when all the other parts of the animal are growing, but it can be seen to become thinner and thinner, until as time progresses, it dries up completely and wears away.'[54]

A 'ductus' is a duct or channel, and the example Galen describes is an important quirk of human development. When we are adults, our blood passes from the right side of the heart through the pulmonary artery to the lungs; after oxygenation it then returns through the pulmonary veins to the left side of the heart, which pumps it through the aorta to the rest of the body. Although linked, the two circulations are distinct; indeed, the blood pressure is significantly higher in the systemic circulation than that which passes through the lungs.

Before we are born the situation is rather different. A foetus in the womb receives all its oxygen from its mother via the placenta. It cannot yet use its lungs, so there is no need for a large volume of blood to pass through them. Most of the circulation therefore bypasses the lungs through two temporary canals: the foramen ovale, a small window between the left and right sides of the heart; and the ductus arteriosus, a short vessel which joins the aorta and pulmonary artery near their origin at the top of the organ. The ductus arteriosus usually closes in the first week after birth, just as Galen observed, and the circulation to the lungs and to the rest of the body are separated. William Harvey noted in the seventeenth century that a large volume of blood passes through this passage during foetal life, and his friend Nathaniel Highmore, the first to accept Harvey's findings about the circulation of the blood, noticed that the closure of the ductus and the foramen ovale coincided with the onset of respiration through the lungs.[55]

In the eighteenth century it emerged that this elegant mechanism did not always work as it should: surgeons examining corpses on the mortuary slab began to find adult hearts in which the foramen ovale had failed to close.[56] In other bodies they observed that the ductus arteriosus had remained open – or patent – well into adulthood. In some cases this defect had no obvious effect on the patient; others suffered shortness of breath, an irregular heart rhythm or stunted growth. Strangely, some physicians believed that those with a patent ductus or foramen ovale were able to breathe underwater. The source of this misconception was Harvey, who observed that foetuses were able to survive in the womb without breathing; he speculated that a patent ductus and foramen ovale might be the physiological mechanism that allowed aquatic birds like ducks and geese to spend long periods of time submerged.[57] It was a neat suggestion, but well wide of the mark: in fact the muscles of diving birds and mammals contain high levels of myoglobin, a protein which stores oxygen and enables them to hold their breath for several minutes.[58]

Patent ductus arteriosus was thus one of the first congenital heart defects to be described and understood, and by the beginning of the twentieth century doctors could also diagnose it with reasonable confidence. In 1898 George Alexander Gibson of the Edinburgh Royal Infirmary wrote about a characteristic noise which could be heard through the stethoscope when examining affected patients. This 'distinct thrill',[59] as he called it, is now known as a Gibson murmur* and is sometimes likened to the sound of a washing machine. Being able to recognise the condition was the essential first step towards treating it, and only a few years later another heart specialist correctly predicted how a patent ductus could be cured.

On 6 May 1907 an American doctor, John Munro, gave a speech to a meeting of the Philadelphia Academy of Surgery. He explained that some years earlier he had been treating a baby girl who subsequently died; during the post-mortem examination he found a large patent ductus, and it occurred to him that it would not have been difficult to repair it: 'The simplicity of the remedy was so striking that I at once made further dissections, and satisfied myself that it would be possible to ligate [tie] the duct provided a diagnosis could be made beforehand.' Munro suggested that artificially closing the ductus would be followed by 'permanent restoration to a normal function of the lungs and arteries',[60] and pleaded with his colleagues not to dismiss the idea out of hand. He was thinking along the right lines, but given the primitive state of anaesthesia at this date it is probably fortunate that no surgeon dared attempt it until many years later.

Although disregarded, Munro's suggestion was not entirely forgotten. In the early 1920s Evarts Graham, professor of surgery at Washington University in St Louis, became convinced that it should

---

* This honour may be undeserved: the phenomenon had already been described in 1874 by a Finn, Osvald Wasastjerna. The tongue-twister 'Wasastjerna murmur', however, might have been a less memorable clinical term.

be possible to cure a patient with patent ductus arteriosus by closing the vessel surgically. He approached the professor of paediatrics at
the St Louis Children's Hospital, explained the problem, and asked his
colleague to send him a suitable patient for operation. To his irritation,
the patient who duly appeared in his office was a fifty-three-year-old
man whose condition was far too advanced to make him a plausible
candidate for surgery. It seems the paediatrician was irked by his junior colleague's effrontery, and had deliberately sent him an unsuitable
patient to ensure that he could not take an unacceptable surgical risk.
Russell Brock later suggested that this 'cruel and stupid' act delayed
the advent of heart surgery in children by fifteen years.[61]

The first surgeon to succeed in closing a patent ductus arteriosus
met similar resistance to the idea, and had to resort to subterfuge in
order to overcome it. In 1938 Robert Gross was thirty-three and a junior surgeon at Boston Children's Hospital. Born with severely impaired
vision in one eye, Gross struggled with depth perception. His father,
who was a piano-maker, helped him develop his hand-eye coordination by employing him in his workshop. Later, when he revealed his
ambition to become a surgeon, Gross senior gave him clocks to take
apart and reassemble; as his fine-motor skills improved, the clocks
got smaller. Remarkably, Gross never revealed this disability during
his career: only after his retirement did he approach a colleague for
advice, and when a congenital cataract was removed from the affected
eye he experienced binocular vision for the first time in his life.[62]

Gross had seen several small children die of a cardiac infection
called acute bacterial endocarditis, a common complication of a patent ductus arteriosus. He was both frustrated by his inability to do
anything for them and attracted to the mechanical nature of the problem. He was convinced that tying off the blood vessel was feasible.
Two other surgeons had by now attempted the procedure, but one had
failed to close the vessel and the other had found when he opened the
patient that the condition had been misdiagnosed.[63] Gross spent many
hours in the laboratory devising a new operation, which he tested
on dogs and then on cadavers. When he was satisfied that he had a

workable procedure he approached his head of department, William Ladd, and explained the proposition. Ladd was unimpressed, telling him to continue his research and explicitly prohibiting him from trying his method on a patient.

Undaunted, Gross bided his time. Ladd was in the habit of taking his annual holiday every August, and as soon as he was safely on a boat to Europe, Gross acted. He selected two patients he thought suitable for operation, reasoning that even if the first died he would have a second chance to demonstrate that the procedure worked. This may seem a curiously unemotional, even callous, approach, but it was entirely pragmatic. Any candidate for surgery would already be gravely ill and would inevitably die if left untreated. If they failed to survive the operation it would prove nothing, since such a high-risk patient faced long odds however perfect the surgery. A single success, on the other hand, would be proof positive that Gross's new operation was sound.

Happily, as things turned out he needed only one. The first patient he chose was Lorraine Sweeney, a seven-year-old girl who had been admitted to the Children's Hospital on 17 August 1938. From early childhood she had been short of breath, and was diagnosed with patent ductus arteriosus. After starting school she began to experience strange episodes in which she became frightened and clutched her breast; when asked what the matter was she would whisper 'something wrong inside of here'. Her mother was alarmed by a loud buzzing noise she could hear emanating from inside the little girl's chest. Her symptoms worsened, and it soon became clear that if left untreated her life would be short.

On 26 August 1938, Gross began an operation that would seal his reputation as one of the great pioneers of paediatric medicine. He was assisted by Thomas Lanman, the most senior member of the surgical staff after Ladd,[64] and Betty Lank agreed to administer the anaesthetic. His colleagues were well aware that they were defying their boss, but were impressed by Gross's steely determination: he was a serious-minded and impressive individual.

It is easily overlooked that anaesthetists were as much the heroes
of these early operations as the surgeons. Their equipment was basic,
and they were being asked to anaesthetise patients more critically ill
than any who had previously undergone surgery, many of them tiny
babies. In the early days of anaesthesia, when the job involved little more than dripping ether or chloroform on to a mask to put the
patient to sleep, it was thought to be an undemanding role, and anaesthetists were typically nurses rather than qualified physicians. Betty
Lank belonged to this caste of nurse-anaesthetists; only in the 1940s
would board-certified physicians (known in the US as anesthesiolo-
gists) take over the job.

With limited equipment to monitor the condition of patients while
they were unconscious, the task of keeping them alive was daunting. But theirs were not the only lives at risk. Chloroform and ether
are both toxic, and ether highly flammable. For Lorraine Sweeney's
operation Betty Lank used a recently discovered anaesthetic agent,
cyclopropane. This was widely regarded as a huge improvement on
the older drugs: when mixed with oxygen it was easily inhaled, it gave
quick and deep anaesthesia, and patients experienced none of the
post-operative nausea associated with chloroform. Unfortunately the
oxygen–cyclopropane mixture had one major drawback: it was dangerously explosive, and thus necessitated extraordinary precautions.
The temperature and humidity of the operating theatre were carefully
controlled; staff were prohibited from wearing silk, wool, leather or
wooden shoes; and electrical equipment could not be turned on or off
during the operation. Anaesthetists were even advised to switch to
another gas if there were thunderstorms in the area.[65] Nevertheless,
accidents still occurred. During an operation for lung cancer at
another Boston hospital a few years earlier a spark had caused a major
explosion, killing the patient instantly.[66] So when Betty Lank admitted
that she was 'scared to death' by the prospect of this operation, it's
possible it was not merely the wrath of Dr Ladd that she feared.

Once the gas had been administered and Lorraine was asleep,
Gross opened an incision on the left side of her chest. After cutting

through the muscle that lay beneath, he severed the cartilage connecting her third rib to the breastbone, and moved the rib out of the way. As air entered her chest through the incision the left lung collapsed, giving Gross a clear view of the heart and its major blood vessels. His fingers were now just millimetres away from the ductus arteriosus, but it would take him more than an hour to find and expose it. In order to do so he needed to dissect the aorta and pulmonary artery free of their surrounding tissue, without causing major bleeding or damaging any of the delicate structures around the heart. In an article written thirteen years later and based on his experience of 412 such operations, Gross emphasised the formidable difficulty of this stage, observing that 'in so crowded a space a single false step can lead to disaster.' In later operations he would devote as much as two hours to this painstaking task.[67]

With the major vessels carefully exposed, Gross could see the ductus joining the pulmonary artery and the aorta. It was only 5 millimetres long, but its 8-millimetre diameter meant that a large volume of blood was passing through it every second. Placing a finger on the heart, he felt an alarming vibration: not just the usual powerful contractions, but an unnatural buzzing that continued even between the heartbeats. He placed the end of a stethoscope on the pulmonary artery and heard a deafening continuous roar that reminded him of steam escaping from some enormous engine. He carefully passed a loop of silk around the ductus and drew it tight. The surgical team waited nervously, watching for any sign that the circulation had been compromised. When three minutes had elapsed without any crisis, Gross decided to tie the loose ends of the silk to close the ductus permanently.

When he did so the worrying vibration disappeared instantly. Relieved, Gross closed Lorraine's chest and sewed up his incision. The operation had been fraught, but the child had withstood the procedure well, and there had never been any threat to her life. The following day Lorraine was well enough to sit in a chair; within forty-eight hours she was walking around the ward.[68]

In their clinical reports surgeons sometimes note that a patient had a 'stormy' post-operative recovery. This is euphemistic, usually indicating a series of unpleasant and possibly life-threatening complications. In Lorraine Sweeney's case the word was appropriate in its literal sense: as she convalesced a dramatic hurricane swept into Boston. When Gross visited her bedside he was pleased to discover that she was in excellent health: her greatest worry was that the wind would knock down the sandcastle she had just built.[69] A little girl on the brink of death had been transformed into a perfectly happy child able to live a normal life.

Not everybody was delighted by this success. Dr Ladd – still on holiday in Europe – read about the operation in a newspaper and was furious at Gross's insubordination. When he first saw Gross after his return to work he asked him if there was anything new he ought to know about. 'Nope, not much, nothing new,' was his junior's reply.[70] Relations between the two men would remain permanently frosty.[71] What perhaps most irritated Ladd was that Gross had been right. All four of his first patients thrived after their operation,[72] and Ladd reluctantly allowed him to undertake more. But things did not go smoothly for long. When the twelfth patient returned from hospital her parents threw a party to welcome her home. In the midst of the celebrations the guest of honour suddenly collapsed and died. A post-mortem revealed that the ligature had cut through the ductus, resulting in massive haemorrhage. After this incident Gross modified the procedure, and instead of closing the ductus by tying it, he began to divide it with a scalpel before suturing the ends. This was a trickier operation, but provided a safer long-term solution.

By 1944, when Alfred Blalock gave a talk to the Massachusetts Medical Society about recent advances in surgery, he could report that Gross had successfully operated on over 60 patients, observing that there were an estimated 20,000 people in the US alone who stood to gain from the procedure.[73] By 1951 the number of patients had risen to over 400, with more than 97 per cent of them cured.[74] Other surgeons reported excellent results with the new operation.

In 1943 a boy aged thirteen was treated in Edinburgh, and five years later was accepted for army service with the top A1 rating for physical condition. He became regimental boxing champion and claimed to be able to run 100 yards in 10 seconds.[75] A short length of silk thread, placed and tied with superlative skill, had turned an invalid into an athlete.

The success of Gross's 1938 operation was one of the developments that emboldened Blalock to develop his Blue Baby procedure. But in the six-year period between these two landmarks another important blow was struck against congenital heart disease. Although both Gross and Blalock were involved in the research behind this development, it was a Swede, Clarence Crafoord, who made the breakthrough.

The aorta is the largest blood vessel in the human body: it's the artery through which freshly oxygenated blood is pumped to all the major organs. About the diameter of a garden hose, it originates at the top of the left ventricle of the heart, ascends for a few centimetres and then curves downwards in a loop known as the aortic arch. It then continues into the abdomen for around thirteen centimetres before splitting into two. Three branches off the top of the aortic arch provide blood to the head and upper limbs; the abdominal aorta supplies the lower half of the body. An unimpeded flow through this crucial vessel is absolutely essential.

In a relatively common congenital abnormality called coarctation of the aorta, a section of the vessel is constricted to a fraction of its normal diameter. Because blood has to be forced through this narrowing, pressure is increased above the constriction and decreased below it. This leads to a striking symptom in which patients have much higher blood pressure in their arms than in their legs. Blood vessels in the thorax often become enlarged as the body struggles to improve circulation to the abdomen, sometimes becoming so swollen that they cause erosion to the ribs. This is a natural compensation mechanism, akin to what happens on a road network when a major route between two towns is closed: vehicles soon start to bypass the

blockage by using smaller side roads, with traffic reaching its destination via a more circuitous route. Similarly, the major arteries are
not the only routes to the major organs: blood can also reach them
via a labyrinthine network of smaller vessels known as collaterals.
The human body has another trick: new collaterals can form between
large vessels, and smaller vessels can enlarge to allow more blood to
pass through them.

Even with these coping mechanisms, coarctation is a debilitating
and life-threatening condition. Sufferers can develop complications
including high blood pressure and heart failure, and without treatment have a life expectancy of just thirty-four.[76] The abnormality was
not regularly diagnosed until enough was known about different congenital heart conditions to distinguish between them. One cardiologist noted in the 1930s that doctors had recently begun to encounter
more cases, though this is probably because they were getting better
at spotting the warning signs.[77] There was no known treatment, and
as late as 1944 one of the most widely used textbooks ventured only
that patients should be protected from infections or undue exertion.[78]
Unknown to its author, a radical cure was just around the corner –
thanks to a discovery made by accident.

By the mid-1930s surgeons in America and Europe were conducting hundreds of animal experiments in order to establish the likely difficulties of surgery on the heart and its major vessels. One thing they
worried about was the effect of interrupting the blood supply to the
rest of the body. They realised that if they needed to cut into the aorta
they would first have to stop blood flowing through it in order to avoid
excessive bleeding. Doing so even for a few minutes would deprive
the major organs of their oxygen supply, which most experts believed
would rapidly prove fatal.

In a series of experiments in 1935 Clarence Crafoord, a surgeon
at the Sabbatsberg Hospital in Stockholm, put this assumption to the
test. Using dogs as his test subjects, he placed a clamp over the aorta
to prevent any blood flowing to the rest of the body. He found to his
surprise that it was safe to interrupt the circulation for as much as

twenty-five minutes, as long as the brain continued to receive an adequate supply.* This he achieved by attaching the cerebral blood vessels to the circulation of a second dog, using glass and rubber tubes.

This result was not at first thought to have any relevance to surgery in human patients, but it turned out to have unexpected significance. Some years later Crafoord was operating on a child with a patent ductus. He used a silk ligature to tie the ductus closed, but when he tightened the thread it cut straight through the walls of the vessel. The bleeding was copious, and Crafoord failed to bring it under control. In desperation he placed a clamp across the aorta to stop all blood flow. This allowed him to close both severed ends of the ductus with sutures, an undertaking which took almost half an hour.[79] Remembering his earlier animal experiments, he was confident that most of the child's organs would not be harmed by such a long interruption to their circulation, but worried that the brain or spinal cord would be irreversibly damaged, causing paralysis or even death.

When the child awoke from the anaesthetic, Crafoord and his team were delighted to find that these fears were unfounded: there was no neurological damage. This set him thinking about coarctation of the aorta, a problem he had discussed with Robert Gross on one of his regular visits to the US. Both men agreed that if the obstructed area was short enough, it should be feasible to cut out the affected section of blood vessel and suture together the two ends. But doing so would involve placing a clamp over the aorta for the duration of the procedure. This would take considerable time, an hour or more, and they believed that cutting off the body's blood supply for so long would inevitably have disastrous results; indeed, Gross had tried the procedure in dogs, and found that many of them suffered partial paralysis.[80]

The fact that his ductus patient had survived for half an hour with the circulation interrupted suggested to Crafoord that this was not the insuperable obstacle it had first appeared, particularly since coarctation

---

* This was not, in fact, an original discovery. The British surgeon Sir Astley Cooper (1768–1841) conducted an almost identical experiment while still a student.

patients tended to have well-developed collaterals which sent blood to the organs via a secondary network of vessels. He asked his colleagues to look out for suitable patients for operation, and in October 1944 was presented with the perfect candidate, a twelve-year-old boy.

On 19 October Crafoord operated. When he opened the boy's chest and exposed the major blood vessels he had a clear view of the curve of the aorta, a tight arch that rose from the top of the heart and then turned downwards. At that point it suddenly narrowed into a constriction which drastically reduced the amount of blood that could pass through the vessel. Crafoord placed forceps on the aorta on either side of this obstruction, clamping it shut. This stopped any blood from flowing through the lower part of the aorta; crucially, the circulation to the brain via the two carotid arteries (which arise from the top of the aortic arch) was not interrupted. A segment of the aorta was now bloodless, and he could cut out the affected section and join the two severed ends. With the heart still beating a few centimetres from his instruments, this was a task requiring immense dexterity and concentration. First he inserted three stitches at equal distances around the diameter of the vessel; with these holding the two cut ends of the aorta together he could then insert fine silk sutures in between them. By the time he had finished, the aorta had been clamped shut for over two hours. This was long enough to be a concern, but Crafoord knew that the brain would not be harmed, and was optimistic that the collateral circulation had been sufficient to sustain the other major organs. When he released the forceps to let blood through the repaired vessel he was relieved to find that there were no leaks: the most dangerous part of the procedure was over.

After an operation lasting six hours, an exhausted Crafoord put the final stitch in the little boy's chest. His patient developed a fever and a chest infection, but soon improved. Two weeks later Crafoord performed the same procedure on a twenty-seven-year-old farmer who had become too ill to work. This too was a success, and when he examined both patients the following March they were in excellent health; the farmer had even returned to work.[81]

Meanwhile in Boston, Robert Gross and his colleague Charles Hufnagel had independently come to the conclusion that it might be possible to repair coarctation by temporarily clamping the aorta. Unaware that Crafoord had already done exactly this, Gross operated on two patients. The first died needlessly after the aortic clamps were removed too quickly, resulting in a sudden change in blood pressure which overwhelmed the patient's circulation. When the operation was next performed, Gross was careful to remove the clamps slowly and the patient made a good recovery. Thinking he had achieved something entirely new, Gross added a postscript about his 'breakthrough' to a paper he had already submitted for publication.[82] When he learned that Crafoord had beaten him to it by a couple of weeks Gross was furious, believing that the Swede had exploited his own research; five years later he banished a visiting surgeon from his operating theatre after finding out that he had been Crafoord's assistant.[83] Such competitions to become the first to perform an operation – to 'establish priority', as it is known – would become a common feature of the next few decades: like the race to put a man on the Moon in the 1960s, these contests would drive progress, but they would also lead to rivalries and bitter disputes.

Being the first matters little, of course, unless the procedure works. Happily, the early operations for congenital heart conditions really did work. One of Blalock's earliest Blue Babies, a boy called Samuel Sanders, went on to become a great pianist, the recital partner of Itzhak Perlman and Mstislav Rostropovich, and lived until 1999.[84] Crafoord was still in touch with his first coarctation patient in 1974, thirty years after his operation.[85] Most spectacularly Lorraine Sweeney Nicoli, whose life Robert Gross saved in 1938, became a great-grandmother, gave an address at Gross's funeral, and was still alive and well in the summer of 2015.

That is not to say that these techniques represented the last word in surgical sophistication. Only a couple of years after the first Blalock –Taussig shunt, Willis Potts in Chicago unveiled a modified version of the procedure which gave still better results.[86] Later, Denton Cooley

– who had been in theatre for Blalock's historic first operation – would refine it further. Despite these improvements, surgeons still yearned to find a cure for tetralogy of Fallot, rather than simply alleviate its symptoms. To achieve this, though, would involve finding a way to operate *inside* the heart; and if such a thing could be done it would also open the way to treating myriad other types of heart disease.

When Albert Blalock died in 1965, Lord Brock, President of the Royal College of Surgeons, wrote that his work had 'inspired and stimulated the advances in cardiac surgery that followed with almost breathless rapidity'.[87] Indeed, within a few years of the first Blue Baby operation the field had been transformed. The era of open-heart surgery was about to begin; and after the brilliant successes of Gross, Crafoord and Blalock, surgeons on both sides of the Atlantic sensed that still greater discoveries lay in store.

3. 'A SENSIBLE HISSING'

Houston, 5 January 1953

In June 1725 a young man from a town in northern Italy visited the house of a local prostitute, only to be seen a short time afterwards hurrying from the building in an agitated state. What happened next was recorded by the great physician Giovanni Battista Morgagni, who served as professor of anatomy at the University of Padua for over fifty years:

> As the woman had not appeared for two or three hours, the neighbours went in and found her dead and cold – lying in bed, in such a posture that it could not be doubted what business she had been engaged in, *especially since manly seed could be seen flowing from her female parts*.[1]

Morgagni's account of this unedifying episode appears in the hugely influential book he published in 1761, *The Seats and Causes of Diseases Investigated by Anatomy*, a compendium of almost 700 autopsy reports. By comparing his pathological findings with the symptoms the patients had experienced before death, Morgagni hoped to improve the rigour

---

* When Morgagni's work was first published in English the section in italics was coyly left in the original Latin. Since modern readers are unlikely to be outraged by this detail I have taken the liberty of translating it.

and precision of diagnosis. In this case he was eager to discover the cause of this young woman's untimely demise, and sent a colleague to inspect the body. In the summer heat there was no time to waste, so the man was instructed to bring back any organs which showed signs of disease. He duly returned with the woman's internal organs and genitals in a bag, and the following day Morgagni dissected them.

When he examined the heart he soon found something amiss. The organ is normally covered by the pericardium, a tough fibrous sac which holds the heart in place within the chest cavity. As well as protecting the heart from infection, it also contains a small amount of fluid which helps to lubricate it during its pumping movements. This time, however, the pericardial sac was not sitting loosely around the heart as it should, but was distended with dark clotted blood. The major blood vessels displayed no outward abnormality, but when Morgagni cut into the largest, the aorta, he discovered why the young woman had died. Near the point at which the artery leaves the heart he found signs of disease: the wall of the vessel had been weakened and ballooned outwards, a lesion known as an aneurysm. This example was the size of a large walnut. It had ruptured, and huge volumes of blood had been pumped into the pericardium and the chest cavity, causing almost instant death. Morgagni ended his autopsy report with an observation that reads as if it were influenced more by morality than medicine, but which was entirely correct:

> When other causes exist, it is not only obvious to reason, but has been demonstrated by dissection, that venereal indulgences greatly tend to accelerate death, by exciting the circulation of blood. They occasion the rupture of latent aneurysms, and the laceration of vessels in the head, which without this or a similar excitation, might have continued to perform their functions much longer—perhaps till old age.[2]

It is quite plausible that the young woman's death was a consequence of her profession: aortic aneurysms are now known to be associated with syphilis, and until the advent of penicillin in the 1940s the majority of cases were seen in syphilitic patients. Some were killed suddenly as the aneurysm burst – 'as instantaneously as if by a pistol-bullet', in the words of the nineteenth-century physician René Laennec.[3] They were the lucky ones: more often the aneurysm would grow, crushing the internal organs, eroding the bones of the spine and ribs and eventually becoming visible through the skin. Patients sometimes died slowly from suffocation, as the aneurysmal sac compressed the windpipe. In 1752 the physician William Hunter was consulted by a corset-maker who had endured the slow growth of his aneurysm for three years, until it protruded through his ribs. Finally it burst as he turned over in bed to cough: 'The blood gushed out with such violence as to dash against the curtains and wall; and he died, not only without speaking, but without a sigh or groan.'[4]

Difficult to diagnose and impossible to treat, from the moment they were first identified in the sixteenth century aortic aneurysms became a doctor's nightmare. A breach in the wall of the aorta is a catastrophe, given the volume and pressure of the blood within, and the fact that it is the only conduit between the heart and major organs. Not only is this 30-centimetre tube vital to life, it is also difficult to reach: the upper part of the aorta is protected by the ribcage, and sits in hazardous proximity to the heart and lungs, while the abdominal aorta is buried deep beneath the viscera, adjacent to the spine. The eighteenth-century medic Henry Mason acknowledged the challenges for the physician: 'As aneurysms in the internal parts of the body are inaccessible, all that can be done for the patient is, to abate the impetus of the blood's motion by a thin diet, and repeated bleeding . . . and the patient at the same time be ordered to refrain from all commotions of body and mind.'[5] This was not treatment but palliative care.

The outlook was not much better two hundred years later in 1952, when the American surgeon Michael DeBakey described aortic aneurysm as 'a fatal disorder, comparable in this respect to cancer'.[6] That would soon change. On the last day of that year a forty-six-year-old sheriff from Arkansas was admitted to DeBakey's Methodist Hospital in Houston. He probably would not have been pleased to be compared with an eighteenth-century Italian prostitute, but from a clinical point of view there was little difference between him and the subject of Morgagni's autopsy – except that the sheriff was still alive. About three months earlier he had suddenly started to suffer severe back pain, which had spread to his lower abdomen and groin. He was diagnosed with an aortic aneurysm, and his doctors were not surprised to learn that he had previously been treated for syphilis.

By the time he arrived in Houston he was in a bad way, physically and psychologically. Like the soldiers forced to live with shrapnel fragments lodged in their chests, he was anxious that his condition could kill him at any moment. An X-ray revealed a large pulsating mass behind his heart – so large, in fact, that it had displaced his stomach and oesophagus to one side, and had started to erode the bones of his spine.[7] The prognosis was dire: no patient had ever survived an aneurysm of this size. And yet three weeks later he would leave Methodist Hospital in excellent health, and be back at work within a couple of months. The operation that cured him was the first in a series of brilliant interventions which both made DeBakey's reputation and prepared the ground for a decade of rapid progress in cardiac surgery. It was also the greatest achievement to date of a medical discipline which had been practised for almost two thousand years – vascular surgery, the surgery of the blood vessels.

Ancient doctors frequently wrote about the blood vessels, although their work was founded on the misconception that the veins and arteries also transported *pneuma*, a vital spirit derived from inhaled air. Nevertheless, a Greek surgeon of the second century AD not only described aneurysms but devised an operation so sophisticated that it enjoyed an unlikely renaissance almost 1,800 years later. Very little is known about Antyllus, whom the great Canadian physician and historian of medicine Sir William Osler described as 'one of the most daring and accomplished surgeons of all time'.[8] In his treatise *On Medicine*, Antyllus distinguished between traumatic aneurysms and those caused by disease, and offered advice on which were amenable to surgery. He ruled out aneurysms occurring in arteries of the neck, armpit and groin as too dangerous to treat, owing to the large size of the vessels involved, but described a procedure which could be used elsewhere in the body. This entailed making an incision in the skin above the artery, dissecting the vessel clear of its surrounding tissue, and using threads to tie it closed on either side of the aneurysm. Finally the aneurysm was slit open to evacuate the blood and any clot trapped inside it, and the empty sac was packed with wadding.[9] This left a section of blood vessel permanently out of commission, but the body would soon compensate for the deficiency; besides, it was better than letting the aneurysm burst. An alternative method was suggested by Antyllus' near-contemporary Galen, who recommended compressing the aneurysm from outside the skin until it disappeared.[10]

These were important contributions, but such methods were only applicable to aneurysms of the smaller arteries which lay near the surface of the body. It was not even known that the aorta was also prone to aneurysm until 1552, when the French physician Jean Fernel observed during post-mortem dissections that they could occur inside the chest. The greatest anatomist of the Renaissance, his contemporary Andreas Vesalius, also described them and is believed to have been the first to diagnose an aortic aneurysm while the patient was still alive.[11]

Treatment was another matter. Ambroise Paré, surgeon to the French king Henry II, described the characteristic sound of blood flowing through an aneurysm as 'a sensible hissing, if you lay your ear next to them'. This noise, known today as a 'bruit', is caused by turbulent flow inside the aneurysmal sac. Where suitable, Paré recommended the operation of Antyllus. But he also asserted that aneurysms deep inside the body were incurable, citing the story of a tailor 'who by an aneurysm of the arterious vein [aorta] suddenly whilst he was playing at tennis fell down dead, the vessel being broken'.[12] Noting that those who suffered such deaths often turned out to have a history of venereal disease, he recommended a diet of 'curds and new cheeses', and taking an infusion of barley water and poppy seeds.

No real progress with treatment was made until the eighteenth century, when the Scottish brothers William and John Hunter turned their attention to the subject. William, the elder of the two, was a physician and anatomist who, in a detailed study of aneurysms which drew heavily on his experience of dissecting cadavers, described the dramatic death of the corset-maker we read earlier. His brother John started his career as William's assistant in his school of anatomy in Soho, and probably became interested in the possibilities of surgical aneurysm repair as a result.[13] William was a figure of great eminence, respected as a teacher and as the leading obstetrician of his generation, but his reputation would soon be eclipsed by that of his younger brother.

John Hunter was not only a talented clinician but also an important experimental scientist who performed pioneering research into transplantation and the placebo effect. His deep interest in the structures of the body and their functions led him to study how anatomy differed between humans and other animals, and over many years he amassed a huge collection of more than 15,000 specimens drawn from several hundred animal and plant species. After his death it was purchased by the British government, and although a large number of items were destroyed in an air raid in 1941 it still forms the core of the Hunterian Museum of the Royal College of Surgeons in London, one of the world's greatest anatomical collections.

Among the museum's artefacts is a memento of one of the achievements that made John Hunter the most celebrated surgeon of his era: a preparation of a blood vessel taken from a human leg following an operation he developed in the 1780s to treat aneurysms. Hunter had frequently performed Antyllus' procedure, but grew frustrated with its failure in aneurysms of the popliteal artery, a blood vessel located deep in the tissue of the thigh. Many surgeons preferred to amputate the leg, which Hunter thought a grotesque admission of failure, and after conducting experiments on dogs he devised an alternative. The first attempt on a human patient was made in December 1785, when he treated a coachman aged forty-five with a longstanding popliteal aneurysm.* His leg was swollen and had turned an unhealthy mottled brown, but despite his discomfort he begged Hunter not to deprive him of his livelihood by amputating.

Hunter began by making an incision along the coachman's inner thigh, and then dissected the artery free. He realised that the conventional method of tying the artery closed just above the aneurysm was doomed to failure, since this section was also likely to be diseased and the ligatures would eventually cut through it, causing major haemorrhage. Instead he attached four cotton ligatures around the artery some distance above the aneurysmal sac, where the vessel was still healthy.† The rationale behind this procedure was simple: if the blood supply to the aneurysm were cut off it would no longer increase in size, the contents of the sac would clot and in time be reabsorbed by the body. After a long convalescence complicated by bleeding and infection the patient was eventually much improved, and by July had returned to his work driving a hackney carriage.[14] Hunter's next three patients fared even better, and five years after the operation were all living normal lives.[15]

The Hunterian operation for aneurysm quickly became the standard procedure for the condition. Hunter's pupil Sir Astley Cooper, the outstanding surgeon of the next generation, called it 'one of the greatest triumphs of our science'.[16] And in 1817 Cooper in turn became the first surgeon to apply a ligature to the aorta, using Hunter's method. His patient was Charles Hutson, a thirty-eight-year-old porter who had been admitted to Guy's Hospital with a swollen groin. Cooper could feel a pulsation in the swelling, a sure sign that it was a grossly distended artery rather than a tumour. He realised that the affected

---

* Hunter's brother-in-law, the surgeon Sir Everard Home, noted that 'what is rather curious, in many recent instances of this disease, the patients have been coachmen and postilions'. Sitting for long periods while travelling along bumpy roads perhaps made them particularly vulnerable to popliteal aneurysm.
† A single ligature might have sufficed, but as Home explains: 'The reason for passing four ligatures was to compress such a length of artery as might make up for the want of tightness, as he chose to avoid great pressure on the vessel at any one part.'

vessel was deep inside the abdomen, making any surgical intervention hugely risky. For several weeks he tried more conservative treatments, including bloodletting and the application of pressure to the swelling. But when the aneurysm began to bleed through the skin he had no alternative but to operate.

Cooper began by administering a dose of opium to his patient – the only pain relief he would receive during this highly invasive procedure – before making an incision in the man's abdomen. That must have been painful enough, but judging by the surgeon's own account of the operation the sequel was truly excruciating: 'Having made a sufficient opening to admit my finger into the abdomen, I then passed it between the intestines to the spine, and felt the aorta greatly enlarged, and beating with excessive force.'[17] After using his fingernail to make space behind it, he then managed to pass a ligature around the vessel to tie it closed. The ends of the ligature were passed between the intestines and left hanging out of the wound to enable further tightening if required. The patient died a few days later, but Cooper had proved that the undertaking was possible, and his daring feat was immediately feted as a landmark in surgery: the patient's aorta, and the ligature Cooper tied around it, can still be seen in the Gordon Museum of Pathology at King's College London.

Few dared to repeat the operation, and though hundreds of articles were written about aortic aneurysm there was no further breakthrough until much later in the nineteenth century, when doctors noticed that some patients improved after the symptoms first appeared. The explanation, they realised, was that blood clots were forming inside the aneurysm, reducing the pressure on its walls. The Scottish physician Alexander Monro, writing in 1827, described one such patient who survived for some time with an aortic aneurysm 'as large as a child's head'.[18] He recommended treating aneurysms by the use of measures intended to promote coagulation inside the sac, such as bloodletting, bed rest, and a simple diet.

Clotting was known as 'Nature's cure' for an aneurysm, and for decades most specialists preferred to take this conservative approach, until the Victorian surgeon Charles Moore pioneered an ingenious operation that was still in use in the 1940s. On 20 February 1863 he was asked to examine a patient with a large aortic aneurysm which had started to protrude through the ribs. Moore knew that surgery was not yet equal to the task of treating the artery itself, and it occurred to him that one alternative might be to harness the body's natural defence mechanisms. Foreign objects in the bloodstream tend to provoke clotting, since they are quickly surrounded and encapsulated by cells called platelets as the body tries to isolate any potential threat. Moore believed that if he could introduce a suitable object into the aneurysm, any blood in contact with it would quickly coagulate. The larger the surface area of this object, he realised, the more blood would clot, and a suitable substance immediately suggested itself: 'If a large quantity of wire could be introduced into the interior of an aneurysm, and disposed about it in coils, a corresponding quantity of fibrin [a fibrous protein involved in clotting] would soon accumulate and increase upon it.'[19]

To Moore's disappointment, his patient – perhaps disturbed at the prospect of being a guinea pig – discharged himself from the hospital, so it was almost a year before he had the opportunity to put his theory into practice. On 7 January 1864 he operated on Daniel D., a twenty-seven-year-old with a gigantic aneurysm which protruded almost three inches from his chest. No incision or anaesthetic were necessary: Moore simply inserted a small tube into the aneurysm and through it threaded an astonishing 26 yards of fine steel wire, which formed coils inside the aneurysmal sac. The patient lived for only four more days: the operation had been too late to save him. An autopsy revealed, however, that the aneurysm was already filled with 'a fibrinous coagulum, enveloping and imbedded in the coils of wire',[20] showing that Moore's theory was sound.

Other surgeons quickly grasped the elegant simplicity of the procedure and continued to use it with a number of modifications. Catgut, silk and horsehair were tried instead of wire,[21] and two Italian surgeons even inserted a large number of watch springs into an aneurysm, an experiment which ended fatally when some of them entered the heart.[22] Copper and silver wire were also used, as much as 200 feet of it, and from the 1870s onwards electric current was sometimes applied to the coils in order to heat them and increase the speed of clotting. In the mid-1930s the American Arthur Blakemore adapted this technique, using a fine wire made of a copper–silver alloy and insulated with enamel. By carefully controlling the current passing through the wire he could heat the coils to 80°C, the optimum temperature for coagulation.[23] His initial results were encouraging – six of eleven patients experienced an improvement in their condition – but after later disappointments his method failed to gain widespread acceptance.

Alternatives were proposed: surgeons tried injecting gelatine and other liquids into the sac to promote coagulation,[24] and others applied ligatures to the arteries coming off the aortic arch in order to slow the flow of blood through the aneurysm. A wide variety of bizarre materials was employed for this operation, including kangaroo tendons[25] and ox aorta,[26] as surgeons tried to find a substance tougher than cotton but sufficiently similar to the body's own tissue that it would not provoke inflammation. One surgeon even wrote to the *British Medical Journal* in 1887 to recommend bloodletting,[27] a treatment which was archaic even then. Such therapies smacked of desperation; a new approach was needed.

Curiously it was a return to ancient medicine, and the method of Antyllus, that revealed the way forward. In January 1888 a young American called Manuel Harris was accidentally shot while hunting rabbits, and two months later was admitted to Charity Hospital in New Orleans with a swollen upper left arm. He was treated by Rudolph Matas, a twenty-seven-year-old surgeon who with his neat goatee and steel-rimmed spectacles had the air and gravitas of a Viennese intellectual. The son of Spanish immigrants, Matas had grown up on a Louisiana plantation and became a considerable scholar, with such a passion for knowledge that the foundations of his house had to be reinforced to prevent the building sinking under the weight of his library.[28] Matas examined his patient and discovered that lead shot had caused a large aneurysm of the brachial artery, the major blood vessel of the upper arm.

Having failed to check the growth of the aneurysm using compression, Matas applied a ligature to the artery, but this too was unsuccessful. With amputation the only alternative, he operated again. After placing a second ligature below the aneurysm, he cut into the sac and removed the clot inside it. He could now see that blood was continuing to seep into the sac despite the ligatures, so he sealed both ends with silk thread before sewing up the external wound. His patient made a complete recovery, but in his report of the case Matas claimed little credit: he pointed out that he had merely been following the example of Antyllus, and that the advent of anaesthesia, 'which allows the operator to cut with a calm and deliberation that were denied his ancestors', had made the operation respectable once more.[29]

Despite its success, Matas did not dare to repeat the procedure for almost fifteen years. But after several similar cases came his way he made an intense study of the problem, and in 1902 described his technique to colleagues.[30] He gave it the name 'endo-aneurysmorrhaphy', an inelegant term for one of the great breakthroughs in vascular medicine. The essence of Matas's operation was that the aneurysm was cut open and the lower edges of the sac folded and sutured together to restore the artery's normal diameter. To visualise the procedure, imagine that a thrifty vascular surgeon buys a cheap garden hose which turns out to have a weak spot in its tubing. Water pressure soon causes the plastic at this weak point to balloon outwards, forming an 'aneurysm'. If this should burst the hose would be ruined, so the vascular surgeon decides to repair it by performing endo-aneurysmorrhaphy. After turning the water off he makes a slit along the bulging section and then sews the sides together so that the tubing is of uniform diameter once more.

Matas had shown that surgeons need not rely on palliative measures to treat aneurysms. But although endo-aneurysmorrhaphy was adopted as the standard technique for treating the peripheral blood vessels it was still too dangerous to use it on the aorta, where the blood flow could not be interrupted for any length of time. He did, however, have one notable but solitary success in treating the condition. In 1923, in an operation reminiscent of Sir Astley Cooper's a century earlier, Matas treated a young woman severely debilitated by syphilis. She had a large aneurysm of the abdominal aorta, which had started to leak. Because it was near the lower end of the vessel, below the kidneys, Matas decided it was safe to intervene. He wrapped two cotton tapes tightly around the aorta, immediately above the aneurysm, so as to prevent any blood flowing through it. This was a radical intervention which shut off much of the circulation to the woman's legs, but Matas was relieved to find that sufficient blood was finding its way to them through other smaller vessels. The aneurysm shrank dramatically, and she lived for over a year before she died from an unrelated bout of tuberculosis.[31]

This method of ligating the aorta was employed by other surgeons, but with mixed results. Until the 1950s there remained no entirely satisfactory treatment for aortic aneurysm, although several new techniques were tested. There was even a brief vogue for wrapping them in cellophane, which appeared to slow their growth. In December 1948 Albert Einstein became the most famous patient to undergo this procedure for a large aneurysm of the abdominal aorta. He did remarkably well, and was able to return to work within a matter of weeks. He remained in good health for another six years; by the time his original symptoms returned in April 1955, surgery had evolved to the point that it might have cured him entirely. His doctors recommended a second operation, but at the age of seventy-six Einstein had had enough, telling the surgeon John Glenn: 'I want to go when I want. It is tasteless to prolong life artificially. I have done my share, it is time to go. I will do it elegantly.'[32] He died peacefully in Princeton University Hospital a few days later.

Indirect approaches to aneurysms had not worked; what surgeons yearned to do was cut them out – a daunting prospect, attended with

formidable risks; but slowly, over several decades, all the major obstacles were overcome. The first step on this long path was taken at
the beginning of the twentieth century by the Frenchman Théodore
Tuffier, an enterprising surgeon who was a pioneer in many fields. In
1901 he was asked to look at a forty-year-old woman who had arrived
at the Hôtel-Dieu hospital in Paris complaining of chest pain. A pulsating tumour the size of a pigeon's egg had recently appeared between
two of her ribs: an X-ray showed that this was merely a small portion of
an aneurysm of the aortic arch the size of a large fist. Tuffier believed
that only an operation could save her, and explained to the woman and
her family that nothing of the kind had ever been attempted before.
Having obtained their consent, on 12 December he operated.

When he opened her chest, Tuffier discovered that the aneurysm
had already eaten into her ribs, its walls were dangerously thin and
it was close to bursting. But there were more encouraging signs: the
aperture connecting this large sac of blood to the aorta was small, and
Tuffier thought it should be possible simply to tie it closed. Carefully
watching the patient's pulse and breathing, he attached a catgut
ligature around the neck of the aneurysmal sac, which immediately
deflated as its blood supply was removed. Thrilled at this sign of success, Tuffier thought it safe to terminate the operation. But he had
made a critical error. Rather than cut the aneurysm out entirely he left
the empty sac in situ, assuming that it would contain any subsequent
bleeding, an insurance policy against future mishap. Alas, this was a
fatal miscalculation: two weeks later the woman died after the tissue
he had left behind became gangrenous.[33]

For the next four decades surgeons largely avoided such direct
approaches to aneurysms, dissuaded by the unsuccessful outcome
of Tuffier's operation. Instead they preferred methods such as wir-
ing them or placing a ligature across the aorta. The results were so
dismal that in 1940 an American expert, Ivan Bigger, was forced to
admit that 'up to the present time, all forms of therapy have yielded
poor results'.[34] But rapid progress in the treatment of congenital heart
conditions in the 1940s would prove to be of crucial importance. Until

Clarence Crafoord's successful treatment of aortic coarctation in 1944, most specialists believed that interrupting the flow of blood through the upper part of the aorta would have rapidly fatal consequences. Knowing that this was not the case gave them new confidence in their ability to attack the vessel directly.

In 1947, Harris Shumacker, a surgeon at Yale, was operating on an eight-year-old boy who had been diagnosed with coarctation. When he opened the patient's chest and laboriously dissected away the tissues around the heart he could see the characteristic narrowing of the aorta, but just below it – and unexpectedly – there was a large aneurysm. With nothing to be gained from abandoning the operation, he clamped the aorta above and below the area of constriction and cut out a 3-centimetre section of the vessel, together with the aneurysmal sac. He then sutured together the two ends of the aorta and slowly removed the clamps to restore blood flow through the repaired vessel. His patient made a good recovery. This was an unplanned aneurysm repair, but thanks to Shumacker's presence of mind and willingness to improvise, it worked.[35]

Shumacker had trained under the Blue Baby pioneer Alfred Blalock, and it was no coincidence that another surgeon who made an early aneurysm repair was also a Blalock protégé. Denton Cooley, who had been present as a young student at the first Blue Baby operation in 1944, had a particularly dramatic first experience. In 1949 he was assisting a senior colleague, Grant Ward, in an operation on a patient who had previously been treated for cancer of the breastbone. During an earlier operation the cancerous bone had been replaced with a metal plate, but this had caused complications. When they removed it to investigate, a jet of blood spurted from the man's chest with such force that it hit the ceiling. Dr Ward quickly thrust his left hand into the chest cavity and stemmed the flow with his fingers. But this was the end of his involvement in proceedings: his right arm was paralysed as the result of a spinal disease and hung uselessly from a splint. After a moment of panic he regained his sangfroid, crisply asking Cooley to help him get his finger 'out of this hole'.[36]

Blood at such pressure could only come from the aorta, and when Cooley peered into the open thorax he saw a large aneurysm which had already burst. This horrifying scenario was far beyond his knowledge or experience so he improvised, using a portion of chest muscle to patch the breach.[37] After several nerve-wracking minutes the fountain of blood had been staunched, and Ward could remove his finger. But this was only a temporary solution: the repair would not hold for long. The two surgeons looked at each other and wondered what to do next. Cooley suggested putting a clamp on the aorta to stop the flow of blood temporarily, giving them a few minutes to sew up the hole. With no viable alternative they decided to go ahead; their patient stabilised and a few hours later was back on the ward. Cooley would go on to repair several other aneurysms at Johns Hopkins using this simple method of clamping the aorta while the aneurysmal sac was excised and the hole in the aorta repaired. The technique was dubbed 'clamp and sew', and was the first successful means of removing aneurysms. And these formative early experiences, operating at the limits of what was known to be possible, were to prove invaluable when he left Baltimore in 1951 to start a new job in Houston.

Today Methodist Hospital is at the heart of the Texas Medical Center, a vast campus of twenty-one hospitals covering more than a square mile. But in 1948, when Michael DeBakey was appointed head of its surgical department, Houston was still a medical backwater. He arrived as the only surgeon in the city with advanced qualifications, and was horrified to discover inexperienced general practitioners attempting complex operations, with predictably awful results. Over the next few years he transformed the department, ejecting incompetent doctors and hiring the most talented young surgeons he could find. Denton Cooley was a great catch: after training with Albert Blalock he had worked with Russell Brock in London, and already had an enviable reputation as a quick and technically brilliant operator.

Cooley's arrival in Houston brought together two of the greatest surgeons of the twentieth century. But they were very different characters. Cooley had been something of a jock at the University of Texas, where he had excelled at basketball and was a prominent fraternity member. At thirty-one he still bore a permanent reminder of these rowdy student days: the initials UT, branded into his chest with a red-hot iron during an initiation ceremony.[38] The affable, laid-back Texan could not have been a greater contrast to DeBakey, a ferociously intense Southerner of Lebanese descent who rose by 4 a.m. and rarely took a day off. A 1965 profile in *Time* magazine called him 'the Texas Tornado',[39] capturing something drastically elemental about him. On his morning rounds he would tear through the hospital, with juniors and students trailing in his wake as he bounded up the stairs between floors. With patients he was gentle and attentive, but subordinates who allowed their concentration to waver for a second could expect a volley of abuse, or banishment from the operating room; on more than one occasion a trainee ejected from theatre for some misdemeanour promptly left the hospital, never to return. Perhaps it was inevitable that these two powerful characters would eventually fall out – and catastrophically – but for over a decade they collaborated on some of the most important work ever done in an operating theatre.

On 11 June 1951, Cooley's first day in his new job, he accompanied DeBakey on his morning rounds. One of the patients, a forty-six-year-old man, had an aneurysm so large that it threatened to break through the skin of his chest. DeBakey asked his new recruit what he thought ought to be done. To his surprise, Cooley replied that he had previous experience of the condition, and that he believed that he could put a clamp across the aorta, remove the aneurysm and repair the blood vessel. Impressed, DeBakey invited him to make an attempt, and when he entered the operating theatre the following day he found that his junior had already succeeded in removing the lesion and was in the process of repairing the aorta. The patient went on to make a full recovery.[40]

In his memoirs Cooley suggests that this operation in June 1951 was the first successful aneurysm repair of its type anywhere in the world. Surgeons, as we have seen, can become obsessed with priority, and this is an interesting example of their determination to come first: DeBakey liked to point out that he had himself performed a similar procedure three years earlier,[41] while his mentor Alton Ochsner reported a successful operation in New Orleans as early as 1944.[42] Such conflicting claims are not uncommon; complicating matters still further, the chief surgeon at a hospital was for many years entitled to put his name to any journal article emanating from his department, whether or not he had personally conducted the operation it reported. This often led to situations where two surgeons at the same hospital took credit for a 'first', with callous disregard for the convenience of medical historians.

Such disputes had not yet tarnished the relationship of DeBakey and Cooley in 1952, when they collaborated on a study of previous attempts to treat aortic aneurysm, including their own. They observed that most surgeons had been 'concerned with palliative rather than curative therapy and the results therefore have been somewhat disappointing'[43] – an understated way of saying that surgery had so far completely failed to find a reliable method of curing this deadly condition. They vowed to adopt a more aggressive approach, one in which the ideal outcome was the total removal of the aneurysmal sac; in other words, a comprehensive cure.

This was the mindset of the two surgeons when the sheriff from Arkansas arrived on New Year's Eve, 1952. Having already established that he had a large aneurysm, they investigated further by taking an aortogram three days later. During this procedure dye is injected into the aorta while an X-ray is taken, allowing doctors to see the outlines of the blood vessels. This showed an extensive aneurysm with a layer of clot on both sides, which had pushed the aorta out of its usual position. But it also revealed a more formidable problem.

Aneurysms come in two main types: sacciform and fusiform. In sacciform aneurysms, a bladder-like swelling arises from a single weak spot in the vessel wall. These were the first to be successfully treated, since if the neck of the sac was sufficiently narrow surgeons could simply clamp it shut and remove the sac. The second kind was far more challenging. 'Fusiform' means 'spindle-shaped', and aneurysms of this variety affect the artery's entire circumference, so that the sac is not a bag attached to the aorta but forms part of the vessel itself. This was what the surgeons saw on the aortogram: removing it would be extremely challenging, since it would entail cutting out a lengthy section of the aorta. Shumacker had managed to remove an aneurysm by excising a few centimetres of the vessel and stitching the ends together, but the example they were now looking at was fully 20 centimetres long. Cutting it out would leave a gaping void where a blood vessel should be; they would have to find a way to bridge this gap.

On 5 January the sheriff was put to sleep with ether and placed on his right side. DeBakey made an incision in his chest and lifted up one of the lungs, revealing the aneurysm. A 20-centimetre section of the aorta had ballooned into a swelling 20 centimetres in diameter, like the distended belly of a snake that has gorged itself. The aneurysm had adhered to the bones of the spine and was awkwardly situated near the point at which the aorta passes through the diaphragm, the tough sheet of muscle separating the thorax from the abdomen. In order to approach the sac, DeBakey had to remove the patient's spleen and then cut through the diaphragm. He injected heparin, an anticoagulant, into the aorta and then placed clamps on the vessel above and below the aneurysm. Next came the job of separating the sac from the tissues around it, without damaging any of the delicate structures to which it had attached itself.

While he applied himself to this task, one of his assistants was examining the contents of a small glass jar: a section of aorta taken from the body of a twenty-one-year-old man who had died in a car crash six days earlier. Shortly after his death it had been excised, placed in a salt solution containing a large amount of antibiotics to prevent infection, and refrigerated. Once the diseased section of the sheriff's aorta had been removed, a graft of this tissue would replace it. The assistant trimmed it to the required length and handed it to DeBakey, who had by now cut out a substantial portion of the aorta, including part of the aneurysm.

The graft was placed in the gap between the two cut ends of the aorta, and working quickly but meticulously DeBakey sutured the graft into position. By the time he had finished, the clamps had been on the aorta for three-quarters of an hour. Gradually, so as not to cause any shock to the patient's system, these were now released, allowing blood to flow through his new aorta for the first time. DeBakey and his colleagues watched carefully for any signs of leakage: despite the high pressure within the vessel, the join was so good that only a few drops of blood oozed through the suture holes. With the circulation restored, they could now remove the rest of the aneurysm and its contents. It was so huge that it left a large cavity in the abdomen, leading DeBakey to worry that the sharp cartilages between the vertebrae, which protruded into this space, might puncture the new graft. So he took the precaution of suturing around the graft a section of omentum, a fatty membrane which normally covers the abdominal contents, to act as a protective bandage.

By the time he had repaired the diaphragm, replaced the rib and closed his original incision, DeBakey had been operating for four and a half hours. The patient was stable, and although his lung partially collapsed the following day, this was quickly treated and he was able to get out of bed six days later. He was transformed: the pain had disappeared and his circulation had dramatically improved. A mere fortnight after undergoing this major operation he was able to go home, and was back at work a month later.[44]

That was not the last that Michael DeBakey saw of the sheriff, however. In August 1962 he returned to Methodist Hospital with lung cancer. An aortogram revealed that the grafted blood vessel was still functioning normally: the operation had been a complete success. DeBakey had given him an extra decade of life, but this time he could do little to help him; he removed the cancerous lung, but the sheriff succumbed to his illness a few months later.[45]

As it turned out, he was lucky to survive so long. Arterial grafts from cadavers – known as homografts – had first been used in 1945 by Robert Gross to repair coarctation, and then to replace an aortic aneurysm by another American surgeon, Henry Swan, in 1949.[46] But problems soon emerged: they had a tendency to deteriorate once implanted, and several patients died after they began to leak. Homografts could only be stored for a couple of weeks, and obtaining them in the first place was difficult. DeBakey and his team were fortunate to have a ready supply of grafts taken from autopsies conducted at another local hospital, having come to an agreement with the state medical examiner[47] – but they were obtained without family consent, an arrangement that would now be deemed highly unethical. Some attempts were made to set up regional artery banks, along the same lines as blood banks, but these efforts foundered when surgeons came to understand that they needed something more durable than tissue from cadavers. DeBakey even experimented with blood vessels taken from other species including horses and giraffes,[48] which have notably tough aortas, but these tissues were rejected by human bodies. He and others had taken great strides forward, but what surgeons really needed was an artificial blood vessel which could be manufactured to order.

In 1901 a young Frenchman, Alexis Carrel, visited Messieurs Assada, a wholesale supplier of sewing equipment in Lyon. He was trying to get hold of some unusually fine needles and thread, and lacemaking equipment turned out to be precisely what he needed. Carrel was already skilled in embroidery, having taken lessons with a local seamstress, Mme Leroudier[49] – but his interest was not in repairing clothes, but human tissue. For the first time (but not the last), haberdashery was to play an unexpectedly important role in the story of vascular surgery.

It was a dramatic political assassination that set Carrel on this path. In June 1894 he was a medical student at the University of Lyon when the French president Marie Sadi Carnot made a visit to the city. As the president left the Palais de Commerce a young Italian anarchist approached his carriage and stabbed him with a dagger. The blade severed one of his portal veins, a major blood vessel supplying the liver, and although he was taken straight to hospital the injury proved fatal. Doctors realised there was nothing they could do for him and watched helplessly as he died slowly from massive blood loss. Lyon erupted in fury, and mobs avenged the president's death by wrecking every Italian café and bar in the city. Carrel was also outraged by the murder, but his reaction was more constructive: realising that the current state of surgical knowledge was inadequate for dealing with such serious injuries, he resolved to do something about it.[50]

At the time of Sadi Carnot's assassination nobody had yet succeeded in repairing a completely severed blood vessel. One of Carrel's professors, Mathieu Jaboulay, was interested in the problem, and in 1895 conducted successful experiments with donkeys and dogs, cutting their carotid arteries and then reuniting the ends by suture.[51] Carrel soon improved his teacher's technique, using tiny needles and fine silk thread coated with Vaseline, which sealed the holes created by each stitch. He then discovered a neat method to join the cut ends of a blood vessel, which he called 'triangulation': the vessel was first united with three stitches, at equal distances around its circumference. An assistant proceeded to pull these threads, stretching the circular cross-section of the blood vessel into a triangle. Sutures could then be placed on the three sides of this triangle, a much easier procedure than attempting to stitch around a circular surface; when the pressure on the three threads was relaxed, the blood vessel returned to its normal shape, with both ends perfectly united.[52] This remains one of the standard techniques of vascular surgery today.

Carrel began this work as a student in Lyon but completed it in America, where he emigrated in 1903. Briefly disillusioned with medicine, his original plan was to become a rancher in Canada, but thankfully he was dissuaded from this course of action and instead found work in a Chicago medical laboratory before moving to the Rockefeller Institute in New York. The lavish resources of the Institute were put at his disposal, and Carrel was able to set up a state-of-the-art research facility. An English visitor recorded his impressions of this unusual place in an article published in 1926:

Carrel's operative theatre is all black; so are the gowns of his assistants and himself. In fact, all is black, with the exception of his operation area. He can get his fine needles made only in England. It takes a month of effort before his theatre sister can thread these needles; the filament of silk is pushed through the eye of the needle obliquely along the shank. The operating theatre for animals is as perfectly equipped as any I've seen for human beings.[53]

In his early experiments on animals Carrel perfected his method of suturing blood vessels, work which would later win him a Nobel Prize. But he soon became aware that there were circumstances in which arteries or veins could not simply be stitched together; it was sometimes desirable to replace an entire section of vessel. His teacher Jaboulay had attempted to transplant a length of artery as early as 1896, but his suture technique was primitive and the operation failed. In 1905, using his more sophisticated method, Carrel cut out part of the aorta of a dog and replaced it with a section of vessel taken from another animal; nine months later it was still alive.

This was an important breakthrough, but Carrel realised that opportunities to perform this operation on humans would be rare, since fresh arteries were difficult to obtain. He proposed two alternatives. Firstly, veins could be used to replace sections of artery: the network of veins in the body provides many possible paths for blood to travel from the extremities back to the heart, so removing a short section of vein from the leg (for instance) causes no long-term problems. This suggestion was prophetic, since the technique is regularly employed today in coronary artery bypass operations. His second proposal was that sections of artery could be removed from cadavers and preserved for future use. In February 1907 he took a section of carotid artery from a dog which had just been killed, placed it in a preserving solution and refrigerated it. Ten days later the blood vessel was transplanted into a second dog. In May 1908, more than a year after the initial operation, Carrel inspected the artery and found that it was still functioning perfectly; in his idiosyncratic English, Carrel observed that 'a vessel transplanted after having been kept in cold storage for a few days or weeks can functionate normally for a long time'.[54]

It was these animal experiments by Carrel that laid the foundations for the use of homografts in aortic repair four decades later; in 1910 he predicted as much, writing that 'it is probable that the aneurysms of the thoracic aorta could be extirpated and the circulation re-established by a vascular transplantation'.[55] But this was only one strand of his research. While still working in France, Carrel experimented with small tubes made of magnesium and even caramel as replacements for sections of artery. Both substances were chosen because they would dissolve over time: Carrel conjectured that by the time the tubes had melted away the body would have laid down new tissue inside them, essentially manufacturing its own new blood vessel.[56] This was little more than an inspired guess, which would eventually be proved correct. Unfortunately Carrel found that they soon became blocked by blood clots, so he tested other materials, using tubes made of glass and rubber coated with Vaseline. These were better, but clots remained a common complication.[57]

Although glass and metal tubes were sometimes used in the treatment of arterial injury during the Second World War, these problems persisted. It was not until 1947 that a better alternative was found. A young American research scientist, Arthur Voorhees, was trying to develop an artificial heart valve, implanting his prototypes in canine hearts. One day he noticed that he had mistakenly placed a silk suture so that it passed into one of the chambers of the heart rather than through the cardiac muscle. Several months later, at autopsy, he discovered that the silk had become covered in what appeared to be normal heart tissue. This made him consider whether the body might lay down tissue over a piece of cloth; if the cloth were fashioned into a cylinder, he speculated that its inner surface might function as a lattice for the formation of a new blood vessel. Putting this theory to the test, he sewed a silk handkerchief into a tube and used it to replace a section of a dog's aorta. Blood passed through the makeshift artery for an hour but then began to leak through the loose weave of the silk, and the dog died.[58]

Still convinced that his idea had merit, Voorhees kept searching for more suitable material. The following year he was working in a military medical facility in Texas, and happened to be given a sample of vinyon-N, a tough polymer fabric used to make parachutes. Working with a senior colleague, Arthur Blakemore, Voorhees conducted a series of experiments in which vinyon-N grafts up to 6 centimetres long were implanted into the abdominal aortas of dogs, and in 1952 was able to report a promising trial involving fifteen animals. It was not an unqualified success, however: several developed clots inside the prosthesis, a difficulty which needed to be overcome before the technique could be attempted on humans.[59] Nevertheless, when his research was published it provoked great interest, and researchers across America were inspired to begin to work on the problem. Voorhees had arrived at an important insight: if the weave of the material chosen for a prosthetic blood vessel was of the right size, fibrin would quickly plug the holes between its threads. Eventually these fibrin plugs would be replaced by fibroblasts, the cells that synthesise connective tissue, and a new endothelium – the inner layer of blood vessels – would be formed. In effect, the fabric functioned as a scaffold on which the body could construct a new artery.

In their attempts to find the perfect material, researchers in the early 1950s fashioned prototype blood vessels from a variety of different synthetic cloths: Orlon, Teflon and nylon were all tried. Michael DeBakey took a close interest in these developments, and one day in 1952 he visited a haberdasher's in Houston to buy some nylon for his own experiments. To his annoyance it was out of stock, but the assistant who served him suggested he try another new material: Dacron. Patented by two British chemists in 1941, and sold in the UK under the brand name Terylene, this was the first polyester fabric. It turned out to be exactly what he was looking for.

DeBakey needed no assistance in making the first Dacron grafts: his mother had taught him to sew as a little boy, and by the age of ten he was making his own shirts.[60] Having borrowed his wife's sewing machine, he cut out rectangles of the material and sewed together the longer edges to make a cylinder. After successful tests on animals, he implanted the first of these home-made arterial prostheses in a human on 2 September 1954. The patient had a large aneurysm of the abdominal aorta, at the point where the vessel splits into two; DeBakey had manufactured a Y-shaped Dacron graft which replicated this bifurcation, and used it to replace the lower section of the aorta and the top part of both the smaller vessels below. The patient survived for another ten years after the operation.[61]

The adoption of Dacron was a major advance. None of the other materials tested could match it: Orlon grafts became misshapen after a few months, while nylon had an unfortunate tendency to break down inside the body.[62] It transpired that Teflon arteries, like Teflon-lined saucepans, were non-stick: their inner surfaces were so smooth that they significantly inhibited atherosclerosis, the deposit of fatty plaques inside the vessel.[63] Unfortunately this otherwise desirable property also prevented new tissue from growing inside the graft. Dacron suffered from none of these drawbacks: a new lining of endothelial cells quickly appeared on the porous inner surface of the cloth, so that the blood was not harmed by contact with synthetic material. But the first Dacron grafts were not wholly satisfactory: because they were made by hand, they had a seam running down one side where the two sides of the fabric had been sewn together, a potential weakness. Approximately 6 litres of blood passes through the aorta every minute, so the graft needed to be as strong as possible in order to contain this high-pressure flow.

One of the earliest patients to receive one was Arthur Hanisch, who travelled from his home in California to be treated for a large aneurysm of the abdominal aorta. Hanisch was a wealthy man, the president of one of America's largest pharmaceutical companies, and after being cured he expected to receive a bill for at least $10,000. But he had not reckoned with DeBakey's quirky charging policy. The surgeon routinely refused payment from teachers and other doctors,[64] and for rich patients sometimes waived his fees, suggesting instead that they make a donation towards the hospital's research projects. This strategy regularly paid dividends, and Hanisch's reaction was typical: astonished by the gesture, he wrote cheques over the next few years for several hundred thousand dollars, many times what he would have paid for his treatment.

Hanisch's support was not purely financial. When DeBakey explained how he needed to improve his fabric grafts, the pharmaceutical magnate revealed that he was also the major shareholder in a sock factory in Pennsylvania. Through this connection DeBakey met Tom Edman, a young textiles researcher who designed a new type of knitting machine, paid for by Hanisch.[65] It produced a continuous tube of Dacron, seamless like a sock, which could be fashioned into grafts of various sizes. These could even be customised to fit the patient's needs: if an aneurysm affected the junction of the aorta and the renal arteries (the vessels supplying the kidneys), a Dacron prosthesis could be manufactured with branches to match the patient's anatomy.

A committee of the American Medical Association had been set up to study the relative merits of different types of fabric graft, and a major study in 1955 concluded that Dacron was the best available.[66] From 1957 DeBakey, Cooley and their colleagues used it exclusively, and by the following year they had treated 737 patients, reporting their results as 'most satisfactory'.[67] Further improvements were to come: Cooley discovered that if the grafts were steeped in the patient's own blood before implantation and then heated in an autoclave, the blood clotted into the pores of the material, sealing it and preventing bleeding. In later years this process was improved by the simpler expedient of impregnating the graft in bovine collagen, the tough protein which makes up most of the connective tissue in animals.

Dacron grafts were first used to treat aneurysms of the abdominal aorta, where the blood flow could be safely halted for long enough to replace the affected section of the vessel. Operating on the thoracic aorta, close to the heart, was a more formidable challenge: the vessel supplies the brain, which cannot be starved of blood for more than a minute or two. One ingenious way round this problem was to attach a graft as a bypass around the diseased section of aorta: only after blood had been diverted into this shunt was the diseased segment removed, ensuring that the circulation was never interrupted. But this was laborious and technically difficult; it was only after the adoption of the heart-lung machine in the mid-1950s that surgeons could cut out and replace entire sections of the thoracic aorta with any degree of security. These machines took over the function of the patient's heart and lungs for the duration of the operation, oxygenating the blood and pumping it through the carotid arteries towards the brain while the diseased aorta was being excised. In the space of a couple of years DeBakey and Cooley succeeded in repairing aneurysms of all parts of the thoracic aorta, proving that no area of the vessel was out of bounds.

Although surgeons continued to experiment with other materials it was not until the 1970s, after the invention of Gore-Tex, that any successful alternative to Dacron was found. Today these polyester tubes are still widely used, although other, non-invasive, methods have also been found to cure aneurysms – a lesion which one recent textbook still described as 'among the most lethal of conditions and the most difficult to treat'.[68]

Two centuries separate the contrasting fates of our first two victims of aortic aneurysm: an Italian prostitute and a sheriff from Arkansas. Our last two will be a king of England and Michael DeBakey himself. George II is the only British monarch known to have died while defecating. On 25 October 1760 he rose as usual at six o'clock and called for his morning cup of chocolate. An hour later he went to his water closet, and shortly afterwards – according to his biographer Horace Walpole – the valet heard a groan and a strange noise 'louder than royal wind', and rushed in to find the king dying on the floor.[69] An autopsy was performed, and the royal physicians found the blood vessels around the heart 'stretched beyond their natural state'; in addition, 'in the trunk of the aorta, we found a transverse fissure on its inner side, about an inch and a half long, through which some blood had recently passed, under its external coat.'[70]

The king had died from a condition known as aortic dissection. Like all arteries the aorta consists of three layers of tissue: in aortic dissection, a weakness develops in the inner lining of the vessel, allowing blood to penetrate into its middle layer. Because arterial blood is at high pressure it can rip the two layers apart for some distance along the length of the aorta; in George's case the vessel had split entirely from inside to out, killing him outright.

Most patients die immediately or within a few hours of an aortic dissection. Some survive the initial episode, although they are unlikely to live for long. In the 1950s the condition was regarded as another type of aneurysm,* and one made particularly difficult to treat by the lengthy sections of the aorta often involved. In July 1954, DeBakey and Cooley effected the first cure of an aortic dissection, repairing the damage by suturing the tear.[71] Although their patient survived they soon realised this method was not ideal, since it left the compromised vessel in situ; with later patients they replaced the affected section with freeze-dried homografts or Dacron prostheses. In the next six years they treated seventy-two patients, three-quarters of whom made good recoveries.[72]

Many people over the next half-century would have good reason to be grateful for this development; one was Michael DeBakey. In 2005 the ninety-seven-year-old surgeon was sitting at home preparing a lecture when he felt an excruciating pain in his chest. An hour later his wife found him lying on a couch in his office. He told her that he knew what was wrong, and that it was serious. In hospital his colleagues confirmed what he had already worked out for himself: he had an aortic dissection. Only too familiar with the poor survival odds for a patient of his age, DeBakey refused consent for an operation. His family and friends were determined, however, and when he slipped into

---

* Aneurysms and dissections are now classified as separate lesions with different underlying causes.

unconsciousness a special meeting of the hospital's ethics committee was hurriedly convened. It concluded that the circumstances were exceptional: DeBakey's assessment of his own chances was needlessly pessimistic, and the views of his doctors and family should be taken into account. The operation was allowed to proceed.

One of DeBakey's most trusted protégés, Dr George Noon, performed the surgery, using techniques pioneered by his patient decades earlier.[73] DeBakey pulled through, becoming the oldest survivor of an operation he invented; a few months later he was often spotted in the hospital gym, obediently following the rehabilitation programme set out by his colleagues. He even returned to work and lived for two more years, dying a couple of months shy of his 100th birthday.

Although this is a book about heart surgery, the organ itself has barely featured in this chapter. Indeed, most people who suffer an aortic aneurysm today will never meet a cardiac surgeon: the aorta is now largely the preserve of vascular specialists. But all the individuals involved in this story went on to make major contributions to the development of heart surgery. The aorta is the largest pipe in an elaborate system of plumbing whose main pump is the heart. And learning how to repair those pipes was an essential prerequisite for fixing the pump itself; barely a decade after the first aortic aneurysm repairs, Christiaan Barnard transplanted his first heart. It was the groundbreaking work of DeBakey and Cooley that made that feat possible.

4. ICE BATHS AND MONKEY LUNGS

Philadelphia, 6 May 1953

Imagine for a moment that you are a mechanical engineer (if you're already a mechanical engineer this won't take much effort). A particularly awkward client has offered you a vast sum of money to design a machine. This is the brief: 'I want a small device, about the size of my fist, which can pump high-pressure liquid at a rate of 5 litres a minute – although it will be required to adjust rapidly and automatically to deliver up to 20 litres a minute when needed. It must have no moving parts, and be capable of running for 80 years without interruption or maintenance of any kind.' You would be compelled to turn down the job: despite years of effort, nobody has ever succeeded in building a pump so reliable. What makes this all the more frustrating is that such a perfect machine already exists: the human heart.

In a lifetime of 80 years the average heart beats around 3 billion times. Mine has done about half of that total so far, pumping the equivalent of 110 million litres of blood (about 44 Olympic swimming pools-full). In 40 years, the closest it's come to misbehaving is the occasional ectopic (mistimed) beat.[*] This sheer reliability is a marvel, but of course

---

[*] This is a common and usually harmless occurrence, and the reason that people sometimes refer to their heart 'skipping a beat'.

it is no accident; the organ has evolved this way for a reason. Our tissues are constantly in need of oxygen, and the 5 litres of blood that pass through our arteries every minute meet that demand. So what happens if the pump stops and the blood supply dries up? Surprisingly, death is not instantaneous. Some parts of the body can survive for half an hour or more: severed fingers can be successfully reattached several hours later.

The brain is more demanding. Such is its need for oxygen that the circulation only has to be interrupted for two minutes before the onset of brain damage, and at normal temperatures most of us will be dead after six minutes. As soon as surgeons began to contemplate repairing heart defects they realised this was a major obstacle to their ambitions. In 1936 the American cardiologist Samuel Levine wrote: 'Until a satisfactory artificial circulation is developed that will nourish the systemic organs and even the coronary arteries, any lengthy operative procedures on the inside of the heart will be difficult or impossible.'[1] Opening the heart meant interrupting the circulation, and this could only be done if some way could be found to keep the delicate tissues of the brain and major organs alive while the heart was unable to provide them with fresh blood. For decades this seemed an insuperable problem.

By the end of the 1940s three congenital heart defects were being treated surgically with great success. Robert Gross had shown that it was possible to cure a patent ductus arteriosus; Clarence Crafoord had pioneered the treatment of coarctation of the aorta; and Albert Blalock's Blue Baby operation had dramatically improved hundreds of cyanotic infants. But the most common congenital condition of all remained beyond the reach of the surgeon. Thousands of babies are born every year with a hole in the heart – a defect in the septum, the tissue wall dividing the two sides of the organ. If the hole lies between the two upper chambers (atria) this is known as an atrial septal defect; if between the two lower chambers (ventricles) it's called a ventricular septal defect.[*] The effects of both are similar: red, oxygenated

---

[*] As we saw in Chapter 2, ventricular septal defect (VSD) is one of the four anomalies found in tetralogy of Fallot.

blood from the left side of the heart mixes with blue, unoxygenated blood from the right side. Because the left atrium and ventricle operate at higher pressure than the right, oxygenated blood is forced into the right side of the heart and pumped back to the lungs, causing the heart to work harder and putting undue pressure on the pulmonary blood vessels. Medics call this a left-to-right shunt: it does not cause cyanosis, because there is no reduction in blood oxygenation. This is the opposite of the right-to-left shunt caused by tetralogy of Fallot, in which unoxygenated blue blood is pushed into the systemic circulation.

A hole in the heart is a simple defect with potentially fatal consequences, and surgeons were deeply frustrated at their inability to treat it. They knew that if they could only gain access to the cardiac interior, smaller defects could be closed with a few stitches, while larger ones could be patched with some suitable material. Actually opening the organ seemed out of the question, so they came up with a number of creative ways of making interventions inside it without doing so.

In 1948 the Canadian surgeon Gordon Murray operated on four children using a clever method that employed connective tissue, the fascia lata, from the thigh. Using a large needle, he passed two or three strips of this material through the heart from front to back so that they lay in front of the defect, and then pulled them taut. His intention was that they would interweave, forming an impermeable barrier across the hole. Murray called this the 'living suture' technique, since the material used was not silk or catgut but the patient's own tissue.[2] Although ingenious, the method was unsatisfactory since the defects were at best imperfectly closed. One child died during the operation, and the other three were not greatly improved as a result.

At least a dozen methods of solving the problem were tested over the next few years, and only a few went any further than the animal laboratory.[3] The most successful was that of Robert Gross, who came up with a truly daring way of gaining access to the interior of the heart, an idea based on simple physics. He realised that if he could somehow attach a funnel to the exterior of the heart and then make a hole in the cardiac wall, blood would not spurt out in great volumes but would simply rise a few centimetres up the funnel. He could then insert his fingers through this pool of blood into the chambers of the heart and perform simple procedures, albeit by touch alone.

After successful animal experiments he designed a 15-centimetre-high rubber funnel, which he called the atrial well. Its lower orifice was 5 centimetres in diameter, the upper aperture 13 centimetres. The base of the funnel was sewn to the cardiac wall, and a 5-centimetre incision made through it to open the heart. This was a dramatic moment, as bright red blood rushed up into the atrial well. Gross was worried that if the pressure were too high it might overflow, but in practice the pool of blood only rose a few centimetres into the funnel. Immersing his fingers into this scarlet reservoir he was able to feel the defect and then repair it. Several of his earliest patients died, but he also had some spectacular successes. One girl of fourteen was transformed: four months after her operation Gross reported that 'she likes to play tennis and engage in other strenuous sports – all of which are entirely new experiences for her.'[4]

This was valuable progress, but it required skill that only a few possessed. Operating blindly in a blood-filled heart, using the two or three fingers that could fit through the atrial well, was a perilous business. A more sophisticated solution was needed, and by the time Gross reported his work in 1953 one had already been found. In September the Philadelphia surgeon John Gibbon revealed his successful use of a machine that would later make open-heart surgery routine.[5] This was a historic moment, but it went virtually unnoticed: Gibbon presented his results at a minor local medical conference, and few of his colleagues knew it had even taken place. Strangely, the inventor of the heart-lung machine performed only a handful of operations before abandoning cardiac surgery for ever.

Despite early aspirations to be a poet, it was almost inevitable that John Heysham Gibbon Jr – known as Jack – would become a doctor. His father was a distinguished surgeon, one of the first in the US to suture a heart wound,[6] and three earlier generations of Gibbons had also been medics.[7] Shortly after becoming a fellow in surgery at Harvard, Gibbon had an idea that would preoccupy him for the next quarter of a century, prompted by his experiences one night in February 1931. A woman who had been admitted to hospital for routine surgery suddenly developed severe chest pain; she had a pulmonary embolism, a life-threatening blood clot in her pulmonary artery. Gibbon's superior, Edward D. Churchill, had her moved to the operating theatre, where a large surgical team spent a sleepless night watching her life ebb away. At eight o'clock the following morning her pulse stopped and an emergency operation was performed, but to no avail. Many years later, Gibbon recalled his frustration during this midnight vigil:

> During that long night, helplessly watching the patient struggle for life as her blood became darker and her veins more distended, the idea naturally occurred to me that if it were possible to remove continuously some of the blue blood from the patient's swollen veins, put oxygen into that blood and allow carbon dioxide to escape from it, and then to inject continuously the now-red blood back into the patient's arteries, we might have saved her life.[8]

This is a concise description of the modern heart-lung machine: a device that removes blood from the patient's body, exchanges its carbon dioxide for fresh oxygen, and pumps it back into the body – temporarily doing the job of the patient's own heart and lungs. Gibbon's early development of such a machine was primarily intended to enable life-saving surgery on patients with pulmonary embolism; it did not immediately occur to him that it might also be a useful aid to cardiac surgery.

When Gibbon began to design his machine two years later he received little encouragement. Dr Churchill was unenthusiastic but reluctantly allowed him to go ahead, while other colleagues were actively hostile to the idea: they were convinced that it would not work, devouring the department's limited resources indefinitely. The only unwavering support came from his research assistant Mary (known as Maly), a talented laboratory technician who also happened to be his wife. Her knowledge, imagination and meticulous experimental technique would be essential to the many years of hard work that followed.

The two main components Gibbon needed were obvious: an artificial lung to oxygenate the blood, and a pump to propel it through the machine and around the patient's body. This simple description conceals a labyrinth of engineering problems. The first of these was replicating the function of the human lung, which allows the red blood cells to swap waste carbon dioxide for fresh oxygen. The organ is highly efficient at gas exchange thanks to its vast network of tiny air pockets, known as alveoli, which give a single lung an internal surface area of around 50 square metres[9] – about the same as the floor space in the average one-bedroom flat. An artificial oxygenator would somehow have to emulate this efficiency without being unwieldy. Then there was the problem of air embolism: bubbles of gas entering the bloodstream. The artificial lung would work by exposing the blood to pure oxygen; if a single bubble of unabsorbed gas reached the body it might enter the vessels of the brain or heart muscle and cause catastrophic damage. The pump presented another challenge: red blood cells are fragile objects, tiny bags of fluid enclosed in a delicate membrane. If roughly handled they can burst, a phenomenon known as haemolysis. Designing a device which combined the necessary delicacy with the power to propel blood to every extremity of the body would be a formidable task. Finally, Gibbon also needed to find a way to prevent the blood clotting, as it normally does when it leaves the body and comes into contact with air.

When he retired to the library to read up on these problems, Gibbon found that many of them had already been investigated by earlier researchers. As early as 1666 the English natural scientist Robert Hooke had suggested that it might be possible to oxygenate blood outside the body. In a series of experiments on dogs, Hooke used bellows to blow air through the lungs. He discovered that inflating and deflating them was not sufficient to keep the animal alive; the air had to be constantly refreshed. In a paper read before the Royal Society, Hooke wondered whether exposing blood to fresh air in a container outside the body might be enough to sustain life; although he proposed an experiment to test this idea, he seems never to have carried it out.[10]

Hooke's contemporary Richard Lower – the first person to attempt a blood transfusion – also investigated the mechanism of respiration. In his meticulous experiments he showed that blood was dark in colour immediately before it entered the lungs, and became bright red as a result of passing through them. This disproved a theory, fashionable at the time, that suggested the heart heated the blood and thereby altered its colour. Lower was in no doubt that blood changed its hue as a result of its exposure to air, and showed that this could be done outside the body by shaking a dish of dark, venous blood vigorously in a dish until it turned a vivid scarlet.[11]

Nobody seems to have thought of putting this discovery to practical use until the nineteenth century. The French physiologist Julien Jean César Legallois was fascinated by the difference between life and death, and in 1813 he speculated about the possibility of reanimating dead animals. He suggested that if the function of the heart were replaced by continuous injection of arterial blood, 'whether natural, or artificially formed', it would be possible to maintain life indefinitely, or even to perform 'complete resurrection' of a corpse.[12] He even speculated that artificial circulation might keep a decapitated head alive, although his attempts to do so in rabbits failed because the blood clotted.

The problem of clotting was partially solved in 1821, when two other French researchers, Prevost and Dumas, showed that beating fresh blood with a whisk removed fibrin, a clot-promoting protein.[13] In the 1850s Charles Brown-Séquard continued the work of Legallois with far greater success, whisking blood to oxygenate it before injecting it into the severed head of a dog: its eyes and muzzle moved, and he concluded that he had restored it to life, albeit briefly.[14] His most celebrated (and gruesome) experiment took place on 18 June 1851, when he attended the execution of a criminal in Paris. The guillotine fell at 8 a.m.; Brown-Séquard then sat beside the headless corpse for the rest of the day, waiting for it to stiffen. By 9 p.m. rigor mortis had set in, and Brown-Séquard began his investigation by carefully amputating the dead man's arm. He later recalled: 'As I wished to inject fresh human blood, and as I could not obtain any from the hospitals at such an hour, I was obliged to make use of my own.' Two friends who had accompanied him to watch the spectacle removed a third of a pint of blood from a vein in Brown-Séquard's left arm, beat it vigorously and filtered it through a cloth, before injecting it into the detached limb. The blood immediately started to ooze out of the severed ends of its arteries and veins, so Brown-Séquard collected and reinjected it, doing so continuously for the next half-hour. At the end of this gory process he found that the muscles of the hand lost their cadaveric rigidity and would once again contract if stimulated.[15]

Further motivation for the development of an artificial circulation was provided by late nineteenth-century research into the functions of the internal organs. Scientists wanted to study the kidneys and liver working in isolation outside the body, which entailed perfusing (continuously injecting) them with oxygenated blood. In 1868 two German researchers, Ludwig and Schmidt, put blood in a balloon filled with oxygen and shook it, before pumping it through isolated organs.[16] They were able to demonstrate that perfused livers continued to secrete bile, and lungs excreted carbon dioxide.[17] A more sophisticated way of oxygenating the blood was invented in 1882 in Strasbourg by Waldemar von Schröder, who bubbled oxygen through venous blood. Bright red blood was produced but the bubbles produced large amounts of foam, which rendered it unusable – a problem that would remain unsolved until the 1950s.[18]

Another device constructed in 1885 by the Austrian researchers Max von Frey and Max Gruber has a good claim to be described as the world's first fully functional heart-lung machine – although it was never used on a living animal. Their apparatus pumped blood into a tilted glass cylinder filled with oxygen, which constantly rotated so that the blood spread out into a thin film covering the inner surface, maximising its surface area.[19] By the time the blood emerged from the bottom of the cylinder it had been oxygenated, and was then pumped into the experimental subject. Von Frey and Gruber never planned to use the device to keep an animal alive, but instead successfully employed it to perfuse the kidneys and hind legs of dogs that had already been killed. The apparatus was simple – and strikingly similar in conception to the machine John Gibbon would invent more than half a century later.[20] Several other artificial oxygenators were constructed around the turn of the twentieth century; most used either the bubble or film techniques, but one invented by the American physiologist Donald Hooker (the uncle of the Hollywood star Katharine Hepburn) employed a rotating flat disc to increase the surface area of the blood, a scheme which would be imitated by later investigators.[21]

When Gibbon began to design his own heart-lung machine in 1933 he had no idea that a Russian scientist had already been working on the problem for a decade. Sergei Sergeyevitch Brukhonenko's interest in the subject was prompted by his experiences as an army doctor during the First World War. He saw many soldiers die from injuries to their major organs which could not be treated because there was no way of doing so without interrupting the circulation. He began his research in 1923, and two years later designed a machine that he called the 'autojector'.[22] It used two pumps to replicate the action of the heart, but the first version of the device did not contain an artificial oxygenator; instead he used the lungs of a recently killed dog. These were placed in a dish and attached to bellows to simulate breathing. The blood passed through them was collected and used to perfuse a living animal.

Brukhonenko used his apparatus to perform a number of impressive and macabre feats. On 18 September 1925 he gave a demonstration to colleagues in which the autojector pumped oxygenated blood through the severed head of a dog, which responded to stimuli and appeared to be aware of its surroundings.* When this research became known more widely it caused a sensation; some speculated that the technology might be used to keep humans alive indefinitely. The playwright George Bernard Shaw declared: 'I am greatly tempted to have my head cut off so that I may continue to dictate plays and books independently of any illness, without having to dress or undress, or eat, or do anything at all except to produce masterpieces of dramatic art and literature.'[23]

On 1 November 1926 Brukhonenko became the first to achieve total cardiopulmonary bypass. He attached the autojector to the major blood vessels of a dog before stopping its heart. For the next two hours the machine took over the functions of the dog's heart and lungs, keeping it alive until unexpected bleeding put an end to the demonstration (and the life of the unfortunate dog). In his account of this experiment, Brukhonenko suggested that in future the autojector might be used 'for certain operations on the arrested heart' – a far-sighted remark.[24] By the late 1930s he had replaced the donor lungs with a bubble oxygenator, but his ambition to apply the machine to human patients was frustrated by the outbreak of war, which brought a halt to his research. In his experiments Brukhonenko used a recently discovered drug, suramin, to prevent the blood clotting, but it was not terribly effective. John Gibbon was lucky in having access to an alternative that was far superior, and which had only just become available: heparin.

One of the surgeons I spoke to while researching this book described heparin as the discovery that made heart surgery possible. Yet this important advance took place in curiously understated circumstances, and the man who made it died in obscurity. In 1915 Jay

---

* A film of this astonishing spectacle was made in 1940 and released in the West as *Experiments in the Revival of Organisms*, introduced by the great biologist J. B. S. Haldane. You can watch it at https://archive.org/details/Experime1940 – though some doubt has been cast on its authenticity.

McLean enrolled at Johns Hopkins Medical School in Baltimore. At twenty-four, he was older than most freshmen, having had a difficult start to life: his father died when he was four, and the family home was then destroyed in the fires that followed the San Francisco earthquake of 1906. When his stepfather refused to fund him through medical school, McLean spent several years working in gold mines and on oil rigs to pay for his education. Such was his determination to become a doctor that he then travelled the 3,800 miles from California to Baltimore and presented himself at Johns Hopkins, even though he had already been rejected by the institution. Impressed by his tenacity, the dean found him a place. Doing nothing to dispel any impression that he was a rather wilful young man, McLean then announced that he would spend his first year in laboratory research, rather than following the standard curriculum.[25] And so he found himself working in the laboratory of Dr William Howell, the world authority on the coagulation of blood.

Howell was investigating a substance extracted from the brain, cephalin, which he believed to be partly responsible for blood clotting. He asked McLean to identify the active ingredient of this mixture, and if possible to refine it. McLean believed the chemical might be found in greater concentrations in other organs, and so also made preparations from hearts and livers. He was curious to find out how long its effect lasted, and so continued to test his samples for some weeks after preparing them. To his surprise, after a while the substance extracted from livers began to inhibit clotting rather than promote it. When he was satisfied that this was not an experimental error he went to tell Howell that he had discovered a powerful anticoagulant. His boss was sceptical, and so McLean gave a simple demonstration: taking a beaker of cat's blood, he stirred in a small amount of the substance. 'I placed this on Dr Howell's laboratory table', wrote McLean forty years later, 'and asked him to tell me when it clotted. It never did clot.'[26]

Howell decided to call the substance heparin, from the Greek word for liver. Having made one of the most important medical discoveries of the twentieth century, McLean's subsequent career was

one of surprising mediocrity: beset by financial and personal problems, he held a few minor academic positions before ending up as a
struggling general practitioner, and was never again involved in meaningful medical research.[27]

. Nobody at first understood the significance of the discovery, which
had little obvious utility: researchers were trying to understand *why*
blood clotted, not prevent it from doing so. William Howell reported
McLean's findings in a paper published in 1918, noting that when dogs
were injected with heparin their blood lost its ability to coagulate, an
effect which lasted for several hours.[28] Eleven years later a physiologist in Toronto, Charles Best, decided to investigate further. A professor at thirty, Best was already well known as one of the scientists who
had discovered insulin in 1921. He and his colleague Gordon Murray
succeeded in producing much purer samples of heparin, and proving
its effect on dogs.[29] They extracted it at first from beef liver, and then
lungs, but when the pet-food industry began to buy these items in bulk
they were forced to move to beef intestines, which slowed down the
pace of their research. The extraction process resulted in some appall-
ing smells, prompting the team's relocation to a farm a safe distance
from the university campus.[30]

In May 1935 Murray injected heparin into a patient and found
that it increased the clotting time of her blood from 8 to 30 minutes.[31]
One of the first to realise the importance of this work was Clarence
Crafoord, the Swedish surgeon who had pioneered the treatment of
aortic coarctation. Having been frustrated in his attempts to treat
blood clots on the lungs, he quickly realised that this drug might be
the answer to the problem.[32] By 1939 heparin was deemed so valuable
that when a consignment was ordered by doctors in England it was
delivered by a navy destroyer rather than being risked on a merchant
convoy.[33]

John Gibbon knew of Best and Murray's research, and when he
designed his first artificial lung in 1934 he was able to obtain heparin
supplies from Toronto. Injecting his experimental animals with the
drug would ensure that their blood did not clot as soon as it left their

bodies. His first device used a vertical rotating glass cylinder as an oxygenator: blood trickling into this container was spread into a thin film and exposed to oxygen before being collected at the bottom and pumped back into the body.[34] Because the artificial lung was too small to use on a large animal, Gibbon chose to experiment on cats. Obtaining them was not difficult: Philadelphia was overrun with strays, and the local authorities were killing 30,000 animals a year. Armed with a piece of tuna and a sack, Gibbon took to the streets at night, returning to the laboratory each time with a fresh supply of feral cats.[35]

The research was laborious, intricate and time-consuming. Mary Gibbon did much of the work, starting early in the morning to prepare the equipment for each day's experiment, a process that took several hours. When it was all sterilised and assembled, she would anaesthetise the cat and connect it to an artificial respirator, before opening its thorax to reveal the heart. Cannulas (tubes) were then inserted into two vessels to convey blood to and from the heart-lung machine. Finally, heparin was injected into the bloodstream to prevent coagulation, and the pulmonary artery was compressed to simulate obstruction by a clot. At this point the heart-lung machine was turned on, and John and Mary began their observations.[36]

After many frustrations and refinements to the equipment, one day in 1935 John and Mary succeeded in their aim. As Gibbon tightened a clamp around the cat's pulmonary artery to prevent blood flowing from its heart to the lungs, the machine came to life and began to take over the functions of both organs. Recalling this moment of elation near the end of his life, he wrote: 'My wife and I threw our arms around each other and danced around the laboratory.'[37] Later that year they succeeded in maintaining the life of a cat for almost four hours while its pulmonary artery was obstructed; without the heart-lung machine this would have killed it in a matter of minutes.[38] The animals often developed complications after the procedure, and some died; but in 1939 Gibbon was able to announce to a surgical conference in Los Angeles that four cats kept alive by the heart-lung machine for up to twenty minutes had all made complete recoveries.[39] One of the surgeons present likened the Gibbons' achievement to 'Jules Verne's dreamlike visions, regarded as impossible at the time but later actually accomplished'.[40]

Like Brukhonenko in Russia, Gibbon was unable to continue his research in wartime, when (to the surprise and alarm of his family) he insisted on volunteering for service. When he returned to civilian life in 1945, his priority was to build a larger machine with the ability to oxygenate enough blood to keep a human alive. He realised he needed specialist engineering help for such a major undertaking, and through one of his medical students gained an introduction to Thomas J. Watson, the chairman of the International Business Machines Corporation, who agreed to construct a machine at the company's expense.[41] In later years IBM would become better known as a manufacturer of computers, but in the 1940s its engineers had wide-ranging expertise in designing everything from punched-card machines to armaments. The first IBM machine was delivered in 1946, a larger and considerably more sophisticated version of Gibbon's prototype. When *Time* magazine interviewed Gibbon three years later he revealed that he had been able to keep dogs alive on this machine for up to forty-six minutes.[42] He also made clear that he now saw this as a means of enabling open-heart surgery: Dwight Harken's wartime feats had demonstrated how robust the organ was, and convinced the profession that it might be possible to go even further by stopping the heartbeat and opening it.[43]

Gibbon knew that the cylinder being used to oxygenate the blood was still not big enough to use on humans; to do so he calculated he would need to construct a machine seven storeys high – an obviously impractical proposition.[44] Then two workers in his laboratory noticed that the rate of oxygenation increased if an obstruction was placed in the bloodstream to produce turbulence. After experimenting with various ways of doing this they replaced the revolving cylinder with a number of screens made from stainless-steel mesh. Six of these screens were suspended in parallel; blood trickled down them in an oxygen-rich atmosphere and was collected at the bottom. This gave the artificial lung a surface area of over 8 square metres, but contained in a unit small enough to fit into an operating theatre.[45]

Perfecting the oxygenator was the most difficult aspect of constructing a machine for artificial circulation; what, then, of the pump, the component which was to replace the heart? Shortly after beginning his research Gibbon had started to use a simple mechanism that propelled the blood without touching it. It had only one moving part: a rotating wheel with three rollers spaced along its circumference. A loop of flexible tubing fitted snugly around the outside of this wheel so that as it rotated the rollers at its edge swept along the tubing, compressing it and moving the blood inside it forwards. Known as a roller pump, this mechanism proved ideal, as it produced a smooth flow without harming the delicate blood cells. Oxygenators have continued to evolve, but in the eighty years since Gibbon first adopted it the roller pump has remained virtually unaltered, and remains a common sight in the operating theatre.

The question of who invented this simple device is a curiously vexed one, and gives some insight into the egos and rivalries of early heart surgery. Michael DeBakey had patented an almost identical pump in 1935 as a tool to facilitate blood transfusions,[46] and later took credit for the invention, pointing out that he had sent Gibbon an early model.[47] But roller pumps were nothing new; DeBakey's version was merely an improvement on an existing design dating back to 1855. In fact, no fewer than eleven similar pumps had been patented before DeBakey's, including several intended for surgical use. This chronology was painstakingly laid out by Denton Cooley in an article published in 1987;[48] a cynic questioning his motives might point out that he was embroiled in a messy thirty-year feud with DeBakey at the time.

By the early 1950s Gibbon felt he was close to being able to use his machine on humans. But he no longer had the field to himself: stimulated by his research, others were trying to build an artificial heart-lung. In April 1951 the Minnesota surgeon Clarence Dennis

made the first attempt to operate inside the heart using bypass, operating on a little girl diagnosed with an atrial septal defect. After successfully attaching her to the machine, Dennis discovered that this
defect was far bigger than expected – so large, in fact, that it proved
impossible to close it, and she could not be saved.[49] Later that year
two successful procedures using similar machines took place in Italy
and the US, though in neither case was the surgeon attempting to
operate on the heart.[50]

John Gibbon waited until he was absolutely satisfied with his
heart-lung machine before risking its use on a patient. The first
operation took place in February 1953, and like Clarence Dennis's
first attempt it was thwarted by an error in diagnosis. The patient was
a fifteen-month-old baby with a failing heart, thought to be caused
by a large atrial septal defect. When he opened the heart he found
the organ enlarged but otherwise normal. He was forced to abandon
the operation, and shortly afterwards she died.[51] Such occurrences
were not uncommon: before the invention of more sophisticated
imaging techniques, cardiologists were largely reliant on X-rays and
the stethoscope, and diagnosis was an inexact science. Surgeons
often cut open a patient only to find an entirely different problem
from the one expected.

Three months after this dispiriting experience Gibbon met a young
woman who would become his most famous patient, an eighteen-year-
old student named Cecelia Bavolek. After a healthy childhood she had
suddenly started to have unexplained episodes of breathlessness and
an irregular heartbeat. In March 1953 she developed alarming symptoms including a fever and coughing up blood, and was admitted to
hospital.[52] After weeks of tests the cardiologists agreed that she had
a significant atrial septal defect. Gibbon believed that he could repair
the hole in Cecelia's heart, and discussed it with the girl and her parents, explaining that he had never before attempted the operation on
a human.[53] Despite the risks, Cecelia and her family agreed, and the
procedure was scheduled for the following month, giving Gibbon time
to prepare his equipment.

The heart-lung machine was a large and elaborate piece of machinery about the size of a grand piano. The IBM engineers had equipped it with electronics to monitor every aspect of its operation, including the temperature and pressure of the blood. These circuits, which resembled the innards of an early computer, were housed in a large cabinet that was filled with nitrogen to prevent flammable anaesthetic gases from entering and causing an explosion.[54] But after the machine had been assembled and carefully checked, one vital ingredient was still required.

Early on the morning of 6 May a queue of bleary-eyed medical students lined the corridor outside Gibbon's operating theatre. They were there to give blood, large volumes of which were required to prepare the heart-lung machine for use. This process, known as 'priming', was necessary because there needed to be blood already in the device at the moment when it was attached to the patient.[55] Once the last donor had left, heparin was added to prevent clotting, and the machine was turned on: when blood had been thoroughly circulated through its tubes and reservoirs it was ready for use.

When John Gibbon began to operate that morning he was not entirely sure what he and his three assistants would find inside Cecelia's chest. He was confident that she had a hole in her heart, but it was not clear whether this lay between its upper chambers (the atria) or the lower, pumping chambers (the ventricles). He began by making a long incision across her chest from one armpit to the other, curving it beneath her breasts to minimise the post-operative scar. He then opened her chest cavity in the space between her fourth and fifth ribs. With a retractor spreading the ribs apart, Gibbon had a clear view of the heart. The right ventricle was horribly swollen, and the pulmonary artery was so enlarged that it vibrated with every heartbeat. To find out what was wrong, Gibbon made a small incision in the right atrial appendage, a small muscular pouch attached to the right atrium. Through this hole he was able to insert a digit and investigate the inside of Cecelia's heart with his fingertip. Immediately he could feel a hole between the two atria – 'as large as a silver dollar', as he later recorded in his operative notes.

With the diagnosis confirmed they could attach Cecelia to the heart-lung machine. She was given heparin, and plastic tubes were inserted into her blood vessels. The first of these was attached to the left subclavian artery, just above the aortic arch; the second was pushed through the right atrial appendage until it reached the venae cavae, the two main veins which return deoxygenated blood to the heart. The machine was now switched on, and began to assist Cecelia's circulation for the first time, though some blood continued to flow through her heart. Almost immediately they noticed a serious problem: blood was leaking from the artificial lung. Insufficient heparin had been added to the donor blood, and clots had started to form on some of the oxygenating screens, impeding flow through the device. After a hurried discussion with his assistant Frank Allbritten, Gibbon decided to continue, tightening a pair of ligatures around the venae cavae to prevent any blood from entering the heart. His machine was now standing in for Cecelia's heart and lungs.

Gibbon made a large incision in the right atrium, revealing a gaping defect in the septum. He intended to close this hole using a patch of tissue taken from the pericardial sac, but Allbritten suggested that it might be easier simply to sew its edges together. Gibbon agreed, and shortly afterwards the final stitch was in place. Once the heart had been closed and sutured, the pump was turned off and the tubes in Cecelia's blood vessels removed. The operation had taken a little over five hours; for twenty-six minutes, Gibbon's heart-lung machine had been the only thing keeping her alive. She was already beginning to come round as Gibbon inserted the last stitch in her chest, and an hour later was talking to her nurses on the ward.[56]

Cecelia made a rapid recovery, and was allowed home within a fortnight. When she returned to hospital in July her doctors found that the operation had been a total success: the septal defect was closed, and she was now able to climb stairs without becoming breathless. Though she was delighted with her improved health, she was also upset by the attention she had received: her name had appeared prominently in newspaper reports of the operation, and journalists had been pestering her and her parents incessantly. Unprepared for such attention, they changed their phone number and refused all requests for interviews.[57] Apart from a few appearances in support of the American Heart Association in the 1960s she avoided public attention, living quietly until her death in 2000.

The operation also took an emotional toll on John Gibbon. When he left the operating theatre he usually wrote a short account of the procedure; but this time he gave the job to his juniors, unwilling to relive the almost unbearable stress it had entailed. For years afterwards he felt a pang of anxiety every time he opened a surgical journal and saw an article about open-heart surgery.[58]

There was another reason for his unease. In July 1953 he operated on two further patients: both were five years old, and neither survived. The first went into cardiac arrest before she had even been attached to the heart-lung machine and died on the operating table; the second had a complex defect which could not be repaired, and succumbed shortly afterwards.[59] This was mere bad luck, but Gibbon was devastated: he had spent twenty years working on a single problem, and had lost three of his first four patients. He announced that he was suspending all cardiac surgery for a year, pending improvements in the equipment. In fact he never operated on the human heart again, handing responsibility for the entire programme to one of his juniors.[60] One could interpret this as the reaction of a disillusioned man, but some of Gibbon's closest colleagues suggest that he had achieved all he wanted to. Two decades working on one problem was enough; it was time to hand the baton to younger surgeons.

The operation on Cecelia Bavolek was by any standards a historic one, but Gibbon was curiously absent from his own triumph. When *Time* interviewed him he explained open-heart surgery vividly ('like drying out a well to do some work at the bottom of it'), but refused to pose for pictures with his machine.[61] Such achievements are normally documented in the international scholarly press, but Gibbon wrote only a short report for the journal of the Minnesota Medical Association. This is one reason for the general sense of anticlimax that followed Gibbon's operation, but there are others. Progress in medicine is not defined by a single success, but by a series of them: one patient cured was not enough to convince the surgical world that the procedure was safe. Many surgeons also believed that Gibbon's research was a dead end, since other, apparently less cumbersome, methods of operating inside the heart were already being developed and were yielding results. Gibbon, it transpired, was not even the first surgeon to perform a successful open-heart operation. That milestone was achieved in September 1952 by John Lewis, a surgeon from the University of Minnesota, who closed an atrial septal defect in a five-year-old girl using a technique completely different from Gibbon's. Instead of maintaining the patient's circulation artificially, he stopped it entirely. Conventional wisdom suggested that this should have fatal consequences, but Lewis had a new surgical weapon at his disposal: hypothermia.[62]

Whereas Gibbon spent twenty years developing his heart-lung machine, hypothermia was being used clinically within five years of the first experiments. The idea was simple: cooling the human body lowers the oxygen requirements of its tissues, so less blood is needed to keep them alive. This increases the length of time for which the circulation may be safely interrupted, giving the surgeon precious minutes in which to operate.

The first person to think of cold as a possible aid to heart surgery was a Canadian surgeon called Wilfred Bigelow. The freezing winters of his native country provided the stimulus for this interest in 1941, when he found himself amputating the fingers of a young man who had fallen prey to frostbite. He was surprised to find that little was known about why frostbitten extremities so often turned gangrenous, and spent some time looking into the problem. A few years later he went to Baltimore to work for Alfred Blalock, and took part in a number of Blue Baby operations. Watching Blalock operate around the beating heart, he realised that surgeons would never be able to cure more complex conditions while the organ was still pumping. And then an idea occurred to him: 'One night I awoke with a simple solution to the problem, and one that did not require pumps and tubes – *cool the whole body, reduce the oxygen requirements, interrupt the circulation, and open the heart.*'[63]

When Bigelow returned to Toronto in 1947 he wasted no time in beginning his research. Surprisingly few people had investigated the effects of prolonged cooling on the human body. In the late 1930s a Philadelphia neurosurgeon, Temple Fay, noticed that cooling cancer cells appeared to inhibit their growth and division. He suspected this might have therapeutic benefit, and began to use refrigeration to treat patients with advanced malignancies. At first he used iced water to chill only the area of the tumour, but then he began to apply it to the entire body, reducing the patient's temperature from the usual 37°C to around 30°C.[64] The results were disappointing, but this study of over 100 patients nevertheless broke new ground: before these experiments hypothermia was generally believed to cause irreversible tissue damage, but Fay had shown that it could be endured for days at a time.

Bigelow's central assumption was that cooling the body's tissues would reduce their oxygen consumption. To test this hypothesis he cooled dogs while monitoring the oxygen levels in their blood. The first experiments took place in a giant freezer cooled to –9°C, but Bigelow and his colleagues soon tired of having to dress up as polar explorers, and instead simply placed the dog in a bath of iced water. The results were surprising: rather than decreasing the dogs' oxygen requirements, it seemed to increase them. Eventually they realised that this anomaly was caused by shivering, which greatly sped up the dogs' metabolism. Once they had succeeded in suppressing shivering through careful use of anaesthetics, they found that oxygen consumption did decline steadily with a reduction in temperature, exactly as predicted.[65]

Over the next few years, Bigelow and his team thoroughly investigated the physiological effects of hypothermia, and found that they could safely cool dogs to 20°C; any lower than this and there was a risk of fibrillation, a dangerous state in which the muscle fibres of the heart stop contracting in unison and begin to spasm chaotically. As the temperature dropped, so did the heartbeat: dogs cooled to 30°C needed only 50 per cent of their usual oxygen intake, and at 20°C this figure fell to 20 per cent.[66] By 1949 they felt they knew enough about the body's response to cold to attempt an open-heart procedure on a dog. The animals were anaesthetised and then cooled to 20°C – at this temperature no further anaesthesia was necessary, since hypothermia alone was enough to keep them unconscious. The chest was opened, and clamps placed on the main cardiac veins, stopping the circulation. Finally an incision was made into the organ and the interior of a living heart revealed for the first time. 'What a thrill to look inside a beating heart!' Bigelow wrote thirty years later. 'What a dynamic, powerful organ.'[67]

He was eager to translate this experience into operations on human patients, but to his frustration did not get a chance to do so: local cardiologists were reluctant to let their patients undergo an untested procedure.[68] Bigelow and his colleagues were crestfallen when they learned that John Lewis had already performed the first open-heart operation using hypothermia, with a Philadelphia surgeon, Charles Bailey, achieving a second success a few months later.

Bigelow's experimental work laid the foundations for cardiac surgery using hypothermia, but the figure who showed its full potential was Henry Swan. Like Bigelow he had served with distinction as an army surgeon in France, and his experience in treating soldiers with terrible injuries to the blood vessels was invaluable preparation for heart surgery. Swan was familiar with John Gibbon's work, but felt that the advantages of the heart-lung machine were outweighed by its cost, complexity and dangers. Hypothermia was simpler, required no complex equipment and entailed minimal expense.[69] At his hospital in Denver, Swan began a spectacularly successful series of operations using the technique. He believed hypothermia could enable surgery on a range of conditions, and deliberately chose cases that were unapproachable by any other method – the only patients on whom he could justify using a relatively unproven procedure. His first fifteen patients included some with an atrial septal defect, but he also attempted to correct cases of pulmonary stenosis – a narrowing of the opening of the pulmonary artery from the heart. Thirteen were improved by their operations, and only one died during surgery.[70]

Hypothermic heart surgery was an extraordinary spectacle, as dramatic as anything seen in an operating theatre since the days when leg amputations were performed without anaesthetic. When the patient had been put to sleep and connected to monitoring equipment and a respirator, they were put in a tepid bath to begin the process of refrigeration. Ice cubes were then added to accelerate the cooling, and the patient was removed when their temperature was still a few degrees above the target of 28°C, since it would continue to drop for some time afterwards. They would then be thoroughly dried and transferred to the operating table. When the chest had been opened and the surgeon was ready to open the heart, artificial respiration would be ceased and blood prevented from flowing into the heart with clamps.[71] The surgeon would then have between eight and ten minutes to complete the procedure before the patient's life would be in danger. In Bigelow's operating theatre the anaesthetist gave a minute-by-minute time check, building to a nerve-shredding climax as the crucial tenth minute approached.[72] Completing a complex repair in these conditions required speed, superlative skill and unwavering self-confidence. Even Swan, who put himself through this experience over a hundred times, admitted he was 'scared to death' every time he operated.[73]

Swan's operations on a wide range of heart conditions represented a new frontier in surgery, and in his article announcing his first fifteen cases he pointed out that he had disproved Stephen Paget's assertion that it would never be safe to operate on the organ: 'Given half a chance,' he wrote, 'the heart keeps beating.'[74] But many were sceptical: it seemed strange to induce one life-threatening condition in order to treat another. Russell Brock, while impressed by Swan's results, declared: 'I cannot bring myself to believe that such a procedure can have a permanent place in surgery,' adding fastidiously that the sight of a bath of iced water in an operating theatre was 'both aesthetically and surgically unattractive'.[75]

The opinion of a respected figure like Brock carried much weight, but criticising a new technique on aesthetic grounds was rather missing the point. A more substantive objection to hypothermia was the fact that it afforded only ten minutes for the surgeon to perform his task. The Amsterdam surgeon Ite Boerema found a way to extend this safe period for up to half an hour by performing hypothermic surgery in a high-pressure chamber similar to those used to decompress deep-sea divers. When patients breathed air at three times normal atmospheric pressure their tissues became saturated with oxygen, radically increasing their ability to withstand circulatory arrest.[76] Several patients were successfully operated on, but his surgeons hated working in a glorified tin can: the high pressure caused ear and sinus pain, and they had to endure slow depressurisation after each procedure had been completed.[77] A few other pressure chambers were built, but their cost and inconvenience outweighed their benefits.

Surgeons uncertain which open-heart technique to disapprove of were spoilt for choice. One arguably even more dubious method was being used – with surprising success – by a colleague of John Lewis in Minnesota. C. Walton Lillehei was another distinguished war veteran who had treated casualties in Algeria and Tunisia before taking part in the Allied invasions of Sicily and mainland Italy in 1943, spending several months encamped at the beachhead at Anzio.[78] He assisted Lewis in the first open-heart procedure in 1952, but soon became convinced that the ten-minute time limit to operations using hypothermia was a fatal flaw. Later that year, two researchers in England discovered that a dog could survive for half an hour with the main blood vessels into its heart clamped shut, as long as a small vein, the azygos, was left open.[79] The blood flowing through this vein represented about 10 per cent of the heart's usual output. The fact that the major organs could survive for so long with so little blood was entirely unexpected, and became known as the azygos flow principle. It considerably simplified the quest for a reliable means of heart-lung bypass, because it reduced the volume that needed to be oxygenated and pumped through the patient per minute.

Lillehei was made aware of this discovery by Morley Cohen, a researcher in his laboratory. Cohen's wife was pregnant at the time, and it occurred to him that the relationship between her and their unborn child was a perfect model for what he was trying to do. In the womb the foetus, unable to breathe for itself, receives oxygenated blood from its mother via the placenta. So, he wondered, could they mimic this arrangement by connecting a large animal to a small one, making one creature breathe and pump blood for both?[80]

Joining the circulations of two animals, known as cross-circulation, was nothing new: in the late eighteenth century the French anatomist Marie François Xavier Bichat connected the blood vessels of two dogs in such a way that the heart of each dog propelled oxygenated blood into the head of the other.[81] In the late 1940s two researchers at Mount Sinai hospital in New York even used a pump to connect a donor dog and a 'patient' animal, on which they attempted open-heart procedures.[82] Cohen and Lillehei repeated these experiments using the azygos flow principle, comparing the results with those achieved using a heart-lung machine. To their surprise the dogs on cross-circulation, which received only 10 per cent of their usual blood supply, not only recovered more quickly but were more likely to survive than those on the heart-lung machine. With results using other methods proving disappointing, they felt they were justified in testing the idea on human patients.[83]

The method would only work when operating on children, since it was necessary for the donor to be bigger than the patient. Lillehei proposed to use parents as donors, given that their blood would usually be compatible with that of their children, and they would almost certainly agree to the procedure. Obtaining approval from the hospital authorities was more fraught; the procedure entailed putting a completely healthy individual – the donor – at risk, and there was considerable resistance to the idea. After much debate a faculty committee eventually gave the go-ahead, and Lillehei operated on his first case on 24 March 1954.

The patient was a thirteen-month-old boy, Gregory Glidden, who had a ventricular septal defect. His father volunteered to act as the donor, and on the morning of the operation both he and his son were given a general anaesthetic. They were placed on adjacent tables in the operating theatre, and tubes placed in major vessels. When the boy's chest had been opened and Lillehei was ready to begin, the venous blood returning to Gregory's heart was diverted into his father's body through a vein in the leg. It then passed through his heart and lungs before being pumped back into the boy's aorta. For the next twelve and a half minutes the father breathed for his son, as Lillehei opened the ventricle and sutured the defect closed. Technically, the operation passed off without a hitch, and the father was unharmed by the experience; but eleven days later the boy died, succumbing to post-operative pneumonia.[84]

Though disappointed, Lillehei and his team were not to be deterred. The following week they operated on another two patients, aged three and five, again using the fathers as donors. These patients made complete recoveries – the first time that anybody had succeeded in closing a hole between the ventricles of the heart. Nineteen of their first twenty-six patients survived, and Lillehei was so confident in the technique that in August he decided to operate on a child with tetralogy of Fallot.[85] Even Blalock and Taussig, the architects of the Blue Baby operation, thought that total correction of such a serious condition was impossible, but Lillehei and his team proved them wrong. Between March 1954 and July the following year, Lillehei operated on forty-five patients using cross-circulation, many of them young children. All had conditions which were previously incurable, and the results were staggering: two-thirds survived, and almost half were still alive more than thirty years later.[86]

Despite the obvious success of cross-circulation, most surgeons had grave reservations about the technique. When Lillehei presented the results of his first three cases at a medical conference, John Gibbon spoke from the floor to articulate the fears he shared with many of his colleagues: 'We are still convinced that it is preferable to perform operations involving an open cardiotomy [opening the heart] by some procedure which does not involve another healthy person. There must be some risk to the donor in a cross circulation.'[87] Indeed there was: although it went unreported, several surgeons with an inadequate grasp of the technique attempted to use it, with disastrous results.[88] In Britain, cross-circulation was deemed so dangerous that it was illegal even to attempt it.[89] One of John Gibbon's junior surgeons, George J. Haupt, remarked that it was the only known procedure which had a potential mortality of 200 per cent.[90]

All forty-five of Lillehei's donors survived, although one nearly died when her heart stopped shortly after the procedure had been completed. The surgeons immediately opened her chest, intending to massage the organ to stimulate a heartbeat, but were hugely relieved when it resumed spontaneously.[91] This near-miss, and the fact that cross-circulation was not suitable for use on adults, persuaded him to try other methods. Two of his departmental colleagues, Gilbert Campbell and Norman Crisp, had been experimenting with an idea first employed by Sergei Brukhonenko in the original version of his autojector: using animal lungs as an oxygenator. Campbell and Crisp used dog lungs to enable heart-lung bypass in operations on children, but most of their patients died.[92] In early 1955 a thirteen-year-old called Calvin Richmond arrived at Lillehei's hospital having been crushed by a truck, which had caused a traumatic atrial septal defect. The boy's family were offered a choice between cross-circulation and using the dog's lung, and chose the latter. A large dog was anaesthetised and one of its lungs removed, placed in a plastic cylinder and ventilated with pure oxygen. Calvin's blood was pumped through the lung for twenty minutes while Lillehei closed three openings between the chambers of his heart. Remarkably, the boy made a complete recovery.[93]

This success was a rare exception. The leading exponent of the method was William Mustard at the Hospital for Sick Children in Toronto, just over the road from Bigelow's department. In 1952 he had operated on seven children with congenital abnormalities using a pump to circulate their blood through a pair of lungs taken from a rhesus monkey: for over an hour these young patients breathed through the lungs of an ape.[94] None survived for longer than a few hours,[95] and when he finally abandoned the method a few years later, only three out of the twenty-one patients were still alive and well.[96]

By 1955 several methods had thus been used to enable open-heart surgery, and all seemed to have significant drawbacks. By the end of the decade, however, there was no doubt about which was the best. Although Gibbon had given up using his heart-lung machine, there were others keen to carry on where he had left off. In Sweden, Viking Björk developed an artificial lung which used rotating discs to pick up a thin film of blood and oxygenate it.[97] And other Americans pursued their own research: John Kirklin from the Mayo Clinic in Minnesota visited Gibbon and with his blessing (and the aid of his engineers) built a replica of his device. An ascetic and exacting individual, Kirklin paid extraordinary attention to detail, and his careful work paid off: twenty-four of his first forty patients survived, and he concluded that the heart-lung machine was a 'reliable and safe' clinical tool.[98]

While Kirklin did much to convince the surgical profession of the merits of the heart-lung machine, the man who turned it from an expensive novelty into an affordable and practical device was Richard DeWall. He had joined Lillehei's laboratory in early 1954 and operated the pumps for many of the early cross-circulation procedures. At Lillehei's request, DeWall looked into the possibilities of artificial bypass, and eventually came up with a scheme radically different from that used by Gibbon.[99] His oxygenator consisted of a 60-centimetre vertical plastic cylinder; blood was pumped upwards through this column, while oxygen bubbles were injected into it through eighteen hypodermic syringes at the bottom. Earlier investigators had been wary of this method of oxygenation, because of the major threat posed to the human body by gas bubbles. DeWall found a simple way of eliminating this risk: a reservoir at the top of the oxygenating column trapped any foam, and then the blood descended through a spiral of tubing, shedding any residual bubbles as it did so.[100]

The simplicity of DeWall's device was revolutionary. The tubing – and the antifoaming agent with which it was treated – came from the dairy industry, and were designed for use with milk rather than blood.[101] None of the parts, in fact, was specially manufactured, and DeWall estimated that the entire apparatus cost no more than $15 to make. Other early heart-lung machines took two full days to prepare, with over 450 glass and metal components to be thoroughly cleaned;[102] DeWall's had no moving parts, could be easily assembled and sterilised, and did not need an army of engineers to maintain it. The first operation using the new oxygenator took place in May 1955, and by the following year he and Lillehei had used it on ninety-four patients, treating a large range of conditions. The results were so good that DeWall's report of these cases stated confidently that 'on the basis of this experience it is predictable that reparative surgery in the open heart is destined to become a major field of endeavour.'[103]

This was the kick-start that open-heart surgery needed: surgeons from all over the world came to watch Lillehei and DeWall at work before returning home to construct their own devices. Soon an even simpler version of DeWall's oxygenator was available: made from two heat-sealed plastic sheets, it cost a few cents to manufacture, could be easily mass-produced, and was intended to be disposed of after a single use.[104] A significant improvement was unveiled shortly afterwards by Willem Kolff, the Dutch-American pioneer of artificial dialysis. Exposing the blood directly to oxygen causes damage to its cells, and Kolff invented a new type of oxygenator in which blood was kept separate from the gas by a semi-permeable membrane. Gas exchange could take place through this protective layer with great efficiency.[105] Kolff's membrane oxygenator was not perfected until the 1970s, but thereafter it became the standard technology seen in operating theatres.

Once the safety of bypass had been demonstrated, the technology was taken up with breathtaking rapidity. Medical circles were abuzz with discussion of the device, referred to in surgical slang as 'the pump'. In 1955 there had been only two hospitals in the world where open-heart surgery was taking place; two years later, when a major conference took place in Chicago to discuss the heart-lung machine, more than 220 clinicians attended.[106] Several different types of device were discussed at that gathering; the following year Russell Brock observed that there were now 'nearly as many varieties of machine as there are of motor-cars'.[107]

A clear consensus in favour of artificial bypass had finally emerged; John Gibbon's dream had come true. But although cross-circulation quickly became redundant, hypothermia did not. Swan continued to use the technique on its own with great success until the early 1960s, but others found that it was a valuable adjunct to the heart-lung machine. The DeWall oxygenator's output was lower than that of the heart, so patients were slowly being starved of oxygen while they were connected to the device, and surgeons had only a limited window of time in which to operate. Hypothermia offered a way of prolonging it. Two Italian surgeons were the first to suggest combining the two techniques in 1953,[108] and five years later a team from Duke University in North Carolina did so in operations on forty-nine patients. Initially the patients were cooled with ice packs or refrigerated blankets, but controlling the temperature in this way proved difficult. The surgeons then adopted a much better method: the blood was cooled by a heat exchanger to around 30°C as it passed through the heart-lung machine, so that the patient's body was chilled from within. Reducing the temperature to the desired level took only a few minutes, and rewarming the blood afterwards was just as quick. The results were promising, with a survival rate of 75 per cent for critically ill patients.[109]

Another new use for hypothermia was discovered by Norman Shumway, a New York surgeon whose work would later lay the foundations for heart transplantation. In 1959 he showed that cooling the heart locally with saline at 4°C made it safe to operate for as long as an hour.[110] Topical or general hypothermia – or a combination of the two – eventually gained general acceptance and remain common techniques today.

A further weapon entered the surgeon's armoury in the 1950s, one which would enable far more radical intervention: stopping the heart. The first suggestion of this drastic measure can be traced back to 1851. A Scottish surgeon, James Wardrop, noted that it was possible to revive apparently dead animals by artificial respiration, and proposed that this might have therapeutic application: 'How far it may ever be expedient to imitate such experiments, and extinguish human life for a while, in order to cure diseases, and restore it again after the disease is subdued, is a matter of grave consideration.'[111]

This was prophetic. A stopped heart would be much easier to operate on than one that kept beating. A little over a century later one of the leading British heart surgeons, Denis Melrose, elaborated on the idea: 'A most valuable contribution . . . to the whole problem of intracardiac surgery would be made if the heart could be arrested and restarted at will.'[112] Building on the observation that potassium salts caused the heart muscle to stop contracting, Melrose experimented on a veritable menagerie of isolated animal hearts: those of dogs, rabbits, a guinea pig, a kitten and a puppy. He found that an injection of potassium citrate into the aorta found its way into the coronary arteries feeding the heart muscle, which quickly stopped beating. A normal heartbeat was restored without further intervention once the chemical had dispersed.[113]

Shortly afterwards Melrose became the first person to deliberately cause cardiac arrest. Once the patient was on bypass the potassium solution was injected, and the heart stopped. The aorta was clamped to prevent more blood from entering the heart muscle, allowing Melrose to operate on an organ that was perfectly still and bloodless. When he finished a few minutes later the clamp was removed, and to the relief of the team the heartbeat resumed spontaneously.[114]

This technique is known as cardioplegia, the Greek for 'heart paralysis'. It was at first regarded with considerable suspicion, with many surgeons concerned that the chemicals would cause lasting damage to the heart muscle. Only a few ventured to use it until a major development in the early 1970s, the consequence of a young biochemist, David Hearse, being invited to watch open-heart surgery at St Thomas' Hospital in London. He was shocked by the primitive measures taken to protect the heart muscle during the procedure, which entailed perfusing the coronary arteries with cooled blood.[115] He decided to look into possible alternatives, and after a few years of research developed an elaborate combination of drugs which greatly improved the ability of the heart to withstand total arrest for ninety minutes or even longer.[116] Hearse's detailed study of the microscopic changes to the cardiac muscle induced by cardioplegia, and the biochemical mechanisms that caused them, showed that the method was safe and indicated the best way of going about it.[117] Variations on the drug cocktail he devised, known as St Thomas' solution, have been a mainstay of the cardiac operating theatre ever since.

Even now, artificial heart-lung bypass is not without its problems. Some of the earliest surgeons to use the pump realised that bringing blood into contact with plastic and other man-made materials inevitably altered its properties. In the 1960s they started to notice a pattern of untoward symptoms displayed by patients who had undergone bypass, which was termed 'post-perfusion syndrome'. In a landmark paper published in 1983 the British surgeon Stephen Westaby stated that 'the damaging effects of cardiopulmonary bypass . . . have contributed considerably to the morbidity and mortality of cardiac surgery over the past 30 years.'[118] This problem still has not been solved: one surgeon I spoke to observed that, paradoxically, any patient kept alive by the heart-lung machine is also being 'slowly killed' by the device. Today bypass is employed for the shortest time possible, and for some conditions new techniques have been invented which avoid its use entirely. But it has become an essential piece of kit: over a million open-heart operations take place worldwide every year.

Despite its enduring shortcomings, John Gibbon's invention was the great leap forward that heart surgery needed, the single greatest advance in the history of the discipline. In 1950 it was possible to use the scalpel to treat only a handful of cardiac conditions. Ten years later the era of open-heart surgery had begun, and there was scarcely a type of heart disease that surgeons had not attempted to correct. In a very short time the heart-lung machine became indispensable. But being able to open the heart was only the beginning: now surgeons had to learn what to do when they got there.

5. RUBBER BALLS AND PIG VALVES

Portland, 21 September 1960

In June 1970 a retired truck dispatcher in Spokane, Washington, fell off a ladder while painting his house and was fatally injured. There was nothing particularly unusual about the death of Philip Amundson: thousands of Americans die in domestic accidents every year. But his survival to the age of sixty-two, and the fact that he was well enough even to climb a ladder, constituted a medical miracle. Ten years earlier he had been a hopeless invalid, unable to walk more than a few steps without getting out of breath. Decades earlier a childhood infection had irreparably damaged one of the valves in his heart, and the organ was now starting to fail. Having exhausted all other options, Amundson's cardiologist told him that his only hope of survival was an experimental treatment developed by a young surgeon, Albert Starr. Animal tests had delivered promising results, but his single human patient had died within hours.

On 21 September 1960, Starr removed Amundson's diseased mitral valve and replaced it with a prosthetic valve, a silicone rubber ball imprisoned in a plastic cage. It worked like a dream: within hours Amundson was sitting up in bed and talking to his nurses. Permanently replacing a human mitral valve was an achievement of unprecedented daring, and doing so with a man-made device made it all the more remarkable. It was a development which promised a cure for hundreds of thousands of patients previously regarded as untreatable, and the hospital authorities knew that the world's media would take an interest. But the operation was kept secret for three weeks, long enough for them to be confident that Amundson would make a full recovery. By mid-October the danger had passed, and the story became front-page news. 'Heart Valve Replaced by Rubber Ball', read a typical headline, accompanied by a photograph of an impassive Amundson holding a model of the device that had saved him.[1]

A handful of surgeons had implanted artificial valves before, with results that ranged from death to mild improvement, but nobody had achieved anything like this success; there was a unique sense of excitement about this operation that suggested it was something special. It had been preceded by two years of promising animal experiments, and Starr was optimistic that heart surgeons finally had a reliable and durable artificial valve which could save the lives of thousands. The device, designed by a retired engineer called Lowell Edwards, exceeded his wildest expectations. Within three years more than 6,000 sick patients had been given one,[2] and many lived for decades. When he died ten years after his operation, Philip Amundson's valve was still working perfectly. But this was not exceptional: in 2014 it was reported that a sixty-seven-year-old woman in Pennsylvania with a Starr–Edwards valve was alive and well forty-eight years after it had been implanted.[3]

Creating an artificial 'spare part' for the heart was a triumph of design and engineering – but even the most sophisticated prosthetic valves are no match for those we are born with. The human heart has four, and their function is simple: to keep the blood flowing in the right direction. Each consists of three tough fibrous leaflets (two in the case of the mitral valve) attached to a ring of tissue, the annulus. The leaflets meet in the centre of the valve aperture like the petals of a tightly closed flower, forming a seal which prevents blood from flowing backwards. When the valve opens these 'petals' rapidly unfurl, allowing blood forward into the next chamber or vessel, before snapping shut to ensure that none flows back the way it came.

The heart is often referred to as a pump, but it's more useful to think of it as a pair of them working in parallel. Pump no.1 (the right side of the heart) sends deoxygenated blood towards the lungs, while pump no.2 (the left side) propels the freshly oxygenated blood to the rest of the body. Each consists of two chambers: a reservoir, known as the atrium, and the pumping chamber, the ventricle.

Every heartbeat has two phases, known as diastole and systole, during which the organ fills and then empties itself of blood. At the beginning of diastole the heart muscle is relaxed, and blood which has completed its journey around the body flows into the right atrium, like water filling a reservoir. From there it trickles through the tricuspid valve into the empty right ventricle. At the end of diastole the muscles of the atrium contract, raising the pressure in the chamber and forcing more blood through the tricuspid valve into the ventricle. A fraction of a second later systole begins and the muscle of the ventricle contracts. This has the same effect as squeezing a plastic ketchup bottle: the contents are compressed, producing an increase in pressure. Increased blood pressure makes the tricuspid valve slam shut, and opens the pulmonary valve. Like ketchup ejected from a squeezed bottle, blood is driven from the right ventricle into the pulmonary artery towards the lungs.

While deoxygenated blood is travelling through the right side of the heart, an essentially identical sequence is unfolding on the left. Freshly oxygenated blood returns from the lungs via the pulmonary veins and arrives in the left atrium. During diastole it flows through the mitral valve into the left ventricle; when systole begins and the ventricle contracts, the valve snaps shut and blood is propelled at high pressure through the aortic valve and into the aorta, to be distributed to the whole body. When the body is at rest this entire process of diastole and systole, known as the cardiac cycle, takes around a second.

If you listen to a healthy human heart you'll hear the familiar rhythmic ba-*boom*, ba-*boom*, ba-*boom*, usually rendered by medics as 'lub-dub'. The quieter first sound, the 'lub', is caused by the mitral and tricuspid valves closing at the beginning of systole; the louder 'dub' is the sound of the aortic and pulmonary valves slamming shut at the end of systole, as the pressure in the two ventricles falls. Sometimes a doctor will be able to hear an additional or anomalous sound through the stethoscope – called a 'murmur' – and this is often evidence of a problem. Among the possible causes of a heart murmur are a valve which has become narrowed and fails to open properly (known as stenosis), or one which no longer provides a tight seal, allowing blood to flow backwards (known as regurgitation).

Repairing or replacing the valves of the human heart was among the most intractable problems of twentieth-century surgery and one which, once countenanced, took more than sixty years to solve. The first suggestion that diseased valves might be amenable to surgical treatment was made by Herbert Milton, the principal medical officer at Kasr el-Aini Hospital in Cairo. In 1897, the year after Ludwig Rehn's first successful repair of a cardiac wound, Milton wrote to *The Lancet* to describe his new method of opening the chest. This was itself of great significance, since the procedure he recommended – splitting the breastbone in order to gain access to the organs of the thorax – is now the incision most commonly used in open-heart surgery. In 1897 there were few operations requiring such a drastic opening of the chest, however, so Milton suggested circumstances in which it might in future be useful, including the removal of foreign bodies from the lungs. 'If once a safe route is established a great field for surgical interference lies open,' he wrote. 'Heart surgery is still quite in its infancy, but it requires no great stretch of fancy to imagine the possibility of plastic operations in some, at all events, of its valvular lesions.'[4]

Why did Milton first think of the valves when considering what operations might be performed on the heart? Partly because they presented the most urgent problem. Specialists in the late nineteenth century knew a lot about valve disorders, their symptoms and the sounds they made when heard through a stethoscope. And there was no shortage of cases: doctors were contending with a veritable epidemic of valve disease, caused by an infection which – in the developed world, at least – has almost disappeared today: rheumatic fever.

The history of rheumatic fever is an interesting example of a disease metamorphosing before our eyes. Pathogens such as viruses or bacteria reproduce at such a rate that mutations can emerge quite quickly, often changing the nature of the illness they cause. When doctors wrote about rheumatic fever in the eighteenth century, the symptoms they described typically included fever and joint pain, or 'rheumatism'. But around 1800 the pathogen appears to have evolved, and started to affect the tissues of the heart; still later, the brain became the disease's main focus, giving rise to the strange involuntary jerking movements known as Sydenham's chorea or St Vitus's Dance.[5] We now know that the pathogen involved is a bacterium, *Streptococcus pyogenes*. This usually causes nothing worse than a sore throat, but in some patients the antibodies produced by the immune system to combat the infection trigger tissue inflammation, causing the symptoms of rheumatic fever. In the developed world the disease has retreated steadily since 1900, but in poorer nations it continues to be a major problem, estimated to cause over 250,000 deaths a year.[6]

The first to make the connection between heart disease and rheumatic fever was David Pitcairn, a Scottish physician working at St Bartholomew's Hospital in London. In 1788 he noticed that patients with rheumatism were more likely to show symptoms of heart disease, and conjectured that the two disorders had a common cause, which he called 'rheumatism of the heart'.[7] The theory came to wider attention in 1812, when William Charles Wells published a detailed study definitively proving the association. Wells had an unusually wide range of interests: he solved the mystery of where dew comes from,[8] and proposed a theory of natural selection almost fifty years before Darwin.[9] One case cited in his landmark paper was that of a young woman who in 1807 died from heart disease a few months after falling ill with rheumatic fever. Inside her heart were found a number of 'excrescences resembling small warts',[10] several of which were on the mitral and aortic valves. These growths, known as vegetations, are a characteristic feature of rheumatic heart disease. Wells's findings were confirmed by many other physicians: in 1909 a doctor at St

Bartholomew's reported that 99 of 100 rheumatic fever patients in his care were also suffering from diseased heart valves.[11]

Rheumatic fever was a common ailment, creating an army of patients with incurable cardiac problems. Particularly upsetting was the fact that a large proportion of them were children – in stark contrast to the situation today, when acquired heart disease predominantly affects the elderly. In 1898 a London physician, Daniel Samways, tentatively offered a suggestion. Writing in *The Lancet*, he predicted that one day mitral stenosis – a narrowing of the mitral valve caused by rheumatic vegetations – might be relieved by 'slightly notching' the valve orifice with a scalpel.[12] Samways felt that if it were somehow possible to gain access to the inside of the heart, making a nick in one of the valve leaflets would increase the size of the aperture and thus increase the flow of blood. His suggestion was barely noticed; but four years later, when the eminent surgeon Sir Thomas Lauder Brunton made a similar suggestion, all hell broke loose.

Mitral stenosis is a distressing condition, causing debilitating breathlessness, fatigue and chest pain. Lauder Brunton's frustration at being unable to ease his patients' suffering was compounded by the realisation that during autopsies it was quite easy to cut open the constricted valve with a scalpel, and it occurred to him that it might be possible to do this on a living patient.[13] He was cautious in his proposal, noting that the operation should only be attempted after it had been tested on animals. Nevertheless, it provoked outrage: an editorial in *The Lancet* noted sniffily that Lauder Brunton had 'proceeded no further than the table of the dead-house in making his investigation', and chided him for proposing a potentially dangerous operation without having first conducted his own experiments to establish conclusively whether it was feasible.[14] There was some support, however: Daniel Samways wrote to back up his colleague, pointing out that the same idea had occurred to him.[15]

Opinion remained divided for some time. The great Rudolph Matas, pioneer of aneurysm surgery, believed the possibility 'not such a chimera as many have supposed'.[16] Ludwig Rehn was discouraging, writing in 1913 that in surgical terms the heart valves were '*noli me tangere*' – out of bounds.[17] Yet he was already out of date, for the previous year two French surgeons had attempted to operate on human patients. Théodore Tuffier tried to ease a case of aortic stenosis using an ingenious and non-invasive method: rather than cut into the heart he pressed his little finger into the wall of the aorta, forcing a pocket of the vessel downwards into the aortic valve in the hope that this would expand its narrowed opening. The patient was improved, though only temporarily.[18] Tuffier's compatriot Eugène Doyen tried something more drastic, inserting an instrument through the wall of the heart in an attempt to dilate a young girl's constricted pulmonary valve; she died shortly afterwards.[19]

One problem surgeons faced was that they could not see what they were doing: opening the heart would remain impossible until the invention of cardiopulmonary bypass several decades later. To get around this difficulty, in the early 1920s two researchers at Washington University in St Louis, Evarts Graham and Duff Allen, invented an instrument for looking at the inside of the heart: the 'cardioscope', a metal tube about the size and shape of a fountain pen, fitted with a lens and a light bulb. The surgeon would make an incision between two ribs to expose the heart, then insert the cardioscope through a small hole made in the cardiac wall. By leaning over the patient's chest and peering through this miniature telescope he could then survey the heart's interior landscape – rather hazily, since blood is opaque and the lens thus had to be in direct contact with whatever the operator wanted to see. It was also fitted with a narrow blade which could be used to cut diseased valve leaflets. Results were mixed: the cardioscope was used to slit the mitral valves of twenty-two dogs, proving that the concept was sound,[20] but when Allen attempted to treat three patients with mitral stenosis in August 1923 they all died. Disheartened, he abandoned his research.

Some months earlier a surgeon in Boston, Elliott Cutler, had performed the first mitral valve operation on a human patient, a procedure he only attempted after several years of scrupulous preparation in the laboratory.[21] Cutler decided that simply cutting a slit in the diseased valve was not enough, since the new incision might heal, and instead wanted to remove a small section of the leaflet tissue. To accomplish this he asked a young research fellow, Claude Beck, to devise a new instrument which he called the cardiovalvulotome. It had a pair of cutting jaws, designed so that they would hold on to the excised tissue and prevent it from getting into the bloodstream.[22] In the spring of 1923 Cutler's colleague Samuel Levine told Cutler that he had found the ideal candidate for operation. She was a twelve-year-old girl with crippling mitral stenosis, the consequence of a bout of rheumatic fever two years earlier. She had been bedridden for six months and her heart was starting to fail: so little blood could pass through the narrowed valve that the pressure on one side had become dangerously high, and as a result the organ could no longer pump enough to the rest of the body.

At 8.45 a.m. on 20 May, Cutler operated. The cardiovalvulotome was not yet ready for use, so instead he used a long thin knife with a slightly curved blade. Suspecting that the heart would cope better with the trauma if it became habituated to gentle handling, Cutler put his hand underneath it and turned it over to look at the other side – perhaps the first surgeon ever to do so. He dripped adrenaline directly on to the heart to make its contractions more vigorous, and then plunged the knife into the left ventricle. He pushed it in until he felt an obstruction which he assumed to be the mitral valve, twisted the blade and made two little nicks in what he hoped were the valve leaflets. Having completed this terrifying procedure completely unsighted, he withdrew the knife and placed sutures at the point where it had entered the heart muscle. The operation had taken a little over an hour.[23]

At first the girl showed worrying signs of complications, but after four days she had made a remarkable recovery. Her doctors were so pleased with her progress that they allowed her out of bed to put in a surprise appearance at the hospital's tenth birthday celebrations, which were in full swing downstairs. Though pleased with her condition, Cutler was guarded about the operation's success. He was not sure what he had done, or whether it would help.[24] Whatever benefit she gained from Cutler's daring work was short-lived, as his patient survived for only two years before dying from pneumonia.[25] The operation did achieve something, though: it proved that a patient could withstand the insult of having an instrument inserted into the cardiac chambers. It was enough to encourage Cutler to persevere, and he went on to operate on seven further patients using the cardiovalvulotome. None survived for longer than a week, and in 1929 he abandoned the operation as too dangerous.[26]

It was the first of many such disappointments: frequently over the next few decades a carefully thought-through idea would result only in failure. Sometimes surgeons wandered down many blind alleys before finding the correct path forward, or allowed themselves to be blinded by their own ingenuity, attempting a procedure long before anaesthetic technique and operating-theatre technology had attained the necessary sophistication. Such setbacks were an inevitable corollary to progress, but they came at substantial human cost. The many patients who died after agreeing to undergo an experimental procedure knew that medicine had nothing better to offer them – but this was scant consolation for their families, who had been given brief hope that their loved one might, after all, get better.

Two years after Cutler's first operation, the London surgeon Henry Souttar tried a different method. Before taking up medicine Souttar had studied mathematics and engineering – experience which clearly influenced his thinking. 'The problem is to a large extent mechanical,'[27] he wrote, and he approached the heart valves as pragmatically as an engineer would a malfunctioning pump. In March 1925 he was introduced to Lily Hine, a sickly nineteen-year-old patient who had grown up in the slums of Bethnal Green, in the sort of insanitary conditions where rheumatic fever thrives.[28] The illness had left her with a mitral valve which was grossly distorted: it would neither open nor close fully, a combination of stenosis and regurgitation.

Souttar felt that he could at least improve the stenosis, and on 6 May 1925 he conducted an audacious operation to separate the fused valve leaflets. Having opened Lily's chest, he made a small incision in the left atrial appendage,* a flap of heart muscle that sticks out from the heart's left atrium. He quickly slipped a finger through the hole and used it to explore the inside of the atrium. He was immediately struck by the wealth of information this simple fingertip examination yielded: by feeling the mitral valve leaflets he could construct a mental picture of their condition, while a rush of blood travelling the wrong way told him that the valve was not closing properly. He had intended to cut the fused leaflets with a knife, but now worried that this would exacerbate the regurgitation. So he improvised, pushing his finger through the valve opening to enlarge it. As he removed his digit from the girl's beating heart there was a terrible moment when a suture slipped, causing a sudden geyser of blood across the operating table. With great presence of mind Souttar checked the flow by gripping the end of the atrial appendage between finger and thumb while an assistant bound it tightly with silk.[29]

Lily Hine was sent to the country to recuperate, and after six weeks claimed to feel much better. The psychological impact of surgery is such, however, that patients often overestimate how much good it has done: Souttar noted that objective tests showed little obvious improvement to her overall condition. And though he was confident that the procedure was sound, he never had an opportunity to repeat it and prove its worth conclusively. Most cardiologists of the era believed (wrongly) that rheumatic fever was primarily a disease of the heart muscle, in which case operating on the valves was futile; London specialists refused to send Souttar another patient.[30] This closed another chapter in experimental heart surgery: without any tangible success to show for their work, the few surgeons who had been willing to countenance the operation decided that further attempts would be futile.

---

* Also known as the left auricle (from the Latin *auricula*), owing to its vague resemblance to an ear.

Many years later Souttar would admit that he had been 'perhaps too adventurous',[31] and indeed history shows him to have been twenty years ahead of his time; it was not until the 1940s that any real progress was made in attempts to repair the heart valves. In 1946 a young surgeon from South Carolina, Horace Smithy, developed a valvulotome, a cutting instrument similar to Elliott Cutler's two decades earlier. It resembled a large metal syringe, with a plunger at one end and a pair of cutting jaws at the other. The jaws were sheathed in the cylinder of the device as it was introduced into the heart; when the surgeon depressed the plunger the jaws would 'bite' out a section of valve leaflet and retain it.

For Smithy the battle against valve disease was deeply personal: he was himself suffering from aortic stenosis, a discovery he made as a medical student when he first used a stethoscope to listen to his own heart.[32] His experiments using the valvulotome on dogs were successful,[33] and when he presented his research at a meeting of the American College of Surgeons in September 1947 it made a big impression: the success of the Blue Baby operation three years earlier had made journalists hungry for further advances in cardiac surgery. One of those who read the newspaper reports was Betty Lee Woolridge, a twenty-one-year-old woman from Ohio. She wrote to Smithy, explaining that she had mitral stenosis and had been given a year to live by her doctors. She begged him to attempt the operation on her: 'Why use dogs when you can use human beings? If anything happened to me you might learn something which could help somebody else.'[34]

Smithy was at first reluctant, but Ms Woolridge was not to be denied. On the last day of January 1948 he operated, cutting out a small portion of her stenotic mitral valve. Ten days later she was well enough to fly back to Ohio, posing for newspaper photographers as she bade farewell to Smithy on the aircraft steps. Smithy was emboldened to operate on six more patients; four survived, but the overall results were disappointing, with only two showing 'slight' improvement.[35]

Smithy's own health was in steep decline, adding a sense of acute urgency to his work. In May he approached Alfred Blalock to ask whether he would consider operating on him; nobody had so far attempted such a procedure on the aortic valve. Blalock was prepared to help, but a trial operation in Baltimore, at which Smithy assisted, was a disaster. One of those present, Denton Cooley, recalled Smithy's reaction as their patient died: 'I looked over at him and saw his face fall. He thought that this was his only chance at having a successful operation for himself.'[36] His last hope had indeed evaporated: Blalock could not be persuaded to repeat the experience, and a few months later Smithy succumbed, aged thirty-four, to the condition he had sought to treat. On 29 October his death was reported under the headline 'Surgeon Dies, Too Weak For Own Cure'.[37]

If only Smithy had survived a little longer! Meaningful progress was painfully close: within a few months three surgeons, working independently and miles apart, made the same important breakthrough in the treatment of mitral stenosis. The first was Charles Bailey of Hahnemann University Hospital, Philadelphia, who had funded his way through medical school by selling ladies' underwear, a crucial sideline, as it turns out: contemplating his wares one morning he was struck by the structural similarity between a girdle and the mitral valve. Suspenders offered firm but flexible support to the stockings, just as the chordae tendineae, tough fibrous strings of tissue, anchor the valve leaflets to muscles on the inner wall of the heart. This insight informed much of his later thinking.[38] A young artist friend helpfully supplied an illustration of a panty-girdle and a mitral valve side by side; his name was Walt Disney.[39]

Bailey, a great admirer of Smithy, had watched his colleague's deterioration with great sadness. At a surgical meeting he listened to his heart and the 'terrible rumble' of the aortic stenosis that would kill him.[40] Bailey needed no reminder of the devastating consequences of valve disease: at the age of twelve he had seen his father die of mitral stenosis, coughing up blood into a basin while his mother did her best to comfort him.[41] Like Smithy, Bailey revisited Cutler's operation, trying to relieve the stenotic valve by cutting a section out of its leaflets with an instrument which acted like a hole punch.

Things did not go well. Four of his early patients died, and one of the hospitals at which he worked banned him from making any further attempts. His other employer, Episcopal Hospital, tried to do the same, but after a heated argument with the head of cardiology Bailey was allowed to continue.[42] On 10 June 1948 he finally had the success he needed. This time he used a new instrument, a knife attached to his forefinger like an extended claw: having inserted it through the heart wall he hooked the blade through the stenotic valve and used it to slit open the commissure, the point where the two leaflets had fused. He then removed the knife and used his finger to dilate the valve further, ensuring it could open fully once more.[43]

The operation saved not only the patient's life – her symptoms were greatly relieved – but Bailey's career. Ten days later she was well enough to travel a thousand miles to Chicago, where Bailey presented her to a room full of impressed surgeons. Evarts Graham, co-inventor of the cardioscope, praised Bailey's ingenuity and made a point that remains as valid today as it was in 1948: 'Unfortunately, as with any new surgical procedure, the pioneers get only the patients who are the worst possible risks.'[44] Like Souttar and Cutler before him, Bailey had only been permitted to operate on those who were at death's door; critically ill patients whose survival prospects were poor even if the surgery went as planned. After years in the animal laboratory Bailey was sure that his procedure was sound; it was only by saving one of these hopeless cases that he could persuade his physician colleagues to send him individuals more likely to survive major surgery. Many later surgeons risked livelihood and reputation as Bailey did, watching patient after patient die before finally proving that a new operation could save lives.

As Bailey travelled to Chicago on 9 June, another surgeon was already repeating his achievement. In Boston, Dwight Harken successfully opened a stenotic mitral valve using a valvulotome.[45] Thinking that he was the first to do so, he hurriedly wrote an article documenting the case, unaware that Bailey had beaten him to it.[46] Three months later, in London, Russell Brock took the bronze medal in this surgical race, performing the first in a series of successful mitral valve operations.[47]

Temperamentally, Brock, Bailey and Harken were quite a trio. Brock was a shy man, but hid this behind a brusque, even abrasive, manner. To his egalitarian American colleagues he must have appeared a throwback to an earlier age, for he belonged to an English tradition which cast senior medics as demigods; his juniors at the Brompton Hospital in London were expected to await his arrival on the front doorstep each morning, ready to conduct the great man on his daily rounds. Harken and Bailey were less intimidating figures, but they simply couldn't stand each other. If they met at a medical conference the tension was palpable, and discussions frequently turned into blazing rows. Bailey had an entertaining explanation for their mutual antipathy: 'My mother was redheaded; my daughter is redheaded. I never was, but Harken was . . . we just tore at each other with the classical vigor of redheaded people.'[48] Many years later they would become good friends.

Though Harken and Brock used a blade to perform their first mitral valve operations, they both subsequently concluded that the Souttar 'finger-fracture' technique of using a forefinger to break open the fused valve leaflets was a vastly superior approach, and adopted it in all their operations.[49] Removing tissue from the leaflets using a punch or valvulotome often rendered the valve incapable of closing fully; rather than curing the stenosis this converted it into regurgitation, which was almost as bad for the patient as the original condition. The designer of the cardiovalvulotome, Claude Beck, who himself went on to become a celebrated heart surgeon, later felt that his invention 'probably delayed the development of the operation for mitral stenosis by some 20 years'.[50]

'In many cases the finger alone splits the valve with an accuracy and speed that no instrument could rival,' Brock observed in 1952, reporting excellent results in a series of 100 operations.[51] Declaring that a 'new field of surgery' had been opened up, Brock suggested that the procedure, which he called mitral valvotomy, was now routine and should be performed wherever there was suitable expertise. Demand was overwhelming: rheumatic fever remained a major concern in the 1950s, with 250,000 Britons believed to be suffering from mitral stenosis.[52] A further improvement arrived in 1954, when the French surgeon Charles Dubost invented a dilator, an instrument even more efficient than the finger at opening a stenosed valve. At its tip were two blunt blades which could be passed into the left atrium and then expanded like an umbrella, pushing apart the fused leaflets.[53] Many other surgeons took up the new operation, and over the next decade thousands of patients with mitral stenosis found their quality of life radically improved as a result.

More challenging still was the problem of mitral regurgitation: there was no easy way to repair valve leaflets so damaged by disease that they would not fully close. Inserting a foreign body in the aperture was one method several surgeons employed to prevent blood flowing the wrong way: Harken suspended small spheres or spindles of Perspex in front of the valve,[54] while Bailey tried an even more difficult technique, sewing the loose valve leaflets together with strips of pericardium.[55] None of these operations was particularly successful: the condition tended to recur, often within a few months. A completely different approach was needed.

As any driver who has endured an unexpectedly expensive afternoon in a garage will aver, replacing a faulty part is sometimes better than repairing it. The first to realise that this applied to hearts as well as engines was Gordon Murray, the Toronto surgeon whose work on heparin proved so vital to the development of open-heart surgery. Murray was working as a junior registrar at the London Hospital in 1925 when Souttar performed his one and only mitral stenosis operation,[56] but what really kindled his interest in the subject was a visit to the laboratory of Cutler and Beck and the opportunity to discuss their work with them.[57]

When Murray began his own research in 1936 he took a radical approach, attempting to create a new mitral valve with spare parts harvested from the patient's own body. In a series of experiments on dogs he cut out the entire valve apparatus, both the leaflets and the chordae tendineae – the stocking and the suspender belt. He also removed several inches of the external jugular vein, a large vessel from the neck; this is one of several major veins which return blood from the head towards the heart, so it is possible to sacrifice one of them without causing serious problems. Having excised this vein graft, Murray then turned it inside out. This was a crucial detail, since the inner surface of veins and arteries, the endothelium, has one particularly desirable property: because it is in constant contact with the bloodstream it must necessarily deter clotting.[58] Murray found a novel way of inserting the section of inverted vein through the cardiac wall and suturing it in place, all without opening the heart. The sling of vein tissue was fixed in position with slight tension, so that when the ventricle contracted in systole the increased pressure would push it flat against the mitral opening, like a newspaper blown against a railing – preventing any blood from flowing backwards into the atrium. Though a number of the twelve dogs operated on died during the operation or shortly afterwards, two survived, apparently quite healthy.[59]

Murray's research was treated with what he described as 'supercilious amusement' by his colleagues, but he was absolutely in earnest, applying the technique to several patients; one was transformed from a bedridden invalid to an enthusiastic golfer,[60] though the fate of the others was not recorded. But there was anger when Murray revealed that he had translated an essentially unproven therapy to humans after such poor results in the animal laboratory; moreover, heart valves were still considered the realm of the physician, not the surgeon. He was summarily banned from repeating the operation.[61]

By the late 1940s, when Murray resumed his research, heart surgery was an established and rapidly advancing discipline. Others were trying techniques similar to those he had pioneered: John Gibbon and his collaborator John Templeton used grafts of venous and pericardial tissue to reconstruct the tricuspid valves of dogs.[62] Murray improved this procedure by wrapping the vein graft around a tendon taken from

the forearm to strengthen the new leaflets, and succeeded in keeping one dog alive for an impressive seven years after surgery. His
human patients did less well: eight of the ten survived, their condition
described only as 'fairly satisfactory'.[63]

But a still more exciting era was on the horizon. While all attempts
thus far had refashioned existing body parts into valve substitutes,
researchers had begun working on a mechanical artificial valve – a
man-made replacement for human tissue. Charles Hufnagel started
his research at Peter Bent Brigham Hospital in Boston, where Elliott
Cutler was still professor of surgery. In 1947 he discovered that it was
possible to insert a tube made from methyl methacrylate (a tough polymer now used as bone cement in hip replacements) into a dog's aorta
so that it acted as an inner lining to the vessel.[64] No clotting ensued;
this was a highly significant finding, as it proved that an artificial valve
made from synthetic materials would be tolerated by the body. A couple of years later a surgeon from Oklahoma City, J. Moore Campbell,
unveiled an experimental device which he had inserted into the aortas of dogs.[65] A hard plastic sphere the size of a pea was confined in
a plastic tube in such a way that when the heart was relaxed the ball
blocked the entrance to the valve; when it contracted, the increased
pressure in the aorta pushed it aside and blood could flow forwards
through the tube.

By coincidence, Hufnagel had hit upon a very similar design for
his own valve – but, unlike Campbell, he took the next leap and used
it to treat a patient. The first person ever to be given an artificial heart
valve was a thirty-one-year-old woman with severe aortic regurgitation. A bout of rheumatic fever at the age of five had seriously damaged her aortic valve, and since her early twenties she had been in
decline, afflicted with chest pain and breathlessness. In September
1952 Hufnagel implanted his valve into the woman's aorta.[66] It did
not replace her diseased one, because the device was too large to be
implanted in its proper anatomical position at the top of the heart. It
was placed instead in the descending aorta, some distance from the
organ; this did not entirely correct the problem, but stopped around 75

per cent of the anomalous blood flow.[67] The patient made a full recovery and was even well enough to work full time, something she had not done for almost a decade.

From the outset it was clear that Hufnagel's valve was a major advance. If suitable patients were chosen they did well, and mortality was low.[68] But it was an imperfect facsimile of human anatomy, and had another serious drawback: it was noisy, emitting a loud click with every heartbeat. Early recipients of the Hufnagel valve could be heard from the other side of a room; one had to give up playing poker because every time he received a good hand the valve started to click violently.[69] Later improvements made it quieter, but not before some patients had become so distressed that they killed themselves, driven to distraction by the incessant ticking inside their chests.[70]

Artificial valves were now a fashionable area of research, stimulated by Hufnagel's success and the arrival of cardiopulmonary bypass, which made it possible to cut open the heart; a bewildering variety of designs was produced and tested, with varying degrees of success. Before the advent of the medical device industry in the 1960s there was little money for research, which meant that most of these prototypes were made in garages or at kitchen tables. The first prosthetic mitral valve ever implanted in a human was a prime example of such a Heath Robinson contraption. It was invented by a surgeon from Sheffield, Judson Chesterman, who was an amateur motor mechanic and based his design on the valves of a car engine. The hospital plumber made him a prototype out of copper, but Chesterman rightly had doubts about placing a metal object inside the heart. The next model was constructed from Perspex by a lab technician, Clifford Lambourne, who polished the valve to the necessary high finish with a silk handkerchief during cinema outings with his wife. On 22 July 1955, Chesterman implanted this device into the heart of a thirty-four-year-old man. The patient died fourteen hours later; although he had become the first surgeon anywhere to place an artificial valve inside the human heart, Chesterman did not pursue his research.[71]

In September 1960, 200 experts from around the world, including many of the most eminent names in heart surgery, gathered at the Edgewater Beach Hotel in Chicago for a conference on the future of the artificial valve. Countless different approaches were discussed, with little consensus reached as to the ideal materials or design. There were many tales of failure; the only success story came from Nina Braunwald, a thirty-two-year-old surgeon at the National Heart Institute in Maryland. One of the first female cardiac surgeons, Braunwald had grown up in Brooklyn and completed her training under Charles Hufnagel. Working with her colleague Theodore Cooper, she set out to manufacture a prosthesis which would closely mimic the appearance and function of the original. She and Cooper took plaster casts of normal mitral valves, and used these to fabricate replicas from polyurethane; artificial chordae tendineae of woven Teflon were then attached so that the leaflets could be anchored to the inside surface of the heart.[72] After successful testing in dogs, Braunwald implanted the valve in five patients with mitral regurgitation. Four died shortly after the operation, but a fifth lived on for three months – the first time a mitral implant had lasted more than a few hours.[73] Among the first to congratulate her on the achievement was Albert Starr, who in his comments after her presentation revealed that he was working on a valve of his own, which he felt had 'much promise'.

In an address drawing proceedings to a close, the conference chairman Dr Alvin Merendino acknowledged the frustration felt by many researchers, but urged them to stay positive: 'Unfortunately, no one unveiled *the valve*. Yet, in all fairness, it must be said that the Conference ends on a note of real encouragement.'[74] His optimism was entirely justified: two weeks later Albert Starr operated on Philip Amundson, and there was little doubt that *the valve* had arrived.

Starr's interest in the problem of valve design had begun serendipitously towards the end of 1958, when a retired engineer called Lowell Edwards made an appointment to speak to him. The elderly man with a Parkinsonian tremor who turned up at Starr's office did not at first impress, dressed in golf kit and trainers and offering some very strange ideas. Edwards explained that he had become interested in the human circulation, and felt that with help from a medical expert he could build an artificial heart. While agreeing that this was an exciting idea, Starr pointed out that ten years of research by surgeons had failed even to produce an artificial valve. So the two men agreed to work together on a less ambitious project: developing a mitral valve prosthesis.[75] As Edwards left his office, Starr wondered whether this shabbily dressed old man who claimed to be a wealthy inventor was a crank; any lingering doubts were banished when he saw Edwards getting into a smart Cadillac parked outside.[76]

Though unconventional, Edwards was anything but a crank. Engineering was in his blood: decades earlier his father, an amateur mechanic, had built a generator – and a steam engine to power it – to provide the first electric light in his town. Inspired by his example, Lowell trained as an electrical engineer before moving into hydraulics. As a young man he developed a machine that used water jets to strip the bark off logs – tremendously useful in Oregon, where the timber industry dominated the local economy. But his most significant invention was a fuel pump for planes flying at high altitude. During the Second World War this booster pump was installed in almost all US military aircraft, and Edwards became a rich man. By the time he met Starr he was living in comfortable retirement, funded by the proceeds of more than sixty patents.[77]

Albert Starr was the younger man by almost thirty years, but there was no sense that he was the junior partner in this new enterprise. Another protégé of Alfred Blalock, at the age of thirty-two he was already an experienced surgeon and a military veteran, having served as a medic in the Korean War and performed more than a thousand operations in battlefield conditions. Starr and Edwards threw themselves into their research, meeting at least once a week to discuss possible materials and designs. They assumed, like most of Starr's colleagues, that a successful prosthesis needed to resemble natural anatomy, and their first prototypes were closely modelled on the human mitral valve, with two leaflets made from flexible plastic.[78] When Starr implanted this device in dogs the results were uniformly poor. The animals died within a couple of days: autopsy revealed that clots were forming on the stitches securing the valve to the heart, and growing until the valve was completely occluded. After several dogs had died Starr had a sudden insight: what if mimicking natural anatomy was a red herring? Maybe haemodynamics – the way the blood flows through the valve – was more important than what the device looked like.

Freed from trying to imitate the real valve, Starr and Edwards looked for an alternative. One obvious precedent was Hufnagel's device, which made no effort to replicate human anatomy; another inspiration was a valve recently investigated by Henry Ellis at the Mayo Clinic in Minnesota.[79] It had no leaflets, but instead used a plastic ball trapped inside a cage of three curved metal struts. The circular base of this valve, which was lined with a ring of cloth, was sewn into the mitral annulus between the left atrium and ventricle so that the cage protruded into the ventricle. When the heart was relaxed and pressure in the atrium was higher than in the ventricle, the ball was pushed to the other end of the cage, allowing blood to flow forwards into the ventricle. As the ventricle contracted, the increase in pressure would push the ball back into the aperture, blocking it and preventing any reverse flow of blood. This was a venerable design, long used by engineers as a valve in a range of applications – it can be traced all the way back to a patent filed in 1858 by one J. B. Williams for an 'improved bottle stopper'.[80]

Working in a shed attached to the summer cabin he owned in northern Oregon,[81] Edwards soon had a prototype and the immediate results were strikingly better: dogs implanted with the device now survived for weeks rather than days.[82] But first attempts are never perfect, and his experiments gave Starr valuable information on where they were going wrong. Edwards had plenty of time to devote to the project, and was able to produce a new prototype valve for testing every few weeks, allowing Starr to assess a wide variety of designs.[83] He implanted these into over forty dogs, with gradual improvement; one, a Labrador called Blackie, survived for thirteen months.[84]

Early in the summer of 1960 the hospital's chief of cardiology, Herbert Griswold, visited Starr's animal laboratory and found it full of healthy, happy dogs with mechanical valves clicking away inside them. Deeply impressed, Griswold urged Starr to transfer his research to humans, pointing out that he had dozens of patients with mitral disease who might benefit.[85] Starr was at first reluctant: he had kept dogs alive with the valve for months, but this was no proof that it would perform adequately for years in a human. If a valve were to last for twenty years it would have to open and close more than 800 million times.[86] Manufacturing a device so durable was at the boundaries of what engineering could achieve. Luckily, Starr's assistants had devised a machine which opened and closed the valve an astonishing 6,000 times a minute, which meant that three weeks of testing simulated forty-three years inside a patient.[87] When they showed Starr that valves put through this ordeal showed negligible wear, with the hard plastic ball virtually unchanged in diameter, he was finally persuaded that the device was ready for human trials.

His first patient was a young woman who had undergone two previous operations for mitral stenosis and was now so unwell that she was forced to spend all her time in an oxygen tent. Starr was pleasantly surprised to find the operation technically much easier than working on the smaller canine heart. When his patient had woken up from the anaesthetic, he and the hospital's chief of medicine, Hod Lewis, went to see her. Starr watched with amusement as his boss bent over the patient with his stethoscope, his moustache twitching as he listened to the unaccustomed click of the device inside her heart.[88] Everything seemed to indicate a successful outcome, until a few hours later she turned over in bed and suddenly died. An X-ray showed that the operation had left bubbles of air inside the heart which had escaped and lodged in the brain, killing her instantly.[89]

When Philip Amundson arrived for surgery, in poor health after two previous unsuccessful operations, Starr vowed that this would not happen again. On 21 September, Starr operated. Once he had opened the chest, he attached Amundson to the heart-lung machine so that the heart could be stopped. He made an incision in the left atrium, exposing the mitral valve. He then cut out the diseased leaflets, leaving just enough tissue to allow him to stitch the new valve in place. Twenty sutures were placed around the diameter of the annulus – tedious work, since they needed to be evenly spaced and placed at just the right depth. Next, the suture threads were attached to the fabric ring at the base of the prosthesis, which could then be gently lowered into place. The heart was allowed to fill with blood, and when Starr was satisfied that no air remained inside he closed his incision and turned off the bypass machine.[90] For the first time in a decade, Philip Amundson had a fully functioning mitral valve.

Amundson made an excellent recovery, the best possible fillip for Starr's confidence in the new device. Of his next six patients only one died; the other five were greatly improved, an excellent outcome given that Starr had been allowed to operate only on the sickest and most hopeless cases.[91] When he presented his results at a surgical meeting early in 1961, Starr admitted that he had at first found the unnatural ball-and-cage valve 'repugnant'; but its success could not be denied, and within months it was being used in hospitals all over America.[92]

It was not long before the Starr–Edwards device had competition. New designs appeared throughout the 1960s, and it became a mark of status for a surgeon to have his or her name attached to a valve: Braunwald, Cooley, DeBakey and Lillehei all received this honour. Some differed from the ball-and-cage pattern, using a free-floating or tilting metal disc to control the blood flow. But none proved as successful as the Starr–Edwards, which continued to dominate the market for years. Though it had triumphantly answered the surgeons' prayer for a simple and reliable artificial valve, it was not without its faults. In particular, it was bulky: it did not work properly in some patients who had an unusually small aorta.

The search for something better led to one of the worst scandals in surgical history. In 1979 a new device, the Björk–Shiley convexo-concave valve, was released on to the market. Within months of the first implantation, reports started to emerge of patients dropping dead without warning. Owing to a production fault a part was prone to coming loose, falling into the bloodstream and causing catastrophic regurgitation, but – disgracefully – almost 86,000 devices were implanted in patients before the faulty models were finally withdrawn from sale. By 2005 more than 600 of them had failed, making the Björk–Shiley valve the most dangerous medical device ever to be used clinically.[93] It later emerged that Pfizer, the company manufacturing the valve, had long known about the problem and hid the evidence from regulators, a transgression which cost it hundreds of millions of dollars in compensation and fines.[94]

This debacle might have destroyed all confidence in the safety of artificial valves, but luckily the Björk–Shiley device already had a successful competitor. In the early 1970s a young entrepreneur called Manny Villafana set up a biotechnology company to manufacture a valve with a novel design. Instead of using a ball or disc to regulate the blood it had two flaps like butterfly wings, attached with hinges to the centre of the valve opening. Villafana chose this 'bileaflet' design not for any scientific reasons, but as a marketing ploy: he reasoned that this would make it radically different from anything already available.[95] Quite by accident, it turned out to be the best commercial decision he ever made. The device proved to be a vast improvement on ball-and-cage models, small enough to fit in every patient and offering a close approximation to the natural valve. First implanted in 1977, and soon imitated by other companies, the bileaflet mechanical valve proved so reliable that it is still widely used today.

Mechanical valves are known to be safe and effective: they last for decades, and patients can expect to live a normal life. Despite all this, fewer are being implanted every year. There is an alternative, one that was being developed in parallel with the Starr–Edwards valve and its successors – and half a century on, it is becoming the option of choice for many patients.

In the 1950s, as surgeons started to appreciate the myriad challenges of designing an artificial valve, Gordon Murray sought another solution. Ten years earlier, Robert Gross had pioneered the use of arterial grafts to treat coarctation, using pieces of blood vessel taken from cadavers to replace diseased sections of the aorta. Murray reasoned that this technique could be modified so that the graft included a functioning valve. In 1955 he operated on a twenty-two-year-old man, inserting an aortic valve taken from the body of a thirty-three-year-old who had died ten days previously.[96] Like Hufnagel, Murray chose to implant it in the descending aorta, deciding that placing it in its anatomically correct position was too technically demanding. His patient's recovery was rapid, and after eighteen months he was able to do hard manual labour. Eight further operations were equally successful, with the grafts still functioning well up to six years later.[97]

Though this was progress, a valve placed in an unnatural position was far from a cure. Murray's grafts were implanted some 10 centimetres from the outlet of the left ventricle: although they reduced anomalous blood flow by around 50 per cent, a significant volume could still travel backwards from the major vessels of the upper half of the body and back into the heart. This residual regurgitation reduced the amount of blood pumped with each stroke, putting the organ under considerable strain. In the summer of 1962 a surgeon in London finally succeeded in placing an aortic graft in its natural position.

Donald Ross was born and raised in South Africa – where one of his classmates had been a certain Christiaan Barnard – before moving to the UK. He was interested in the idea of transplanting valves, but realised that without some method of preservation, suitable grafts would be difficult to come by; surgeons could not rely on a suitable donor having died in the previous week. He learned of the work of two researchers in Oxford, Carlos Duran and Alfred

Gunning, who had found that if the valves were immersed in ethylene dioxide and freeze-dried they could be stored for long periods at room temperature.[98]

The first implementation of this useful technique happened more or less by accident. During an operation on 24 July 1962, Ross was attempting to repair the badly diseased aortic valve of a middle-aged man when, in his words, 'the whole thing finally disintegrated and went down the sucker.'[99] This was a calamity, since mechanical valves were not yet available in England. In desperation, Ross sent a colleague to get one of his experimental freeze-dried grafts and sewed it into the patient. This was merely a temporary measure: Ross intended to replace the homograft with a mechanical valve as soon as he could get hold of one. But that proved unnecessary, as the patient made a good recovery and lived for another three years. In his subsequent report Ross made a more radical proposal, suggesting that an even better replacement for a diseased aortic valve would be the patient's own pulmonary valve, which could itself be replaced by a homograft. Though this might seem a complication too far, there was solid logic behind it: the two valves are almost identical, and although the pulmonary valve operates at lower pressure than the aortic, research had shown that when it was transplanted into the aorta it quickly thickened to compensate.[100] Another five years passed before he put this plan into action, but the operation – known as the Ross procedure – quickly proved its worth. It was particularly effective with children, because the new aortic valve grew with the patient; many surgeons still use the procedure today.

Unlike many new techniques the use of freeze-dried homografts became an immediate success, and dozens more patients were soon operated on. There was much excitement about the development, which seemed to promise the most satisfactory solution to valve disease. But after a few years, patients started to return to hospital showing signs of valve failure, and when samples were examined under the microscope they showed worrying signs of deterioration. Homografts were not the answer after all.[101]

One of those watching with interest was a young doctor in Paris, Alain Carpentier. Destined to become one of the world's great cardiac surgeons, Carpentier had developed a taste for innovation during his training, when he had come into the orbit of Robert Judet, a pioneer of the artificial hip. After some agonising he decided to specialise in cardiac surgery, excited by the rapid pace of developments in the field. In his first valve operations Carpentier used the Starr–Edwards prosthesis, but regular complications drove him to look for alternatives. He performed the first homograft implantation in Paris, but French law – which required a forty-eight-hour delay between death and recovery of a donor valve – made it virtually impossible to ensure that the grafts were safe to use.[102]

Most parts of the body cannot easily be transplanted, since alien tissue is soon detected by the immune system and attacked, a phenomenon known as rejection. The heart valves, though, are peculiar in that they are composed largely of collagen, a tough fibrous protein generally ignored by the immune system. This simplified the implantation of homograft valves, since grafts were unlikely to provoke rejection. It also raised an intriguing possibility: why not use grafts from another species? Animal collagen was no more likely to prompt an immune response than human tissue, and that way valves could be grown to order and made available wherever and whenever they were needed. These would be known as xenografts – from the Greek 'xenos', meaning 'foreigner'.

For two years Carpentier and a colleague, Jean-Paul Binet, experimented with xenografts from various species. But which to use? What was needed was a valve of a suitable size which was anatomically similar to a human's. The best match came from a gorilla they autopsied at Prince Rainier's private zoo in Monaco. But the idea of breeding gorillas for their heart valves was patently ridiculous, and they found eventually that three animals were required to offer a variety of sizes: lambs provided a small valve, pigs a medium one, and calves the largest.[103] In September 1965 they inserted a pig valve into the heart of a forty-seven-year-old patient in Paris, the first of eighty such procedures. Although the early results were excellent, degradation of the valve remained a problem, with many patients falling ill after two or three years. Carpentier had been using a mercury-based solution to preserve the grafts, and decided to look for a substance that would protect them for longer.

This was a chemical problem rather than a medical one, and Carpentier began his search by investigating the aldehydes, a group of compounds used in embalming and to tan leather. After working his way systematically through more than fifty of them, Carpentier alighted upon glutaraldehyde, a molecule already used in micros-copy to 'fix' biological specimens in their pristine state for examina-tion. When applied to valve tissue, Carpentier found that it not only made it invisible to the immune system but also strengthened it.[104] After experiments showed that inflammation tended to appear at the junction between human and pig tissue, Carpentier began to mount the grafts in a polymer cloth frame; the addition of this man-made material created a composite graft for which Carpentier coined the term 'bioprosthesis' – an artificial device constructed from biological material.[105]

One further improvement lay in store, courtesy of a Swedish sur-geon, Åke Senning, who had been working on a different approach. Dissatisfied with the rapid deterioration and unpredictable avail-ability of homograft valves, he decided to make his own from scratch. After removing the diseased valve he used strips of fascia lata, tough tissue from the patient's thigh, to construct a replace-ment.[106] These worked well, and using the patient's own tissue made rejection impossible. But each valve had to be painstakingly con-structed leaflet by leaflet, an operation requiring terrific deftness. It was Donald Ross who realised that much time and effort could be saved if the fascia lata valves were constructed outside the body and mounted in a frame, which could then simply be sewn in place. Using this technique he was able to construct replacements for the aortic, mitral and tricuspid valves – sometimes using two or three in the same heart. The initial results were outstandingly good,[107] but within three years the grafts started to fail, and Ross's collaborator, the Romanian-born Marian Ionescu, started to look for a longer-lasting substance.

Ionescu realised that it was not necessary to use the patient's own tissue; the success of porcine xenografts had proved that even valves from a different species could be well tolerated by the body. Building on Carpentier's work, he used glutaraldehyde to preserve bovine pericardial tissue, the tough membrane surrounding the heart in cows. Once treated it was then cut into strips and fashioned into a valve with three leaflets, fastened into a cloth-covered wire frame.[108] This new technique immediately opened a world of possibility: valves could be constructed well in advance, in a range of sizes, and stored more or less indefinitely at room temperature. A surgeon in need of a replacement valve could simply pick one of a suitable size off the storeroom shelf. Bovine pericardial bioprostheses would prove even more durable than pig valves, lasting up to twenty years without deterioration.

By the 1980s surgeons had two excellent alternatives for patients suffering from serious valvular disease: the mechanical valve or the bioprosthesis. But the two are not interchangeable. Although mechanical valves can last a lifetime, they introduce foreign materials into the body, increasing the risk of sudden blood clots. To mini-mise this danger, patients must take anticoagulant drugs for life. Tissue valves, on the other hand, are unlikely to cause clotting problems but have a maximum lifespan of around twenty years. In practice this means that younger patients are generally given a mechanical valve, while the elderly are more likely to receive a bioprosthesis.

Why, then, is curing valve disease not now simply a matter of selecting a suitable device and implanting it in the patient? That was indeed standard practice for many years, but today's clinicians do everything in their power to avoid using devices they spent decades perfecting. Strange as that may seem, it is because surgical philosophy has evolved in parallel with technology. The heart valves we are born with have been perfected by millions of years of evolution, structures unmatched by even the most sophisticated prosthesis. Why replace the ideal valve with something inherently inferior?

This was the question Alain Carpentier asked himself one evening in 1967 as he left work at the Hôpital Broussais in Paris. Walking through its venerable arch to the street outside, he noticed that it resembled a mitral valve: the iron gates were the leaflets, anchored to the firm 'annulus' of the stone arch. It occurred to him that if the structure were partially destroyed, a decent architect would have little difficulty in rebuilding it, using some sort of physical support to restore the original geometry of the gates: 'Obviously a surgeon would do the same for the mitral valve!'[109]

Carpentier's insight would transform the treatment of valve disease.In many cases of mitral regurgitation, he realised, it should be possible to reconstruct rather than replace the diseased valve. His aim was to support the distorted annulus by implanting a firm ring around it, bringing together the leaflets so that they would meet in the centre of the valve and once more provide a tight seal. After testing several different designs, Carpentier concluded that kidney-shaped rings worked best.[110] The new operation was known as annuloplasty, and in the years that followed its introduction Carpentier made an intensive study of the many ways in which valves could be distorted by disease. The result was a new range of techniques which could be used to repair the mitral valve: cutting out superfluous tissue, tightening floppy leaflets with sutures or even moving the chordae tendineae. This new arsenal in the battle against valve disease is sometimes known as 'the French correction', a pun coined by Carpentier himself.[111] After thirty years of experience it was apparent that it offered something that no prosthesis ever could: a cure. A tissue valve is merely a temporary measure, while a patient with a mechanical device faces a lifetime on prescription drugs. In

Carpentier's words, 'It is only cured if you make the effort to reconstruct the valve, to restore the mobility, to reshape the orifice as it should be, as designed by God Himself.'[112]

Surgeons have often been accused of playing God; many decades spent battling the ravages of valve disease finally taught them that imitating His works is sometimes preferable to replacing them.

6. METRONOMES AND NUCLEAR REACTORS

Stockholm, 8 October 1958

On 6 April 1964, while in Los Angeles filming the Billy Wilder comedy *Kiss Me, Stupid*, Peter Sellers had a massive heart attack and was rushed to hospital. At the age of thirty-eight the British actor was one of the biggest stars in Hollywood: *Dr Strangelove*, the film that would earn him his first Oscar nomination, had just been released, and his surprise marriage to Britt Ekland a few weeks earlier meant that his name was seldom out of the gossip columns.

When he arrived at Cedars of Lebanon Hospital, Sellers was still conscious and his condition appeared relatively stable, but over the next twenty-four hours he suffered eight cardiac arrests. Medical staff told journalists that he was near death, and a guard was posted at the door of the intensive care unit to deter unwanted visitors. At one point his heart stopped for almost two minutes; he was immediately whisked off to a room containing a gleaming new piece of equipment, a large metal cabinet covered with knobs and dials. The hospital's chief of cardiology, Eliot Corday, picked up two leads, plugged them into the machine and attached them to the actor's chest with small suction cups. Sellers's unconscious body jerked periodically as pulses of electric current surged through it, and shortly afterwards his heart was beating once more; any longer and the result would have been brain damage or death.

This life-saving apparatus was an artificial pacemaker, and it supplied regular pulses of electricity which prompted his damaged heart to beat when it was unable to do so by itself. Sellers remained attached to it for three days, clinging tenuously to life, but he did eventually recover. After several months of recuperation he was well enough to return to work, though in later years he would suffer many more heart attacks – he once said that 'I'm trying to give them up; I'm down to two a day'[1] – before another finally killed him in 1980. But he had been lucky: without the pacemaker, invented only a few years earlier, that first cardiac arrest in 1964 would also have been his last.

A lot has changed in the half-century since those events in Los Angeles. Pacemakers are no longer a luxury owned by a few hospitals but the most common medical device in the world, with 250,000 given each year to American patients alone.[2] The behemoth sitting by Peter Sellers's hospital bed has been superseded by tiny objects that can be implanted into the body: the smallest available today is the size of a large pill and is inserted directly into the heart via a vein in the leg.[3] They listen constantly to the heartbeat, correcting any disturbance in cardiac rhythm so subtly that their owners do not even know it is happening. And since the 1980s thousands of lives have also been saved by an implantable defibrillator, a device capable of reversing cardiac arrest by imparting a powerful electric shock, entirely automatically.

John Gibbon spent more than fifteen years perfecting the heart-lung machine, but his experience was relatively painless when compared with the tortuous development of the pacemaker and defibrillator. Both devices were conceived and then abandoned by visionaries who found that the world was not yet ready for their ideas, before being reinvented years later when medical thought had moved on. Though they differ fundamentally in their operation, the pacemaker and defibrillator are both predicated on the interesting fact that the heart is not merely a pump, but a pump controlled by electricity. This crucial insight was learned only after generations of scientists had tried and failed to answer a perplexing question: what causes the heart to beat?

In the first decade of the sixteenth century Leonardo da Vinci had suggested that the organ was made of muscle, an insight that explained its movements as nothing more than repeated muscular contractions. But whereas we can flex a bicep at will, the cardiac muscle contracts sixty times a minute without our telling it to; somehow it acts independently of the conscious mind. It was not at all clear why this should be the case. Several theories were put forward and then rejected: some believed that the brain stimulated the heartbeat via the nerves known to connect the two organs, while others suggested that an innate quality of the cardiac muscle, known as 'irritability', caused it to contract spontaneously.

The first inkling that there was a completely different mechanism at work came with the discovery that electric current affects the way the heart operates. In the eighteenth century, when the properties of electricity became a preoccupation of natural philosophers, it was not long before anatomists began to experiment with its effects on human tissues. Doctors (and a good many charlatans) attempted to cure all manner of disease with 'medical electricity', applying current to whichever part of the body was affected. A physicist from Geneva, Jean Jallabert, noticed that passing electricity through a muscle made it contract, and also found that it caused the heartbeat to accelerate.[4] This observation was confirmed by John Wesley, the founder of Methodism, who as well as being a minister and theologian was an amateur physician and an enthusiastic proponent of electrical medicine. In his 1760 book *The Desideratum: or, Electricity Made Plain and Useful*, he recorded this messy sounding experiment: 'Open a vein in a person standing on the rosin [an electrical insulator], and the blood will fly out to a certain distance. But let him be electrified, and it will spin out with a much greater force and to a far greater distance.'[5]

Wesley may even have performed the first electrical cure of a heart arrhythmia. In 1757 he was approached by Silas Todd, a forty-eight-year-old schoolmaster who had suffered from heart palpitations for seventeen years. Wesley passed an electric shock through his chest, noting that his patient 'has been ever since perfectly well'.[6] The episode is strikingly similar to the modern technique of cardioversion, in which an electrical impulse is used to correct certain types of tachycardia, disorders in which the heart beats too fast.

Still more dramatic was the story of Catherine-Sophie Greenhill, a three-year-old girl who on 16 July 1774 fell out of a first-floor window on to the pavement outside her parents' London home. An apothecary called to the scene found that her heart had stopped and declared her dead, but a neighbour called Squires – apparently an amateur scientist – arrived twenty minutes later with an electrostatic generator, with which he passed electricity through various parts of her lifeless body. When he applied it to her chest the pulse reappeared, and the child began to breathe again – possibly the first use of cardiac defibrillation.[7]

Medical electricity fell out of favour in the 1850s, when doctors found that the extravagant claims made for the treatment were not supported by clinical results.[8] But just as medics were abandoning its therapeutic use, researchers discovered that electricity played an essential role in the human body. In 1856 the Swiss anatomist Rudolf von Kölliker connected a galvanometer – an instrument for measuring current – to a frog's beating heart and demonstrated that each contraction of its muscle was accompanied by a tiny pulse of electricity. He also noticed something even more significant: when he attached the nerves of a frog's leg to the cardiac wall, the leg twitched just before the heart began to contract, suggesting that the electrical impulse not only preceded the muscle contraction, but also caused it.[9]

This hinted at a possible mechanism for cardiac action, but placing electrodes directly on the heart was not a practical method of studying electrical activity in living patients. Thirty years later the British physiologist Augustus Waller developed a way of doing so without breaching the skin. He attached electrodes to the front and back of a patient's chest and connected them to a capillary electrometer, a device which used a thin column of mercury to measure electric potential. When he examined the mercury through a microscope he found that it moved slightly with each beat of the heart. These movements could be turned into a graph representing electrical changes over time, recognisable today as a rudimentary electrocardiogram. The first ever ECG, taken from a patient at St Mary's Hospital in London, was published in a medical journal in 1887.[10]

One of those present on this historic occasion was a young Dutch doctor called Willem Einthoven. He immediately grasped its significance, while realising that the unwieldy apparatus gave results too inexact to be useful. After several years of research he unveiled a much-improved device, which he dubbed the 'string galvanometer'. Signals from the chest electrodes were passed through a silvered quartz thread suspended in a magnetic field. Even tiny voltages would cause this to be deflected, and the degree of deviation was then measured photographically.[11] This gave results far more precise than Waller's mercury column, allowing Einthoven to observe features of the wave produced by the heartbeat that had never been seen before. His research was published in 1906, but few took much interest in his work until four years later, when he revealed that by installing a cable between the hospital and his laboratory he had been able to study the heartbeat of a patient a mile away.[12] Einthoven won a Nobel Prize for his invention, which for the first time made it possible to describe the electrical activity of the heart – and to diagnose disturbances in its rhythm with great accuracy.

As Einthoven was preparing his first results for publication the mystery of what makes the heart beat was finally solved. A decade earlier the Swiss cardiologist Wilhelm His had spotted a previously unnoticed bundle of muscle fibres which extended through the septum between the two sides of the heart. He realised that the purpose of this specialised tissue was to conduct electrical impulses from the right atrium to the two ventricles, causing them to contract – the first physical evidence of a conduction circuit inside the heart.[13] By 1906 a number of similar fibres had been identified, but the source of the electrical signals remained unknown. It was finally discovered that summer by a medical student, in the unlikely surroundings of a farmhouse in the Kent countryside. Martin Flack, the son of the local butcher, was assisting the anatomist Arthur Keith in his research in an improvised laboratory in his drawing room. While Keith and his wife were on a bicycle ride one afternoon Flack dissected the heart of a mole, and found a 'wonderful structure' high in the right atrium.[14]

The tiny bundle of nerves Flack saw through his microscope was not much to look at, but it represented the final piece of a puzzle that had mystified the greatest scientific minds for centuries. His 'wonderful structure' was the sinoatrial node, the heart's natural pacemaker and the origin of the signals that make it beat. Once or more a second the SA node fires out an electrical impulse that propagates through the heart muscle, causing the atria to contract. A fraction of a second later the electrical signal reaches a similar bundle located in the wall between the two sides of the heart, the atrioventricular node, which in turn sends out an impulse that makes the ventricles contract and eject their load of blood.

The sinoatrial node is the heart's orchestral conductor, and the muscle fibres contract in time to its beat. Like a real maestro, it can change its tempo as circumstances demand: responding to nerve impulses from the brain and hormones in the bloodstream, the pacemaker increases the heart rate when we exercise, and reduces it when the body's oxygen needs have returned to normal.* The network of electrical connections responsible for the heartbeat is complex – so complex that it is still not fully understood. Disease or old age can cause the conduction pathways to break down or make new, anomalous connections, disrupting the electrical signal and provoking arrhythmia – a disturbance in heart rhythm. The voltages involved are tiny, measured in millivolts, but this microscopic electrical system regulates the cardiac rhythm with precision. Finding out what makes the heart tick was a crucial breakthrough that helped doctors understand the manifold ways in which it can go wrong; but it would be some years before they found a way of translating this knowledge into an effective treatment.

*

---

* Changes in heart rate caused by stress, strong emotion or stimulants such as caffeine are also mediated by the same mechanisms.

The Australian Mark Lidwill is perhaps unique among medical pioneers in being better known for catching a fish. On 8 February 1913 he became the first person in the world to land a black marlin, a powerful saltwater species capable of swimming at 80 mph and much prized by game fishermen. The 70-pound specimen he caught that day in the waters off Port Stephen was donated to the Australian Museum, where its skeleton still resides today.[15] His monster catch managed to overshadow his invention the same year of an anaesthetics machine that was used in most of Australia's hospitals – and, fifteen years later, his creation of the world's first artificial pacemaker.

What interested Lidwill was what happened to the heart as it failed. He was one of the first to use the ECG to find out how its electrical signals changed as a patient died, and noticed that death was often preceded by a breakdown in the cardiac conduction system. He knew that applying electricity to the heart muscle made it contract, and concluded that it might be possible to help an ailing heart by artificial means.[16] With a colleague from the University of Sydney he designed a machine intended to provide an artificial stimulus for the heart in cases where the sinoatrial node had stopped producing its electrical signal. His device, which was plugged into a lighting socket, had two electrodes: one was attached to a pad on the skin, and the other was a needle which was plunged into the heart. Regular pulses of electricity were then passed through this circuit to stimulate the cardiac muscle. His first patient was a baby born without a heartbeat at the Crown Street Women's Hospital in 1926; after the usual resuscitation methods had been tried without success, Lidwill thrust the needle of his pacemaker into the ventricle and switched it on. The heart immediately responded, and ten minutes later when the machine was turned off it was beating normally. The child made a full recovery, and when Lidwill reported his research at a medical conference in 1929 he expressed confidence that his device could save many lives: 'There may be many failures, but one life in fifty or even a hundred, is a big advancement where there is no hope at all.'[17]

It is curious, then, that Lidwill's advance did not lead anywhere. His research went almost unnoticed, and seems to have come to a halt when his collaborator left the Sydney maternity hospital. One of the few investigators aware of his work was Albert Hyman, an American cardiologist whose interest in the problem of cardiac resuscitation began during his first week as a surgical intern in 1918. The twenty-five-year-old doctor was on duty when a middle-aged man was admitted to his hospital in Boston with a broken leg. As Hyman examined him the man's heart stopped beating. The emergency-room medics inserted a long needle through his chest to inject adrenaline directly into his heart – a technique that had recently been adopted to treat cardiac arrest. The heart began to beat again, but a few minutes later its rhythm became unstable and then stopped entirely, with further injections proving futile. Hyman was desperate to understand what had happened in the minutes leading up to his patient's death, and in particular why the heart had restarted and then stopped again. For the next five years he kept meticulous notes every time he witnessed a similar case, hoping to spot something that might lead to an effective treatment.[18]

Adrenaline was not the only substance injected into the heart on these occasions: many others, including caffeine and camphor, were also tried. Hyman noticed that the choice of drug made no difference to the chances of success, and inferred that it was the prick of the needle, rather than the chemical injected, which prompted the muscle to contract.[19] His first thought was that a simple puncture with an empty needle would be as effective as any other method, but this rarely kept the heart beating for more than a few minutes. To keep it going for any length of time several pricks would often be required, which might cause serious damage. Instead he conceived the idea of an electrical stimulus conveyed to the heart muscle through a needle. A pulse of electricity would have the same effect as a needle prick, and it could be repeated once a second or more, until the muscle had recovered enough to produce its own contractions.

With his brother Henry, an electrical engineer, Hyman constructed a machine which he called the 'artificial pacemaker'. Like Lidwill's device, it was intended as a temporary stand-in for the patient's own sinoatrial node in cases where the cardiac conduction mechanisms had broken down. It was powered by a small generator, which had to be hand-cranked every six minutes, and used two electrodes, one of which was a needle inserted into the heart. The device could be adjusted to various rates, providing between 30 and 120 electrical impulses per minute.[20] It was tested on a dog called Electra, whose heart was artificially stopped and restarted no fewer than thirteen times. 'The dog that died thirteen times' became a minor celebrity, and was adopted as a pet by one of Hyman's assistants.

When he presented his work at a conference in 1932, Hyman had only used his pacemaker on a few patients, and his work aroused little enthusiasm. Though his colleagues remained unconvinced, the media took a close interest in a device that seemed to offer the possibility of bringing the dead back to life. By the following year Hyman had succeeded in reviving sixty patients from cardiac arrest,[21] and a series of newspaper headlines reported his achievements to fascinated readers. Particularly sensational was the story of a New York millionaire in the final stages of heart disease who summoned Hyman to his bedside. He told the doctor that he knew he was about to die, but needed to live long enough to pass on some confidential information to his son, who was travelling from the other side of the country. A few hours later he went into cardiac arrest; the long pacemaker needle was inserted through his chest, the electric impulses switched on, and after fifteen minutes the patient regained consciousness. The son duly arrived, and was able to speak to his father while the machine continued to stimulate a heartbeat; twenty-four hours later the millionaire died.[22]

This anecdote has a whiff of journalistic embellishment to it, and some of the contemporary reporting seems even more dubious. Implausibly, it was claimed that three Cuban soldiers shot dead in battle had been restored to life by the pacemaker.[23] In the 1930s, when a stopped heart was believed to be the very definition of death, recovery

from cardiac arrest was nothing short of resurrection, and many people were eager to know whether Hyman's patients had experienced
any intimations of an afterlife. To answer such queries he commissioned a clergyman to interrogate those 'raised from the dead', who
reported – disappointingly – that they remembered nothing about it.[24]
Nevertheless, suspicions lingered that there was something immoral,
even sacrilegious, about Hyman's work, and he received angry letters
accusing him of interfering with God's handiwork.[25] Initial excitement at his invention turned to disapproval and horror: one possible
reason was the release in 1931 of *Frankenstein*, starring Boris Karloff as
an unnatural creature constructed from human corpses and given new
life by the miracle of electricity. Another was the antics of Dr Robert
Cornish, a young researcher who claimed to have resuscitated dogs
after they had been asphyxiated, using artificial respiration, injections
of heparin and a table that rocked like a seesaw to restore their circulation. In 1934 Cornish wrote to the governors of three US states asking for permission to revive the corpses of prisoners after execution
in the gas chamber. His request – which was denied – aroused general disgust, and may have turned public opinion against those who
claimed to bring the 'dead' back to life.[26]

Hyman persisted with his work despite the hostility directed
against him, and in 1936 he replaced his original bulky apparatus with
a battery-powered model the size of a large torch.[27] His efforts to find
a manufacturer failed, and a German researcher who tested the pacemaker found that he could not even use it to revive a rabbit.[28] Although
Hyman continued to use the device until the early 1940s, he could not
persuade other doctors that it was safe and effective, and his invention
faded into obscurity.

What exactly do we mean when we refer to 'cardiac arrest'? Most
people understand the term to mean a stopped heart, but it's a little
more complicated than that. A patient is in cardiac arrest if their heart
abruptly ceases to pump blood around the body – a lethal condition
unless speedily treated, often killing within minutes. It is not the same

thing as a heart attack, in which an interruption to the organ's blood supply causes sudden damage to part of its muscle. Heart attacks can lead to cardiac arrest, but there are many other possible causes, including blood loss, drug overdose, hypothermia or a pre-existing heart condition. Cardiac arrest does not necessarily mean that the heart is entirely motionless; the term is a rather vague one which encompasses several distinct eventualities. The pacemaker was developed in order to treat patients who were in a specific type of cardiac arrest known as asystole, in which there are no contractions and all electrical activity has ceased. This would not work in the majority of cases, however, since asystole is a comparatively rare form of cardiac arrest. Much more common is a type called ventricular fibrillation, in which the muscle goes into a sort of spasm, destroying the heartbeat and preventing the organ from pumping. To treat this condition required a rather more dramatic approach.

In 1849 two German physiologists, Carl Ludwig and Moritz Hoffa, performed an experiment which entailed passing a strong electric current through the heart of a live dog. To their surprise the powerful contractions of the cardiac muscle ceased and were replaced by a strange quivering which halted the circulation, killing the animal. This was ventricular fibrillation, but the significance of the observation did not become apparent until several decades later, when the introduction of electrical power to major cities provoked a new dread of electrocution – a strangely disproportionate fear, given that gas lighting caused far more fatalities.[29] Little was known about the mechanism of death by electrocution, and so researchers set to work investigating how it killed, and whether the process could be reversed.

In the early 1890s Jean-Louis Prévost and Frederic Batelli, two scientists at the University of Geneva, made a useful discovery. They repeated Ludwig and Hoffa's experiment, but instead of watching their experimental dog die, Prévost and Batelli managed to revive it. They found that imparting a second shock of much higher voltage banished the fibrillation from the heart – in other words, defibrillated it.[30] Their work was repeated ten years later in the United States by Louise

Robinovitch, a physiologist so devoted to the subject that her doctoral research had involved electrocuting a very large number of rabbits. She was the first to appreciate that the defibrillating electrodes should be applied only to the thorax, so as to exclude the delicate brain structures from the circuit,[31] and even designed a portable defibrillator for use in ambulances.[32] This was truly groundbreaking work, and yet it was largely ignored by the medical establishment: whether because of her sex or her temperament, Robinovitch was regarded as something of a maverick.[33]

Her findings had already been forgotten by 1925, when the managers of a large American electrical company became alarmed at the number of employees dying while working on high-voltage power lines, and asked a team at Johns Hopkins medical school to look into the problem. Their conclusions confirmed those of Prévost and Batelli thirty years earlier: when a dog was given an electric shock of around 110 volts, its heart went into ventricular fibrillation. This could be reversed by a much more powerful shock – they used 2,200 volts – which caused the heart to stop entirely for a few seconds before resuming its normal beat.[34] One of the researchers, the electrical engineer William Kouwenhoven, designed a defibrillator to impart such shocks whenever needed, apparently unaware that Robinovitch had already done so twenty years earlier.

Kouwenhoven's defibrillator and Hyman's pacemaker, both invented in the early 1930s, were superficially similar, so it is important to distinguish between them. Each employed electricity to stimulate a heartbeat, but they performed very different functions. I've described the sinoatrial node as the heart's conductor, in charge of an orchestra whose players are the organ's muscle fibres, but it may help to extend that analogy a little. Imagine that an orchestra is in the middle of a concert when the conductor unexpectedly puts down her baton and walks off stage. The players suddenly have no beat to follow, so they stop playing and the music grinds to a halt. They are in a state of musical asystole – nothing is happening. But the situation is rescued by a member of the audience, who produces a metronome, places it on the absent conductor's music stand and sets it going. This is all the players need to resume their performance: the loud and unvarying *tick* of the metronome may lack the fine nuance of a proper conductor, but it's enough to keep the music going. Like the metronome, Hyman's pacemaker provided an artificial beat that the cardiac muscle fibres could follow.

The defibrillator was designed to cope with another problem: ventricular fibrillation, in which the muscle fibres have lost all coordination and are contracting at random. This time the conductor is not the problem: the orchestra, rather than falling silent, have lost concentration and are now improvising wildly. Instead of playing as an ensemble they all do their own thing, resulting in deafening cacophony, while the conductor's increasingly desperate gestures from the rostrum are ignored. Suddenly there is a blinding flash and a bang: a member of the audience has set off a firework in the auditorium. The players are so startled that they stop playing. There is silence for a moment, and the conductor finds that she now has their undivided attention; the performance can resume in an orderly manner. Kouwenhoven's defibrillator, like the firework, offered a sudden shock to the system: a high-voltage pulse of electricity that abolished all muscle activity for a second, allowing the natural pacemaker rhythm to establish itself once more.

If you've watched a lot of medical dramas you might have been misled into thinking that a defibrillator can be used to reverse any type of cardiac arrest. We're all familiar with the scene: a patient lies stricken in an intensive care bed, surrounded by worried faces. Suddenly an alarm goes off and the camera zooms in on the ECG, which briefly goes haywire before the trace settles into a featureless flat line, the machine's regular 'bip, bip, bip' replaced by a monotone '*beeeeee*'. The medics spring into action, placing defibrillator pads on the patient's chest, shouting 'Clear!' and unleashing a powerful shock that makes the whole bed jerk. Several more attempts are usually obligatory to wring every drop of suspense out of the situation, but eventually the heart springs back into life and everybody breathes a sigh of relief.

The scenario is not only hackneyed but utterly implausible. Medics distinguish between 'shockable' and 'unshockable' arrhythmias, and asystole – indicated by the flatlining ECG – is one of the unshockable varieties, so a defibrillator is no use in treating it.* The more commonly encountered ventricular fibrillation, on the other hand, is shockable, so a defibrillator will often be effective in restoring a natural heart rhythm.

Kouwenhoven's work attracted the attention of Claude Beck, Elliott Cutler's former research student, who was now a surgeon in Cleveland. Like most members of his profession he was familiar with the problem of ventricular fibrillation, which sometimes arose when the heart was handled. Those unlucky enough to encounter this complication were helpless as they watched the cardiac muscle begin to seize: nothing they did would restore it to a natural rhythm. In its disordered state the heart could eject only a fraction of the usual volume of blood, and within a few minutes the patient would be dead.

In 1937 Beck outlined the advantages of the defibrillator to a meeting of surgeons, but his presentation made little impression. He installed one of the machines in the Cleveland Clinic and attempted to use it on a few patients, but by the time he applied the electrodes to their hearts the fibrillation was well established, and brain damage had already set in.[35] It was not until 1947 that he had his first success. The patient was Dick Heyard, a fourteen-year-old boy who was undergoing surgery for pectus excavatum, a deformity in which the thorax has a concave appearance. After an uneventful operation the boy's heart abruptly stopped as Beck was closing his chest. 'The patient was apparently dead,' he recorded. Outside the operating theatre Dick's distraught mother was told that her son's heart had stopped beating, and she sank to her knees in prayer.[36]

Beck hurriedly reopened the incision and began to massage Dick's heart, squeezing it rhythmically with a gloved hand. He continued

---

* This is a fatal flaw in the plot of the 1990 thriller *Flatliners*, in which Kiefer Sutherland, Julia Roberts and Kevin Bacon play medical students who investigate near-death experiences by stopping and restarting each other's hearts.

doing this for forty-five minutes; to get a sense of what this must have been like, imagine standing at a table squeezing a tennis ball every second for three-quarters of an hour – but with somebody's life depending on it. After what must have seemed an eternity, the ECG finally showed that the heart was alive, but in ventricular fibrillation. Beck applied the defibrillator electrodes to the heart and passed a shock of 110 volts through it. It continued to quiver feverishly, so he tried again. Suddenly all activity ceased, and for a second it stood stock still. Then a rapid but feeble heartbeat appeared; as Beck continued to massage the heart the contractions grew stronger, and after twenty minutes he was able to close the wound in the boy's chest.[37] A month later Dick returned home. 'Boy Who "Died" Is Alive Through Prayers', read a headline in the local newspaper,[38] which seems a little unfair on Beck.

While the defibrillator slowly became an accepted surgical tool, the pacemaker, which had been invented and abandoned twice, seemed a medical dead end – until 1949, when Wilfred Bigelow became the third person to stumble upon the idea. Then several years into his hypothermia research, he seemed to be making good progress, cooling dogs to well below their normal temperature in order to perform experimental open-heart surgery. But his team had encountered an infuriating problem. Sometimes when a dog was being cooled to the target temperature, its heart would stop without warning, and resist all attempts to restart it. Bigelow watched this happen in his basement laboratory one morning. His first feeling was exasperation: instead of operating on the dog, he and his team would have to spend the day trying (and probably failing) to revive it. As he looked at the quiescent heart, Bigelow was struck by how healthy it looked. He gave it an experimental prod, and to his surprise it responded with a vigorous contraction. Intrigued, he poked it repeatedly; each jab provoked an apparently normal heartbeat.[39]

Bigelow reached the same conclusion as Hyman: perhaps a small electric shock would have the same effect. He approached the Canadian National Research Council, who put him in touch with an electrical engineer, Jack Hopps. Hopps had been working on a new technique for pasteurising beer, a subject close to his heart, and accepted the new assignment reluctantly. But he soon became fascinated by Bigelow's idea, and when another surgeon in his team, John Callaghan, came across a description of Hyman's pacemaker they had confirmation that they were on to something. Hopps visited Kouwenhoven's laboratory to learn about the defibrillator and what he had discovered about the conduction pathways of the heart, and not long afterwards he developed a pulse generator, a table-top unit that produced a regular electrical impulse.[40] Bigelow hoped that the pacemaker would keep his dogs alive while they were being put in deep hypothermia, but the first trial was a failure: the first animal went into cardiac arrest at 17°C, and nothing would revive it. Disheartened, he tested the device on rabbits and dogs at normal temperatures and found that the pacemaker consistently succeeded in restarting a stopped heart. Once the heart was beating the device could even be made to override its native rhythm, giving the surgeon control over the heartbeat and allowing him to dictate its rate, between 60 and 200 beats per minute.[41]

In their early experiments they used a needle electrode similar to that used by Hyman, but Bigelow and his colleagues realised that this method was unnecessarily laborious. They developed a catheter electrode, a wire which could be inserted through a vein and navigated through the blood vessels towards the heart. This allowed the pacemaker to be used without opening the chest, considerably simplifying the operation. Bigelow became convinced that it was suitable for use on humans, and Callaghan employed it in treating five patients with severe cardiac arrhythmias. To their frustration the treatment had no effect; Callaghan later realised that the electrode had been placed in the wrong part of the heart. Two inches lower and it would have worked – a small distance, but one that made the difference between life and death.[42]

In October 1950 Callaghan gave a presentation about this work to a meeting of the American College of Surgeons. A week later he received a letter from Paul Zoll, a cardiologist at Beth Israel Hospital

in Boston, asking for further details of the pacemaker apparatus.[43] Zoll
saw the device as the possible solution to a problem. Earlier that year
he had treated a woman who was suffering regular Stokes–Adams
attacks, episodes of unconsciousness caused by temporary cardiac
arrest. These are a sign of heart block, a problem with the conduction pathways which prevents the electrical signal from the natural
pacemaker from reaching all of the heart muscle. Zoll was unable to
do anything for her, and was deeply upset when she died three weeks
later.[44]

During the Second World War, Zoll had worked with Dwight
Harken in his army hospital in Gloucestershire, watching him take
fragments of shrapnel out of soldiers' hearts, and had noticed how
sensitive the cardiac muscle was to external stimulation.[45] He reasoned that an electrical stimulus might prevent sudden death in heart
block patients by keeping the organ pumping during periods when its
natural rhythm disappeared. After animal experiments using a signal
generator similar to that developed by Hopps and Callaghan, he discovered that it was not necessary to place electrodes directly on the
heart: if a higher voltage was used, they could be attached to the skin
of the chest. This was much quicker and safer, and still gave him full
control of the animal's heartbeat.

The first patient treated with the external pacemaker was a
seventy-five-year-old man who arrived at the Boston hospital on 28
August 1952. His cardiac rhythm was unstable, resulting in regular
Stokes–Adams attacks, and the medics struggled to keep him alive
with adrenaline injections directly to the heart – thirty-four of them
in just four hours. Eventually they decided to use the pacemaker, and
electrodes were placed on his chest. It kept him alive for twenty-five
minutes, but then his heartbeat faded to nothing and the doctors
admitted defeat. The following month a second patient, a sixty-five-
year-old man, was admitted to the hospital in severe heart failure. On
his sixth day there he had the first of several episodes of cardiac arrest,
and he too was connected to the pacemaker. Regular electric shocks of
up to 130 volts were passed through his chest. At first the device was

needed only occasionally, but on the fourth day the natural rhythm disappeared entirely and it had to be used continuously. For more than two days his heart was kept beating by regular shocks, ninety of them every minute, from the large box at his bedside.[46]

The subsequent recovery of this patient was a watershed. Physicians and the public alike were impressed: 'Plug Failing Hearts into AC Outlet', suggested one dangerously simplistic headline.[47] But heart block was a fairly rare condition, so it was not immediately obvious that the pacemaker would often be needed. Zoll didn't know it, but the development of open-heart surgery would soon make his device an essential item for all cardiac operating theatres.

The first person to appreciate this was a pathologist from Chicago, Maurice Lev. In the early 1950s, around the time that Walton Lillehei was performing the first of his open-heart operations using cross-circulation, Lev pointed out to him that working inside the organ was likely to provoke heart block. 'What's that?' asked Lillehei. Lev explained that cutting and stitching cardiac tissue would probably disrupt its conduction pathways and affect the heartbeat. This was much like an orchestra trying to rehearse in a hall where the lighting only works intermittently: while the lights are on the players can follow the conductor's beat, but as soon as they are plunged into darkness they can see nothing and stop playing.

Lev was soon proved right. Many of Lillehei's early patients had ventricular septal defects, holes in the wall between the two ventricles. Repairing them entailed placing sutures perilously close to conductive tissue, and seven of his first seventy patients developed heart block as a result. All of them died.[48] Lillehei found that a drug called Isuprel reduced the mortality rate to 50 per cent, but this was still unacceptably high. When he heard about Zoll's work he realised that a pacemaker might be the answer, and tried the method on several of his patients. It did succeed in keeping them alive, but there was a problem. The device imparted a 60-volt electric shock every second that it was turned on. This could be exquisitely painful, and for patients reliant on the machine day and night it caused significant distress. One patient who was on a Zoll pacemaker for several weeks killed himself by disconnecting the device, preferring death to an apparently endless torture.[49] Others developed skin burns and blisters at the electrode sites; given that Lillehei's patients were mostly children, this was deeply unsatisfactory.[50] In animal experiments his colleagues found that if the electrodes were placed directly on the heart a much smaller current was required, so small that the patient would not even notice it. Lillehei adopted this technique in early 1957, attaching electrodes to the heart after completing each operation. The results were striking: mortality from heart block dropped from 40 per cent to 2 per cent.[51]

As he soon discovered, there were some drawbacks to this life-saving therapy. Children who were wholly dependent on a device plugged into a wall socket could not easily be moved: a simple trip to the X-ray department entailed trailing an extension lead halfway across the hospital. That was inconvenient, but when a major power cut hit Minneapolis on 31 October 1957 the disadvantages of a mains-powered pacemaker became painfully apparent. For three hours, doctors ran around administering drugs to patients as they desperately tried to keep their hearts going. Miraculously all survived, but Lillehei knew he had to find a way to prevent the scenario from arising again.[52]

The obvious solution was a portable battery-powered device. Lillehei asked a physics student to design something, but several months later the undergraduate admitted that he had made no progress. Irritated, Lillehei bumped into Earl Bakken, an electrical engineer who was often in the hospital maintaining operating theatre equipment. He told him about the problem and asked whether he thought he could make one for him. Bakken accepted the challenge, and went home to do some tinkering in his garage. These unassuming premises were the headquarters of Medtronic, a two-man company he had founded with his brother-in-law a few years earlier. Business was slow, and as well as mending broken medical equipment Bakken often found himself moonlighting as a TV repair man. Rooting around in the messy workshop, he unearthed an old issue of *Popular Electronics* magazine. He remembered an article giving instructions for constructing an electronic metronome, a simple circuit using only a few basic components which when attached to a loudspeaker would produce regular clicks at an adjustable rate. Bakken realised this was just what he needed, made a few tweaks to the original circuit and put it in a small box with a battery.* A few weeks after being given the commission he delivered the first portable pacemaker to a delighted Lillehei.[53]

Bakken assumed that the new device would require months of animal testing, so when he returned to the hospital the following day he was shocked to see a young patient already wearing his prototype on a strap around her neck, with wires poking through an incision in her chest. He sought out Lillehei, who told him that a quick test in the animal laboratory had shown that it worked, so he saw no point in waiting any longer before using it.[54] Bakken was sent back to his garage to make more of them, and within a few months it became quite ordinary to see one of Lillehei's young patients wandering the corridors with the vital equipment dangling from a holster over one shoulder.

The impact of this development was spectacular. 'Not only has the threat of sudden death in these patients been removed, but their physical and emotional development has been dramatic,' Lillehei wrote.[55] Children reliant on the pacemaker could get out of bed and even go home. Most would only need it for a short period, until their heart rhythm returned to normal, but it could be left in place for many months if necessary. Although Lillehei had only envisioned it as a post-operative measure, he soon found it was effective in patients who developed heart block in old age or as the consequence of a heart attack. Bakken had to take on extra staff to meet the demand, and several thousand units were sold over the next few years. Many patients returned to work after years as invalids, and could lead active lives: one newspaper reported the story of Carl Baker, a thirty-eight-year-old

---

* Strangely, Bakken was not the only person to be thus inspired. Adrian Kantrowitz, a surgeon in Brooklyn, independently adapted the same metronome circuit for a pacemaker implanted into a patient in September 1961.

engineer who was able to play golf and go hiking with his pacemaker strapped to his waist.[56]

But the device was far from perfect. Being permanently connected to a box of electronics is not terribly convenient if you want to take a shower or go for a swim. The pacemaker wires were fragile: one patient regularly turned up at Bakken's office on a Monday morning having broken one while dancing at the weekend.[57] The most serious problem was infection, since the leads emerged from the body through what was in effect a permanent wound in the skin. The only way to prevent this complication would be to implant the entire unit – electrodes, leads and the pacemaker itself – inside the body, though few researchers thought this practical, or even possible, in 1958.[58]

One person who did not share this pessimism was the Swede Åke Senning. A protégé of Clarence Crafoord, Senning was fascinated by engineering and helped to develop the first heart-lung machine and defibrillator in Scandinavia.[59] His introduction to cardiac arrhythmia was a painful one: as a boy he managed to electrocute himself with a table lamp, causing a brief episode of ventricular fibrillation that caused him to feel as if his heart had stopped.[60] Senning was a regular visitor to the US and had talked to Bigelow and Lillehei about their work. With the help of a technician from a local electronics company, Rune Elmqvist, he began his own pacemaker research at the Karolinska Hospital in Stockholm. Senning and Elmqvist began by constructing a device much like Bakken's, but Senning was acutely aware of the drawbacks of an external pulse generator and wanted to create something small enough to implant under the skin.[61]

Such a thing would have been unthinkable only a couple of years earlier, but technology was entering an exciting new era. The pacemakers of Bigelow and Zoll had used vacuum tubes, large and unreliable components that had to be housed in a bulky casing. The transistor, an amplifying and switching device invented in 1947, consumed far less power and was a fraction of the size, making it possible to miniaturise electronic circuits. The first mass-produced transistor radio, the Regency TR-1, went on sale in late 1954; promotional material described it as smaller than a cigarette packet or martini glass, comparisons that surely say something about the preoccupations of advertising executives in this era. Using the silicon transistor, only just available in Sweden, Elmqvist was able to build a pacemaker that fitted in the palm of the hand.

Senning was in no hurry to use Elmqvist's invention on a patient, but on 6 October 1958 he found himself with no other choice. That day Else-Marie Larsson, an 'energetic, beautiful' woman, walked into his laboratory and asked him to implant a pacemaker into her forty-four-year-old husband, Arne. Some weeks earlier her husband had contracted hepatitis after eating oysters in a restaurant, and the infection had spread to his heart. Now he was suffering up to thirty Stokes – Adams attacks a day, with Else-Marie watching helplessly at his bedside each time his heart rate dropped to a paltry twenty per minute. Senning explained that he was still conducting animal experiments and did not yet have a pacemaker for human use. 'So make one,' was her imperious reply.[62]

Her zeal was irresistible. To be on the safe side, Elmqvist assembled two pacemakers, simple electronic circuits each using a pair of transistors. He encased them in epoxy resin using a Kiwi shoe-polish tin as a mould, producing an object roughly the size and shape of an ice-hockey puck.[63] On the evening of 8 October Senning operated, attaching electrodes to Arne's heart muscle and tucking the pacemaker into a pocket behind the abdominal muscles. All seemed well at first, but at 2 a.m. it abruptly stopped working. After a frantic dash to Elmqvist's lab to pick up the spare, Senning replaced the faulty unit the following morning, and this time there were no alarms: the pacemaker worked as expected, and Larsson suffered no more Stokes – Adams attacks. Every week or so the battery ran down and had to be recharged. In a futuristic touch this was done wirelessly: a coil strapped to Larsson's chest transmitted power by electromagnetic induction to a smaller coil embedded underneath the skin.[64]

The pacemaker remained effective for only six weeks, but that was long enough to see Larsson through the crisis.[65] He was well enough to manage without a pacemaker for the next three years, though the underlying heart block was still there. In 1961 his condition deteriorated again and Senning implanted a third device. There would be a further ten by the end of the decade, and when Arne Larsson died in 2002 he had received twenty-two pacemakers in total, and outlived the surgeon who saved him.[66] His contribution to the development of the pacemaker went further than being its first guinea pig: a trained electrical engineer, Larsson also became involved in improving the device.[67]

At least half a dozen people have been described as the 'inventor' of the pacemaker, but Rune Elmqvist surely has a strong claim to the title. The simple device he constructed may have lasted little more than a month, but it was the first to be implanted inside the body; more to the point, it gave its first patient forty-four extra years of life. A few months later a slightly improved model was implanted into two patients in London by the surgeon Harold Siddons: one continued to work for ten months, an impressive demonstration of its capabilities.[68] The fact that these successes predated the work of the American engineer Wilson Greatbatch – 'inventor of the pacemaker', according to the front cover of his memoirs[69] – does nothing to diminish his achievement, for he was the first to produce a device which lasted not months, but years.

Another electrical engineer by training, Greatbatch began his career producing machines for an animal laboratory at Cornell University. He became interested in the problem of cardiac pacing after a chance conversation with two brain surgeons in 1951, and was immediately sure that electronics would provide a solution. A few years later he stumbled across one by mistake: while assembling a device to monitor heart rates in laboratory animals he accidentally inserted the wrong component, and found that the resulting circuit produced a periodic electrical pulse.[70] This was not at all what he had been intending, but he immediately realised that it might be used as the basis for a pacemaker. Greatbatch struggled to interest clinicians in his idea until early 1958, when he finally met a surgeon who was receptive to his ideas.

William Chardack, the chief of surgery at the Veterans Administration Hospital in Buffalo, was instantly swayed by Greatbatch's conviction that modern electronics made a long-term implantable pacemaker a realistic prospect. Chardack believed that a device using a mercury cell – a power source invented during the war – could last for at least a couple of years before needing to be replaced.[71] Encouraged by the surgeon's enthusiasm, Greatbatch left his job and sank $2,000, his life savings, into the project.[72] His first pacemaker was, in appearance at least, similar to Elmqvist's. Measuring 6 centimetres in diameter and just 1.5 centimetres thick, it was covered in epoxy resin which was then coated in a thin shell of silicone rubber.[73] Its first success came in June 1960, when Chardack implanted one into the chest of Frank Henefelt, a seventy-seven-year-old with complete heart block. In the months before the operation Henefelt's heart rate dropped to thirty-two per minute, causing regular blackouts. One particularly nasty fall resulted in a skull fracture, and he took to wearing a football helmet around the house.[74] After implantation he was completely cured, with a healthy heart rate of fifty-five; the helmet was set aside and he was able to resume a normal life. The next two people to receive a pacemaker had similarly happy outcomes, and suddenly patients were beating a path to Chardack's door and asking to have one of his 'heart-stingers' implanted.[75] The wider medical profession, often slow to embrace such technology in the past, soon realised that a fully implantable pacemaker was a real step forwards, a treatment that allowed patients to put months or years of ill health behind them.

In October 1960 Greatbatch sold the patent for his invention to Earl Bakken's firm, Medtronic.[76] This was something of a gamble, since an independent expert had recently concluded that the potential market for the device was tiny, estimating that no more than 10,000 pacemakers would ever be needed in total.[77] By the turn of the millennium 600,000 were being sold *every year*,[78] and Bakken's struggling business-in-a-garage had been transformed into a multinational corporation with more than 85,000 employees.[79]

After many false starts and much scepticism, the pacemaker was finally accepted as an effective therapy. But it was not without its deficiencies: in early patients the voltage required to stimulate the heart tended to increase over time until the device ceased to have any effect, a problem eventually solved by the introduction of a new type of electrode*. Another weakness was the leads, which tended to fracture until better materials and methods of construction were discovered. Battery life was a major concern: Greatbatch had estimated that his pacemaker would last five years or more,[80] but early patients were lucky if their device lasted eighteen months. It would be another decade before a really durable power source became available; but in the meantime there was a still more formidable problem to be solved.

The first implantable pacemakers were unsophisticated objects that did only one thing: emit a pulse of electricity roughly every second to stimulate the ventricle, ticking away like a metronome until the battery ran down. The rate was preset and could not be changed, so the patient's heart rate did not vary between rest and exercise. The device also took no account of the heart's underlying rhythm, raising the possibility that the artificial pacemaker might 'compete' with the signals from the natural one. In the worst-case scenario this might even induce ventricular fibrillation and death. What was needed was a pacemaker which did not interfere with naturally generated muscle contractions. The answer was a beautifully ingenious piece of engineering, a device that listened to the heart as well as sending it instructions. The basic mechanism was invented as early as 1942, although without any idea of its application to pacing. Two New York cardiologists investigating heart

---

* The first electrodes were 'unipolar': a single wire was placed on the heart, which meant that the electrical current needed to travel through a large area of the body back to the pacemaker to complete the circuit. The newer 'bipolar' electrodes contained both terminals of the circuit in a single lead so that the current had only 1 centimetre or so to travel, greatly reducing the energy required.

block placed an electrode on the atrium to detect the natural pace-maker impulse. This was then sent to a circuit which amplified the signal and returned via another electrode to the ventricle.[81] In cases of total heart block – where the electrical signals from the atrium never reach the ventricles – the device provided an artificial diversion, bypassing the electrical blockage.

In 1957 two researchers in Boston, Moses Judah Folkman and Elton Watkins, took the first step in turning this idea into a clinical solution. They experimented on twenty-four dogs, surgically producing heart block so that the atrial signals failed to reach the ventricles and giving them an unnaturally slow heartbeat. They then attached them to a miniature transistor amplifier, a device that picked up the tiny electrical signal from the atrioventricular node and magnified it fifty-fold. This amplified signal was enough to prompt ventricular contraction. It was like giving night-vision goggles to the members of an orchestra trying to play in a pitch-black auditorium: previously unable to see the conductor, they could now follow her beat. The beauty of the device was that it permitted a normal rhythm rather than imposing an artificial, unchanging one: the heartbeat varied with exercise, between 90 and 130 beats per minute. 'The dog is frisky and eats well,' they reported – it had been returned to full health.[82]

This was not a complete solution, since the device would only stimulate the ventricles if the natural pacemaker consistently produced an impulse. Some hearts are so damaged that the sinoatrial node fails to do this. To deal with this scenario, a Miami cardiologist, David Nathan, conceived a device that combined a pacemaker with an atrial-impulse amplifier. An electrode placed on the atrium 'listened' constantly for a signal, amplified it and passed it on to the ventricles; if no impulse was detected, an artificial pacemaker circuit stimulated the heart muscle until the natural signal returned.[83] A New Jersey surgeon, Victor Parsonnet, hit upon an even better solution three years later: his 'demand' pacemaker monitored the ventricles rather than the atria, and only came into action if it noticed that the heartbeat had dropped below 69 per minute.[84] Parsonnet's device did not entail a potentially dangerous operation to attach electrodes to the heart: instead, they were passed up through a vein via an incision in the groin. This technique, originally described by Bigelow's colleague John Callaghan, had been rediscovered in the early 1960s and soon became the method of choice when implanting pacemakers.

An extra level of complexity arrived in 1971 when a Massachusetts electrical engineer, Baruch Berkowitz, developed a pacemaker that acted not just on the ventricles but on the atria as well. This so-called 'bifocal' pacemaker monitored cardiac activity and, when required, stimulated both chambers in sequence, making the heart-beats more efficient by increasing the volume of blood ejected with each stroke.[85] In little more than a decade the pacemaker had evolved from a simple metronome for the heart into something far more sophisticated.

But the device still had an Achilles heel: its longevity. Wilson Greatbatch's estimate of a five-year lifespan for the first implantable devices proved hopelessly optimistic. The weak link was the mercury-cell battery, which generally lasted no longer than eighteen months. Many patients only discovered this when their old symptoms recurred, and their doctors had no way of predicting when the units would fail. At one hospital in London, doctors took to placing a medium-wave radio next to their patients: regular clicks from the loudspeaker indicated that the pacemaker was still functioning.[86] Many possible alternatives to the unreliable mercury batteries were tested: in 1960 a Birmingham surgeon, Leon Abrams, developed a pacemaker with a power pack outside the body, which transmitted power to its electrodes wirelessly via coils.[87] Others tried to harness the natural movements of the patient's body, using a mechanism like that of a self-winding watch to generate electrical power.[88] Eventually the search for the perfect power source led to one of the odder innovations of medical history: a nuclear-powered pacemaker.

In 1968, Victor Parsonnet wrote to the United States Atomic Energy Commission, asking for help in developing a long-lasting power source. The Commission was keen to improve the image of nuclear technology by employing it in small-scale – and demonstrably safe – civilian applications, and had already developed plutonium-fuelled generators to power lighthouses and space probes.[89] AEC scientists agreed that it should be feasible to design a nuclear battery small enough to power a pacemaker. The device they created was compact and simple: a thin wire of plutonium-238 was encased in a titanium capsule. As the plutonium decayed it threw out alpha particles which collided with the walls of the capsule, creating heat that was converted to electricity by a component called a thermocouple – the same technology that later powered the Voyager space probes. In 1969 a pacemaker containing a nuclear cell was successfully implanted into a dog called Brunhilde[90] – the researchers apparently did not think it an ill omen to name her after a Wagnerian heroine who dies in a blazing inferno.

After exhaustive tests the nuclear pacemaker was finally implanted into a human patient in France in April 1970. Three months later Constance Ladell, a fifty-six-year-old mother of four from Barnet, became the first person in Britain, and the third anywhere in the world, to receive one of the devices. The day after her operation, which was reported in the *Evening Standard* under the headline 'Atom Heart Mother Named',[91] members of the rock band Pink Floyd were in a BBC radio studio rehearsing for a live performance of their latest, as yet unreleased album. Mulling over possible names for the work, the lead singer Roger Waters was flicking through the evening paper when he spotted the story. 'How about that, lads?' he said, pointing at the headline. The LP was duly released as *Atom Heart Mother* – the first and only number one to be named in honour of a cardiac device.[92]

By 1975, around 1,400 nuclear pacemakers had been implanted without a single battery failure.[93] In Britain the Atomic Energy Research Establishment at Harwell was awarded a government contract to produce pacemaker batteries, one of the largest civilian applications for nuclear technology.[94] And the results were phenomenal; designed to have a ten-year lifespan, the devices proved even more durable. Dozens lasted for twenty years or more, and one implanted in 1973 was still working thirty-one years later.[95]

There were obvious concerns about placing a plutonium cell inside the human body. If just a millionth of a gram of fuel were to reach the bloodstream it would prove fatal, so it was necessary to take stringent safety precautions. The triple-walled titanium capsule was designed to withstand an aeroplane crash or the impact of a bullet, and every device was government-registered to ensure its whereabouts were known.[96] Neither of these drastic scenarios was ever put to the test in real life, but when a nuclear pacemaker was inadvertently incinerated in 1998 the capsule survived intact, with no escape of radiation.[97] In this respect they proved far safer than conventional devices, which had an unfortunate tendency to detonate when heated: in 1977 a crematorium in Solihull was badly damaged by a series of explosions caused by a mercury-cell pacemaker that had accidentally been left inside a body.[98] As a result of that incident, regulations were introduced to ensure that devices were removed before cremation, but a survey in 2002 found that half of all UK crematoria had experienced explosions caused by cardiac pacemakers.[99]

The heyday of the nuclear pacemaker was brief, and the reasons for its decline were unrelated to its safety record, which was impeccable. In 1972 Wilson Greatbatch and his colleagues invented a lithium-iodine battery with a lifespan of ten years. It was smaller and far cheaper than the nuclear cell, and had none of the practical difficulties associated with radioactive substances. It was an obviously superior solution to the problem of battery life, and has remained the standard pacemaker power source ever since. It also made possible the development of another type of device that emerged in the 1970s: the implantable cardiac defibrillator, or ICD.

*

The science of cardiac resuscitation had come a long way since Claude Beck first defibrillated a patient during an operation in 1947. Eight years later Paul Zoll designed a defibrillator which could be used on the closed chest, without the need for an incision.[100] But these early models used alternating current, which damaged and burned healthy tissue – to such an extent that, as Dwight Harken put it, 'you could smell the patient's heart cooking'.[101] The Boston cardiologist Bernard Lown and Baruch Berkowitz showed that direct current was far safer, and their new type of defibrillator, first used in 1961, was a huge advance. It was not only able to resuscitate patients without a pulse (those in ventricular fibrillation), but could also be used to correct less serious types of arrhythmia in which the heart continued to beat, but in a disordered fashion.

Lown named this treatment 'cardioversion'. The first patient to receive it was a sixty-three-year-old woman who arrived at Peter Bent Brigham Hospital after a heart attack. She had tachycardia (an unnaturally fast heartbeat) which failed to respond to drugs. Lown decided to attempt cardioversion, and the patient was given a powerful electric shock lasting 2.5 milliseconds. Her heart was immediately restored to its natural rhythm. 'The patient was awake within two minutes and was quite startled by the newly found sense of well-being,' Lown recorded.[102]

Another method of resuscitation that arrived at about the same time was, by comparison, startlingly low-tech. In 1960 William Kouwenhoven, the inventor of the modern defibrillator, wrote that 'anyone, anywhere, can now initiate cardiac resuscitative procedures. All that is needed are two hands.'[103] The technique he and two colleagues had discovered – or rather rediscovered, since similar research had been undertaken in Germany in the 1880s and then forgotten – entailed compressing the chest rhythmically with the hands. This was a vital addition, since it meant that heart-attack victims could be brought back to life even if they collapsed miles from the nearest hospital. In retrospect it is strange that such a simple method, one which is now taught to millions of amateur first-aiders every year, was introduced years after the invention of the defibrillator.

Another realisation dawned on the medical profession in the 1960s: some hearts were, as Claude Beck put it, 'too good to die'. 'Almost every physician has had experiences in which death occurred, and when the heart was examined the damage was inadequate to explain death,' he wrote.[104] A heart attack was not necessarily a fatal event, merely a process that could often be reversed. This was a profound insight that revolutionised the care of cardiac patients. In 1961 a senior registrar at Edinburgh Royal Infirmary, Desmond Julian, proposed a new type of ward for those who had suffered a heart attack, with twenty-four-hour nursing, electronic monitoring and resuscitation equipment.[105] It was not long before these coronary care units started springing up around the world: first in Australia, then hospitals in America and Canada followed suit.[106] Studies published a couple of years later showed that such wards drastically reduced mortality among cardiac patients. This was good news for those already in hospital; but many patients with serious arrhythmias were well most of the time and could not be kept permanently on a ward. What could be done for them?

This was the question the cardiologist Mieczysław Mirowski asked himself in 1966 when an old friend and colleague dropped dead from ventricular tachycardia while having dinner with his family.[107] The condition from which he suffered had been diagnosed weeks earlier and responded to drug therapy, but everybody knew it could recur at any time. Mirowski wondered how his death could have been prevented, short of keeping him permanently in hospital. And then an idea occurred to him: would it be possible to miniaturise a defibrillator, make it work automatically and only when needed, and implant it in a patient?

This was a hugely ambitious project, but Mirowski was a man of exceptional tenacity. A Polish Jew, he grew up in Warsaw and was fifteen when the German army captured the city in 1939. Rather than submit to wearing the yellow star of David he set out on a six-year peregrination through eastern Europe and Russia, living on his wits and covering more than 6,000 miles. When he finally returned to Warsaw in 1945 his entire family, and their home, had disappeared. He went on to study medicine in Poland, France and America, where he worked for Helen Taussig at Johns Hopkins, before finding a job as a cardiologist in Israel. It was there that he conceived the idea of an implantable defibrillator, but his hospital lacked the requisite technical resources to get the project off the ground. It was not until 1968, when he moved to Sinai Hospital in Baltimore, that he was able to make any progress.[108]

There he joined forces with an electronics expert, Morton Mower, who had coincidentally had the same idea for an implantable device. Defibrillators were bulky objects, and Mower was at first sceptical that it would be possible to shrink one to the necessary size. But they soon realised that placing electrodes directly on the heart substantially reduced the voltages necessary to defibrillate, and hence the size of the electrical components involved. A rudimentary prototype was ready by 1969 and was implanted successfully in dogs.[109] Like others before him, Mirowski encountered considerable resistance to the idea, and at least one journal rejected his first paper on the subject.[110] When it was finally printed in 1970, Bernard Lown – the leading authority on defibrillation – was scathing in his response. He suggested that the device was likely to give unnecessary shocks, with possibly fatal results: 'That the heart will be injured is certain; the only uncertainty is its extent.'[111] Another specialist described the proposed device as a 'bomb inside the body'.[112]

Prevailing opinion was so hostile that Mirowski and Mower were unable to raise funding for their project, and at first had to pay for their own equipment. Their situation eased somewhat after they reached agreement with a small medical technology firm, Medrad, to develop the device in partnership. The research was demanding and dangerous, involving electrical currents of thousands of volts. Mower narrowly escaped electrocution when one accidental discharge leapt from the electrode he was working on into a bowl of water six inches away.[113]

Making the device small enough turned out to be relatively straightforward; the main difficulty was how to make it recognise a serious arrhythmia. There was no room for error: a single unnecessary shock to the heart could kill the patient. At first Mirowski used a blood-pressure sensor, but this proved unreliable.[114] The team eventually adopted a method that entailed continuous analysis of the heart's electrical activity, using a mathematical formula called a probability density function to identify the chaotic state characteristic of ventricular fibrillation.[115]

By 1975 they had a working model, which was implanted in dogs. To convince the sceptics, Mower and Mirowski made a short film of the device in action. It showed a normal dog being put into ventricular fibrillation with an electric shock and collapsing as its heart stopped pumping. A few seconds later its unconscious body jerked as the automatic defibrillator went into action, zapping its moribund heart back to life. Shortly afterwards it was awake and got back to its feet.[116] Long-term testing followed, with five dogs given the implantable cardiac defibrillator for periods of up to three years.[117] By late 1979 Mirowski felt that they were ready to put the device into a human.

The first ICD was implanted in an operation at Johns Hopkins on 4 February 1980. The patient was a fifty-seven-year-old woman who had had a heart attack eight years earlier. She had suffered regular episodes of arrhythmia ever since, and on one occasion had only survived because she collapsed on the steps of a hospital, where a defibrillator soon brought her back to life.[118] Mirowski watched as the surgeon, Levi Watkins, attached electrodes to her heart. One was passed through a vein to the right atrium; the other was a rectangular patch that was placed on top of the pericardium. The device itself was placed in a pocket under the skin of the abdomen and then connected to the two electrode leads. This first implantation was an unqualified success: when Mirowski reported the procedure five

months later the patient was still alive and had suffered no more episodes of fibrillation.[119]

Within a year of this landmark operation sixteen patients had
received an ICD. The device could be tested by artificially inducing a
dangerous heart rhythm, and in the vast majority of cases the device
quickly corrected the problem.[120] Many cardiologists remained suspicious of the innovation, however, and over the next few years Mirowski
and his colleagues produced an avalanche of clinical studies to demonstrate that it was both safe and effective. The earliest model was
only able to detect ventricular fibrillation, but by 1983 Mirowski and
Mower had produced a second-generation device – a cardioverter-
defibrillator – which was also able to convert dangerous tachycardias
into a normal heart rhythm.[121]

One early concern about the ICD was its effect on the patient –
how painful would it be to receive a shock of several hundred volts
to the heart? A few early units malfunctioned, imparting a series of
shocks at regular intervals and causing great distress. But when the
ICD functioned normally, patients reported that the sensation was
generally no worse than being given a firm punch in the chest.[122] And
such temporary discomfort was certainly bearable if the alternative
was cardiac arrest and death. When Mirowski began his research,
most of his colleagues believed that there were few patients who
would benefit from such a device. By the mid-1980s it was painfully
apparent that sudden cardiac death was a problem of epidemic pro-
portions – there were thousands of patients whose hearts were in danger of going into a life-threatening arrhythmia at any moment. By 1985
sufficient patients had received the device for researchers to establish whether it was effective in preventing death. The results were
stunning. If left untreated, up to 66 per cent would be expected to die
within a year; but mortality among those who had been implanted
with a device was just 2 per cent.[123] As evidence in its favour piled up,
the medical establishment finally accepted the ICD without reserva-
tion. It had taken twenty years to convince them. The inventor was
fond of quoting his 'three laws of Mirowski': 'Don't give up; don't give

in; and beat the bastards.'[124] There could be no better vindication of his
bloody-mindedness.

By 2009 more than 250,000 ICDs were being implanted every
year worldwide.[125] The current models are vastly more sophisticated
than those of the 1980s, treating a greater range of arrhythmia and
often combining the functions of an ICD and pacemaker in one unit.
The latter has also been transformed: modern pacemakers are fully
programmable, tailoring their response to the needs of the patient,
and record all cardiac activity so that doctors can analyse it in detail,
with data transmitted to a computer wirelessly or even over the
internet.[126]

Today's devices can even be controlled remotely, a fact that provided a chilling plot twist for the TV drama *Homeland*. In an episode
broadcast in 2012, terrorists discover the serial number of the US vice
president's pacemaker and are able to hack into it, accelerating his
heartbeat until he goes into cardiac arrest and dies. Astonishingly, the
scenario is not as far-fetched as it at first appears. In 2008 a group
of researchers investigated the security of wireless-enabled ICDs and
discovered that they were able to take control of them using equipment available on the high street – though a would-be assassin would
have to be standing next to their victim in order to be successful.[127] Nor
was this just a theoretical risk. Vice President Dick Cheney was given
an ICD in 2001 after many years of serious heart trouble. Six years
later the device was replaced with one with wireless capability, and
his cardiologist Jonathan Reiner immediately became worried that it
was vulnerable to malicious attack. At his request the manufacturer
altered its software to disable the function, ensuring that the vice
president would not be the first ever victim of a uniquely futuristic
crime.[128]

The development of the pacemaker and then the ICD was a triumph of technology over disease. In the nineteenth century countless patients suffered from mysterious heart palpitations that
eventually killed them. Today's cardiologists do not use such vague
terminology, and can identify specific arrhythmias and usually treat

them – frequently by implanting an electronic device. This is often a palliative measure given to those who have already suffered a major heart attack. But – as the old adage goes – prevention is better than cure; what if it were possible to identify those at risk of such an event and somehow prevent it? Even as the pacemaker was being perfected in the 1960s another front was opening up against heart disease – one which relied on the old-fashioned virtues of the scalpel and superlative surgical skill.

7. 'STRONG AND PECULIAR SYMPTOMS'

Cleveland, 19 October 1967

Conventional wisdom – and an old proverb – tells us that words will never hurt us, yet on 16 October 1793 the celebrated surgeon John Hunter was killed by an insult. At a bad-tempered meeting of the governors of St George's Hospital in London he became involved in a row about student admissions. Unpleasant words were exchanged, and Hunter grew so irate that he rose from the table and walked out. As he entered the next room he turned to a colleague as if to speak to him, groaned, and fell down dead.[1]

To one of his friends, at least, his death came as no surprise. Edward Jenner, who would later attain everlasting fame by discovering vaccination against smallpox, had realised a decade earlier that Hunter was seriously ill and that his ailment would probably kill him – but decided against raising it on the grounds that 'it must have brought on an unpleasant conference between Mr Hunter and me'.[2] Hunter had himself first noticed worrying symptoms in 1773, and thanks to the meticulous notes he was in the habit of taking about his own health we know what they were. They began with stomach pain, then his face took on a deathly pallor; he struggled to breathe and realised that he could not feel his own pulse. Taking Madeira, brandy and ginger had no effect, but after some time the discomfort finally receded.[3]

Over the next twenty years he experienced many such episodes, with increasing chest pain and inability to tolerate even minor exertion. In the months before his death he was unable to dress or eat dinner without feeling an intolerable weight on his chest.[4]

It's clear from these descriptions of Hunter's illness – chest pain, exacerbated by exercise – that he was suffering from angina pectoris, a symptom of coronary heart disease. It was recognised even millennia earlier: the Ebers Papyrus, an ancient Egyptian medical text dated to around 1500 BC, describes chest pain radiating down the arm and warns that the symptom often betokens imminent death.[5] A thousand years later a famous Indian surgeon, Sushruta, discussed a symptom which he called 'hritshoola', pain above the heart aggravated by exertion and eased by rest.[6] These descriptions were, however, vague, and it was not until the eighteenth century that the ailment acquired its modern name.

The doctor who called it angina pectoris (literally, 'choking of the breast') was William Heberden, a friend and colleague of John Hunter. In 1772 he described 'a disorder of the breast marked with strong and peculiar symptoms', which he had observed in over a hundred patients:

> They who are afflicted with it, are seized while they are walking (more especially if it be up hill, and soon after eating) with a painful and most disagreeable sensation in the breast, which seems as if it would extinguish life, if it were to increase or to continue; but the moment they stand still, all this uneasiness vanishes.[7]

After a year or so the condition tended to worsen so that sufferers experienced pain even at rest. Most of those Heberden examined were men in late middle age, and eventually 'the patients all suddenly fall down, and perish almost immediately'. He had no idea how the condition might be treated, or of its cause: post-mortem studies of its victims revealed 'no fault in the heart, in the valves, in the arteries, or neighbouring veins, excepting some small rudiments of ossification in the aorta'.[8] The importance of this apparently minor finding eluded Heberden, but in 1775 a similar observation was made by the botanist and physician John Fothergill on examining the body of 'H. R.', a rather overweight sixty-three-year-old man who after three years of angina pain had died suddenly while in a violent fit of rage. The heart was found to contain a number of hard plaques, but most significantly, 'the two coronary arteries, from their origin to many of their ramifications upon the heart, were become one piece of bone.'[9]

The importance of this pair of vessels can barely be overstated. Seventeenth-century anatomists named them the coronary arteries (from the Latin *corona*, a crown) because of the way they encircle the heart as a wreath does the head. The coronaries receive their blood via two openings, the coronary ostia at the base of the aorta, and branch out into a network of vessels entwined like tendrils around the heart, which provide the cardiac muscle (the myocardium) with freshly oxygenated blood. Despite their small diameter – 4 millimetres at maximum – they receive as much as 5 per cent of the body's total blood flow, because the myocardium, the muscle that never rests, has an extraordinary thirst for oxygen. In most parts of the human body, about 25 per cent of the oxygen in the blood is removed as it passes through the tissue; the heart's metabolic demands are such that it extracts up to 80 per cent of the available oxygen from its blood supply. During heavy exercise it consumes four times more than the brain, despite being only a fifth of its weight. Given the vital function of the coronary arteries, any blockage impeding the flow of blood to the heart can clearly have catastrophic consequences.

Fothergill's findings were confirmed shortly afterwards by Edward Jenner during an autopsy on the body of another angina patient: while dissecting the heart his knife struck an object so hard that it damaged the blade. His first thought was that some plaster had fallen from the ceiling, but then he saw that the coronaries had become 'bony canals'.[10] He became convinced that coronary artery disease was the cause of angina pain, but when John Hunter started to suffer the same symptoms Jenner decided against making his theory public. It was not until twenty years later that his conjecture was proved correct: a post-mortem on Hunter's body showed that his coronary arteries had turned to 'bony tubes'.[11]

Not all were persuaded, however. When the theory appeared in the first book on angina, written by Caleb Parry and published in 1799, one reviewer challenged it, noting that 'we have more than once hinted a suspicion that the heart is not the organ originally affected'.[12] This scepticism was understandable, since autopsies showed that the dramatic calcification of the coronaries was present in some angina sufferers but not others. Conversely, some hearts with extensive coronary lesions came from individuals who had never suffered from angina. This made it difficult to assume a definite causal relationship between the two, and debate over the nature of the disease would continue for well over a century.

Parry's advice for the angina patient was little more than a counsel of despair, warning against strenuous exertion such as 'loud talking, violent laughter, and every strong effort'. He recommended salt-water enemas, peppermint water and opium, while acknowledging that even these would provide little relief.[13] Therapy had progressed no further by 1855, when the French physician Duchenne de Boulogne described angina as 'the most terrible malady which can endanger a man's life, for having tortured him for some time it almost invariably kills him'.[14] This is no exaggeration: in its advanced stages angina pain can be excruciating, and many sufferers have an overpowering sense that death is imminent. Medicine could offer no respite until 1867, when the young Scottish physician Thomas Lauder Brunton discovered that inhaling a few drops of amyl nitrite from a cloth gave rapid pain relief. When he tested the drug on a patient at St Bartholomew's Hospital who had been enduring angina attacks lasting up to an hour every night, the man's pain disappeared completely in less than a minute.[15] The mechanism of its action remained unknown for some decades, but amyl nitrite was later identified as a vasodilator – a chemical that relaxes and temporarily widens the blood vessels.

Though some progress had been made in alleviating the symptoms, physicians were little closer to understanding angina's cause. At the beginning of the twentieth century there were many theories: some believed it was a disorder of the spine or nerves,[16] others that it was definitely a stomach problem.[17] The leading British cardiologist, Sir James Mackenzie, suggested that weakness of the cardiac muscle was to blame.[18] But another group of physicians were becoming increasingly confident that coronary artery disease was the culprit, as Jenner had first suspected. They would eventually be proved right, aided by the careful work of a researcher in Chicago, James Herrick, who was interested in coronary thrombosis, the formation of clots in the coronary arteries.

Most physicians believed that coronary thrombosis was inevitably fatal: if anything obstructed the arteries it would starve the heart muscle of blood, causing more or less instant death. Herrick found that this was not necessarily true, showing that several of the hundreds of hearts he examined at autopsy had coronary arteries which had been obstructed for many years before death. It must often be possible, he concluded, for blood to find an alternative route through the extensive network of connections in the coronary circulation, or for new vessels to form in response. Crucially, he also suggested that 'slight angina attacks . . . may well be due to obstruction of small coronary twigs' – tiny branches of the vessels.[19] This would explain why autopsies often failed to find coronary disease in those who had suffered from angina – the disease might be diffuse: spread through the smaller vessels, rather than concentrated in the readily visible larger branches. When he announced his findings to a meeting of the Association of American Physicians in 1912, Herrick later recalled, his presentation 'fell flat as a pancake'[20] – and it would be almost a decade before his ideas were generally accepted.

Slowly, the relationship between coronary artery disease, angina and heart attacks was becoming clear. The coronary arteries, it turned out, are particularly susceptible to atherosclerosis, a process in which a hard, fatty deposit is laid down on the inner surface of the blood vessel. As the plaque grows it obstructs the vessel, impeding blood flow to the heart muscle. If the occlusion is severe, a region of the myocardium becomes starved of oxygen, or ischaemic, causing the pain of angina. Plaques may also provoke the formation of a thrombus or clot, causing a sudden obstruction so severe that a large area of myocardium dies. This is a myocardial infarction, also known as a heart attack – if a large area of the muscle is affected it will cause cardiac arrest and death, but smaller infarctions may have comparatively minor effects.

Herrick could only suggest using drugs to treat angina patients, but he also made a prescient remark which hinted at the eventual solution: 'The hope for the damaged myocardium lies in the direction of securing a supply of blood through friendly neighbouring vessels so as to restore so far as possible its functional integrity.'[21] More than fifty years of surgical effort would be expended in the pursuit of this apparently modest goal.

With the medical profession yet to reach a consensus on what the condition was or what caused it, the first operations to treat angina aimed to reduce the symptoms rather than effect a cure. In late nineteenth-century France there was a brief vogue for the notion that many common diseases were attributable to disorders of the nerves. The physiologist Charles-Émile François-Franck suggested in 1899 that angina might be treated by sympathectomy, an operation which entailed cutting through one of the nerve clusters near the spine. The procedure had become fashionable for treating a range of disorders, including Graves' disease, epilepsy, glaucoma and 'idiocy'[22] – though probably without much benefit. He believed that angina was caused by the irritation of a specific nerve at the base of the neck; severing it ought to cure the condition.

Nobody attempted to test this theory until 1916, when the Romanian Thoma Ionescu became the first person to treat angina surgically. His patient was a thirty-eight-year-old man who enjoyed a dual career working in the law courts and singing in a church choir. This evidently did little for his moral wellbeing, since he was also syphilitic, alcoholic and a heavy smoker. When he arrived at the Coltea Hospital in Bucharest he was diagnosed with angina, and on 2 April Ionescu operated, using a local anaesthetic so that the patient remained conscious throughout. The procedure, which the surgeon described as 'very delicate, but not at all difficult', involved severing a large nerve at the base of the neck. As Ionescu grasped the nerve to pull it free of its anchorage near the spine, the patient cried out, saying that he could feel 'electric vibrations' running along the fingers of his left hand. He soon recovered, however, and within a few days was well enough to go home.

In the chaos of wartime Ionescu soon lost touch with his patient, and resigned himself to the possibility that he might never learn whether the operation had been successful. To his delight, four years later the man reappeared, having sought out the surgeon to thank him for curing his symptoms. He reported that he had felt no more pain and was back at work. Nor had he curtailed his vices: 'I have not even broken off my friendly relations with Bacchus,' he told Ionescu, 'since my job demands it.'[23]

Sympathectomy was subsequently adopted in several European and American hospitals, with Walter Coffey and Philip Brown, two surgeons from San Francisco, reporting 'brilliant successes' in their attempts to relieve angina.[24] By now, however, most experts agreed that they were treating the symptom, not the cause: severing nerves made the patient's life more comfortable by preventing pain signals from reaching the brain, but did nothing to treat the underlying disease.* Researchers started to look for a better operation.[25]

An alternative was tried in the early 1930s with some success. Like sympathectomy it was an 'indirect' operation, since it made no effort to attack the coronary arteries directly. It entailed simply cutting out the thyroid, the large hormone-secreting gland in the neck

---

* In many cases it was highly effective. The operation is still sometimes performed today for patients with severe angina which cannot be treated by any other method.

which – among other things – regulates the speed of the metabolism. Surgeons had noticed that when patients with an overactive thyroid who also had heart disease were treated by excision of the gland, their cardiac symptoms often improved. Removing the thyroid slowed the metabolism, which in turn reduced the heart muscle's need for oxygen. This led Elliott Cutler, the pioneer of mitral valve surgery, to speculate that the same might be true for patients who had heart disease but no sign of thyroid disorder.[26]

The first test took place at the Peter Bent Brigham Hospital in Boston in June 1932, in an operation performed by Cutler's colleague John Homans, who removed a large portion of the thyroid from a fifty-three-year-old painter whose angina was getting progressively worse. When he left hospital some weeks later he still experienced occasional angina, but the attacks were less frequent.[27] This and other encouraging early results emboldened Cutler to try the more radical operation of total thyroidectomy, in which the whole gland was removed.[28] The procedure was often successful, and some surgeons adopted it as their preferred treatment for patients with severe and intractable angina. But they knew they were avoiding the real challenge, the impaired blood supply to the heart muscle; and while Cutler and his colleagues in Boston were developing their thyroid hypothesis, Claude Beck was at work in his Cleveland laboratory, trying to attack the problem directly.

Beck's interest in the possibilities of surgical intervention on the heart had emerged a quarter of a century before he became the first person to use a defibrillator in 1947. In the early 1920s he began a series of more than 1,200 experimental cardiac operations, concentrating on myocardial revascularisation – the creation of an artificial blood supply for the heart muscle. But the crucial insight came from an observation he made a decade later during an operation in November 1934. The patient had survived a heart attack, causing a large area of dead tissue on the myocardium which Beck was attempting to remove. A section of the scar had become attached to the pericardium, and when he cut through this adhesion Beck noticed that it bled briskly.[29] This surprised him: when scar tissue forms inside the body it often sticks two adjacent structures together, but Beck had never heard of this process creating new blood vessels as well. He spoke to a colleague, the pathologist Alan Moritz, who told Beck that he had seen the same thing in four hearts with pericardial adhesions. Moritz wanted to know how these new vessels communicated with the rest of the circulation, so he injected them with a jet-black solution of soot to see where it would go next. To his surprise, it seeped out all over the myocardium: the newly formed vessels had infiltrated the heart muscle, like the roots of a plant in moist earth.[30] Intrigued, Beck wondered whether it might be possible to initiate this process deliberately, thereby creating a new blood supply for the heart.

After a long series of experiments on dogs, Beck hit upon a promising procedure. By early 1935 he felt ready to try it on a patient, and in February the perfect subject presented himself. Joseph Krchmar was a forty-eight-year-old former coal-miner from Ohio. Five years earlier he had started to suffer from angina, forcing him to take up less strenuous work on a farm. The attacks became so severe that he could not get out of bed and had an overwhelming sense that he was about to die. In this desperate condition he readily agreed to an operation, though Beck told him cautiously that it was a 'thousand to one' chance that it would work. On the morning of 13 February he was wheeled into an operating theatre at Lakeside Hospital, accompanied by his wife Laura, who insisted on watching the procedure.[31]

Beck began by making an incision in the pectoral muscle on the left side of Krchmar's chest. Then he cut open the pericardium and roughened its inside surface with a file, before scraping off the epicardium, the layer of protective tissue coating the heart muscle. As he did this the heart began to beat unpredictably, and Beck was forced to pause repeatedly to make sure it did not go into a fatal spasm. He then sutured two sections of pectoral muscle, complete with the large artery supplying it, to the surface of the heart and closed the chest. The surgeon hoped that new blood vessels would soon appear between this muscle graft and the myocardium, bringing more oxygen to the heart and relieving the angina pain.

Krchmar remained in hospital for three months; when he finally left, Beck recorded that 'The worried expression has left him, and he has a fine spirit.'[32] It wasn't just his mood that had improved: the angina attacks were banished. The only side-effect was weakness in the left arm, caused by the loss of pectoral muscle, which ruled out a return to manual work. Though Krchmar survived for another fifteen years, this physical diminishment meant his story was not an entirely happy one. Deprived of his livelihood, his chances of finding a job during the Depression were slim, and he was forced to live on benefits. Two years after his operation he told an interviewer he was not sure it had been worthwhile,[33] and newspapers were quick to point out the absurdity that a society capable of such medical marvels could not provide Krchmar with something so basic as a job.[34]

While Beck was trying to create an artificial cardiac blood supply in his laboratory at the edge of Lake Erie, another surgeon was conducting parallel research on the greyhound racing tracks of south London. Laurence O'Shaughnessy was in his early thirties and already one of the leading British thoracic surgeons when he began to investigate the possibilities of myocardial revascularisation. Shortly after beginning his experiments he had a chance conversation with a dog-racing aficionado, who told him about Mick the Miller, a celebrated greyhound which had been forced to retire through ill health in 1931. O'Shaughnessy learned that the breed was particularly prone to heart failure, and that there were many dogs which might benefit from the treatment he was trying to develop.[35]

O'Shaughnessy's idea mirrored Beck's, except that instead of grafting a muscle to the heart he used the omentum, an apron of fat which sits in front of the intestines. He had already used this tissue in operations on the throat, and noted its excellent blood supply and propensity for forming new vessels wherever it was attached. To test the procedure, O'Shaughnessy first needed to replicate the effects of coronary artery disease in a healthy greyhound. So he tied off one

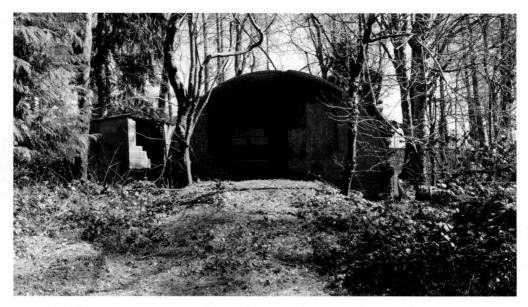

The last remaining Quonset hut on the site of the US 160th General Hospital in Gloucestershire. During the Second World War Dwight Harken used one of these ramshackle buildings as an operating theatre, removing shrapnel fragments from the hearts of more than 50 soldiers without a single death.

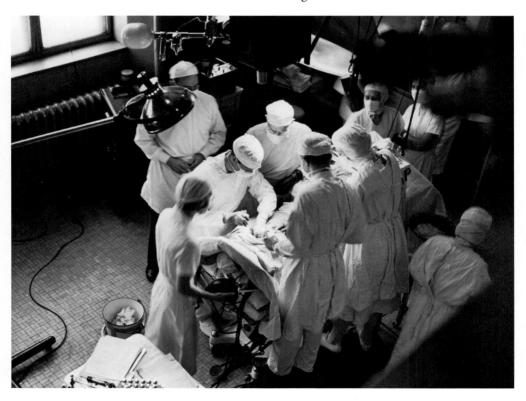

Alfred Blalock (centre) performs a Blue Baby operation at Johns Hopkins Hospital in Baltimore. Vivien Thomas is standing behind him.

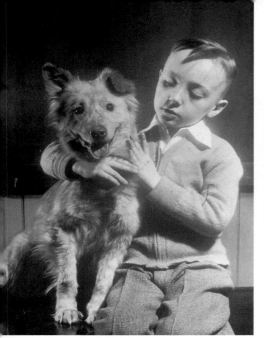

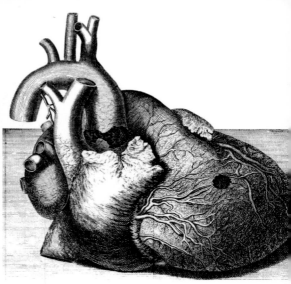

Michael Schirmer, aged five, with Anna the experimental dog. Schirmer lived for another 69 years after undergoing the Blue Baby operation in 1945.

The heart of King George II, who died suddenly while using the royal lavatory in 1760. The dark area visible at the base of the largest blood vessel, the aorta, is the catastrophic rupture believed to have killed him.

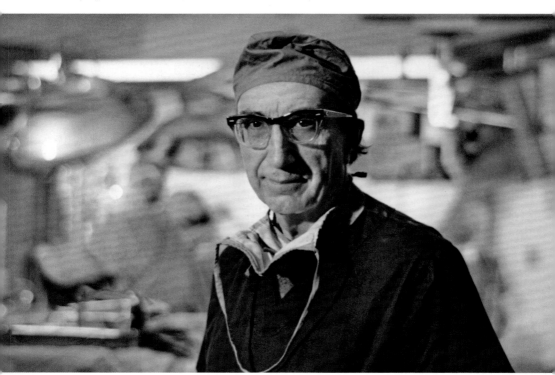

Michael DeBakey, one of the most innovative and prominent figures in cardiac surgery, whose extraordinary surgical career spanned more than six decades.

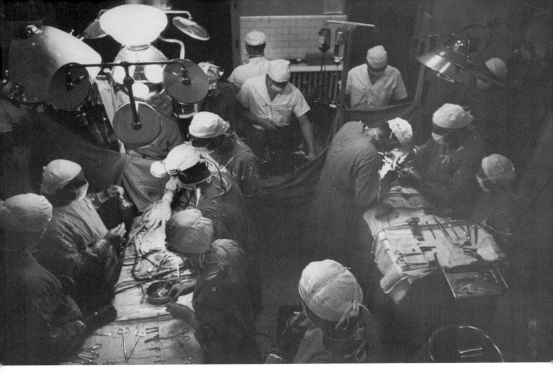

C. Walton Lillehei (left, wearing headlamp) performs open-heart surgery in 1954 using cross-circulation. The life of his five-month-old patient, Marsha Gilliam, is being sustained by the heart and lungs of her mother on the right. Marsha is still alive at the time of writing.

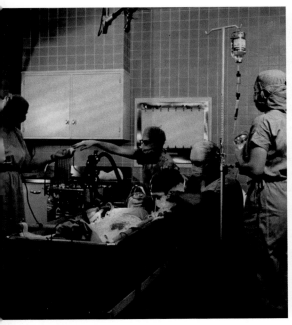

A patient being cooled to 28°C in an ice bath in preparation for hypothermic open-heart surgery at the US National Institutes of Health in 1955.

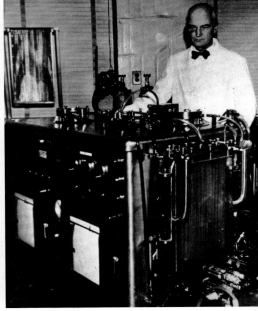

John Gibbon with the second model of the Gibbon–IBM heart-lung machine.

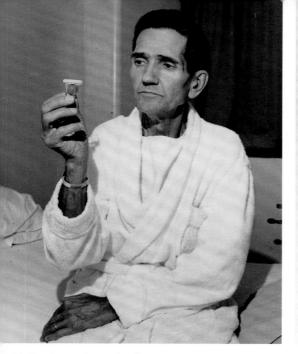

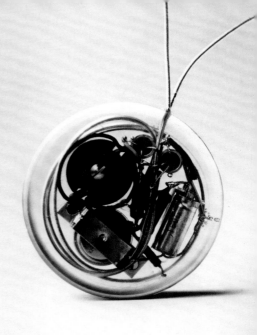

Philip Amundson, the first patient to receive a Starr–Edwards artificial valve, examining the simple device that saved his life.

The world's first implantable pacemaker, constructed by Rune Elmqvist and implanted in 1958. It was approximately 55mm in diameter and 25mm thick – the dimensions of the shoe polish tin Elmqvist used to encase it in plastic.

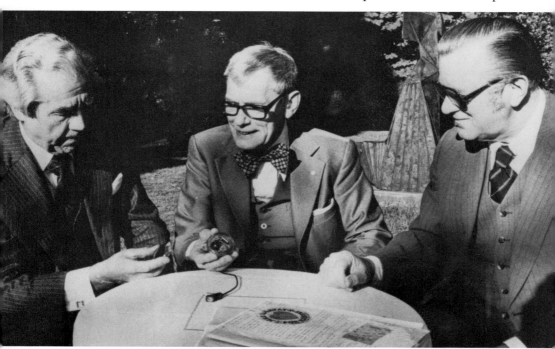

Left to right: the surgeon Åke Senning, Rune Elmqvist and Arne Larsson, the recipient of the first implantable pacemaker, at a reunion marking the twentieth anniversary of the operation.

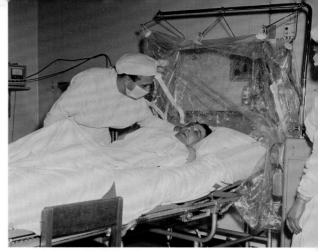

The world's most famous patient: Louis Washkansky is examined by Christiaan Barnard shortly after receiving a new heart in December 1967.

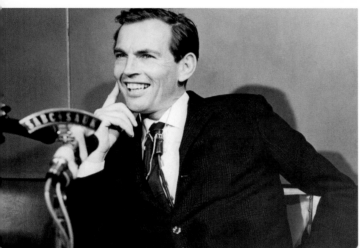

A relaxed Christiaan Barnard faces the press. His charisma and good looks helped make him the instantly recognisable poster boy for the early transplant era.

Gerald Scarfe's uncompromising take on Barnard's feat articulates the fears of many who saw organ transplantation as a modern form of bodysnatching.

The cartoon's captions read:
Patient: But Doctor – I don't think I'm dead.
Doctor: Don't worry you soon will be.

The placard on the patient's bed reads:
Symptoms *Sore Finger*

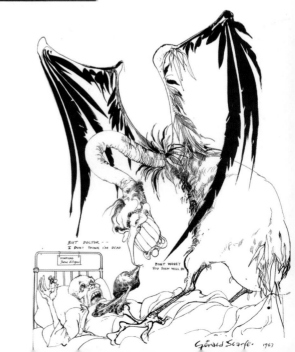

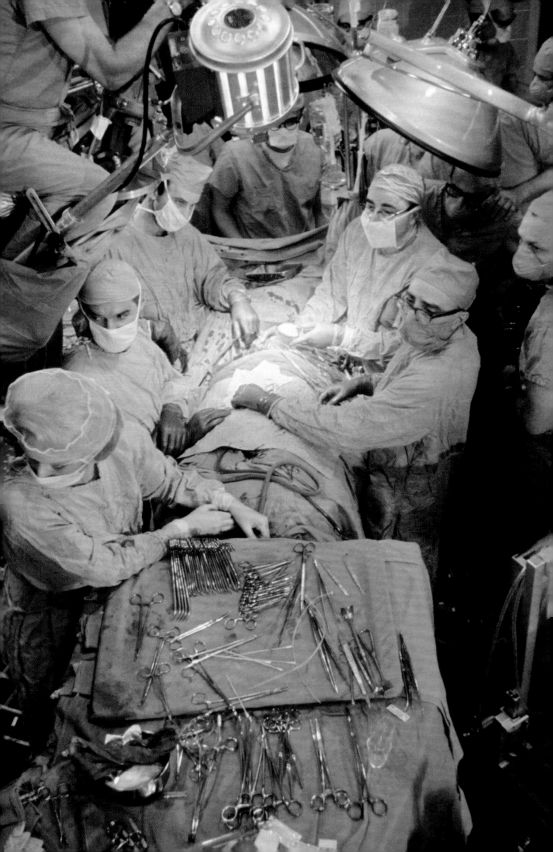

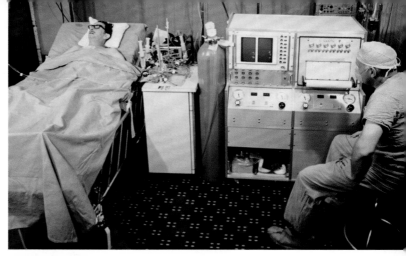

Right: Haskell Karp, the recipient of the first total artificial heart. The control console for the device is on the right.

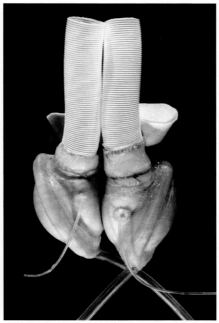

Left: The artificial heart that was implanted into Haskell Karp by Denton Cooley on 4 April 1969. The original device is now in the collections of the National Museum of American History in Washington, D. C.

Opposite page: Michael DeBakey (front right) during the operation to implant an LVAD into Marcel DeRudder in April 1966. Such groundbreaking and complex procedures often involved a huge team of specialists.

'Even though I have an artificial heart, I still love you.' Barney Clark, the first recipient of a permanent artificial heart, with his wife Una Loy. He survived for 112 days after implantation.

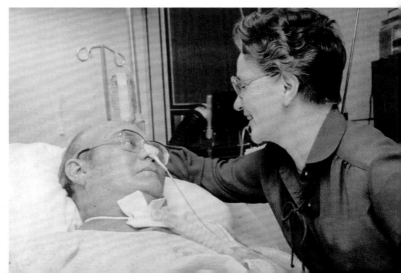

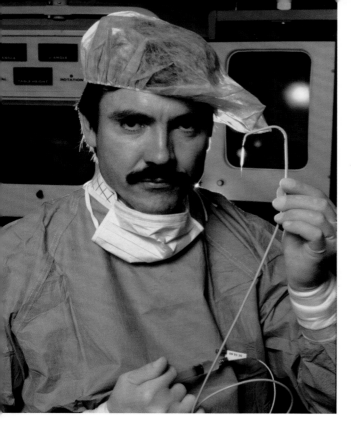

Andreas Grüntzig brandishing the balloon catheter he invented in 1977, which made it possible to perform percutaneous interventions on the coronary arteries. Grüntzig and his wife both died in 1985 when the light aircraft he was piloting crashed during a storm. He was 46, and his wife only 29.

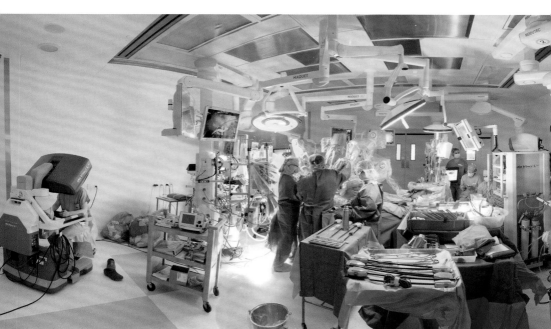

Robotic cardiac surgery in progress at Jewish General Hospital in Montreal. The surgeon, Dr Emmanuel Moss, sitting at the console on the far left, controls the plastic-covered robotic arms above the operating table in the centre of the picture.

of the coronary arteries to reduce the blood flow to its heart muscle, which left it struggling to complete a circuit of the track. The next day he attached a graft of omentum to the affected section of its heart wall; five months later the dog was able to run just as well as it had when healthy.[36]

The following year O'Shaughnessy moved on to human patients. He tried several alternative approaches, some of which did not involve the omentum: one used an abrasive paste to provoke adhesions between the pericardium and heart, and another entailed suturing part of the lung to the cardiac surface.[37] In every case the rationale was the same: to attach a new source of blood to the ischaemic heart muscle, in the hope that new vessels would sprout between them. By 1938 he had operated on twenty patients: six died, but most experienced some degree of relief from their angina.[38] O'Shaughnessy's efforts were brought to a halt by the outbreak of war, when he volunteered as an army surgeon; in May 1940 he was struck by a shell fragment during the evacuation of Dunkirk and killed. News of his death took some days to reach London, where his brother-in-law George Orwell was anxiously scouring the railway stations for any sign of him.[39] The loss of this gifted surgeon at the age of thirty-nine was a huge blow to the medical world – and, arguably, to literature. In 1947 Orwell was diagnosed with tuberculosis, which was to kill him three years later. Nobody would have been better equipped to treat him than O'Shaughnessy, the country's leading expert in the disease.

Beck and O'Shaughnessy's first operations were among the most daring yet performed upon the heart, but Dwight Harken's wartime triumphs would soon show that even more radical procedures were feasible. When Beck was able to resume his work in 1945 he modified his original technique, using grafts of fat and pericardial tissue rather than pectoral muscle. Powdered beef bone or asbestos was first sprinkled on the surface of the heart, to provoke inflammation and the growth of new vessels.[40] He continued to use this procedure (the 'Beck

I' operation) until the 1950s, although in 1948 he unveiled an alternative, the 'Beck II'.

This procedure took an entirely different approach. Beck turned his attention to the coronary sinus, the large vein which collects deoxygenated blood from the myocardium and returns it to the right atrium. He was interested in the possibility of using the vessel as a direct route to the heart muscle – in effect, turning it from a vein into an artery. This was achieved in two stages. In the first operation a vessel was harvested from the patient's arm, and used to make a shunt which delivered oxygenated blood from the aorta to the coronary sinus. At a second, a few weeks later, he used a ligature to reduce the diameter of the sinus, a crucial step which increased the pressure in the vessel and reversed the flow of blood.[41] In a normal heart, blood percolates downwards from the coronaries and through the myocardium before collecting in the coronary sinus at the bottom of the heart; after the Beck II operation the reduced circulation through the diseased coronaries was augmented by a new supply flowing backwards through the sinus. In Beck's hands this was a notable success: in 1957 he reported that in his last seventy-seven patients the mortality had been zero.[42] But it was a major and dangerous undertaking, entailing at least two separate operations, and few other surgeons were willing to take it on. 'Patients who have been operated upon recommend the operation to others who have the disease,' Beck wrote. 'They cannot understand why [it] has not gained greater acceptance by the medical profession.'[43]

Beck performed more than 5,000 experimental operations over thirty years in developing his procedures,[44] so the note of exasperation is understandable. But, as his peers pointed out, there was no objective proof that the operations worked. Yes, the majority of patients said they felt better, but was the effect real or merely psychological? There was as yet no way of measuring blood flow to the myocardium directly, so Beck could only assess his results by his patients' subjective impressions. Besides, by the late 1950s something better had come along.

That was thanks to the Canadian Arthur Vineberg. He began his experiments in 1945, and spent the next seventeen years trying to persuade his colleagues at Royal Victoria Hospital in Montreal that his method really worked. Vineberg realised that when there was a serious blockage to a coronary artery, attaching other structures to the cardiac surface (the lung, omentum, muscle and even the small intestine[45] had been tried) would not deliver anything like enough blood to the parched myocardium. His approach was more radical: he wanted to create an artificial third coronary artery. After a series of animal experiments he finally found a way of doing this, one that involved some radical replumbing. His intention was to find an artery which could be removed from its usual function without damaging tissues elsewhere in the body, and reroute it so that it provided a substantial supply of blood to the heart muscle.

The vessel he chose was the internal mammary artery. There are two of these, running in parallel inside the ribcage down the middle of the breastbone, supplying blood to the chest wall between the collar bone and the navel. Vineberg knew that sacrificing it would have little effect on nearby tissues, since plenty of blood would still reach them from an extensive network of collaterals. He began by freeing the artery from its position in the chest wall and cutting through it; the bleeding end was then fixed in a tunnel excavated in the wall of the heart. It was a crude measure, and its first results were not especially promising. But when Vineberg examined the body of the eighth dog to undergo the operation he found something truly exciting: after four months the artery implanted into its heart muscle had sprouted new vessels. Dye injected into it flowed directly into the coronary circulation, indicating that the procedure had successfully created a new blood supply to the myocardium.[46]

The transition from canine to human subjects had the most disappointing start possible in April 1950 when the first patient died two days after the operation. At autopsy it transpired that both of his coronary arteries were totally blocked by clots, but the new graft was still functional.[47] Vineberg's second attempt, six months later, was far more positive. His patient was a fifty-four-year-old oil worker who was living on a liquid diet because solid food resulted in intolerable angina. By the time he left hospital in December he was eating normally, completely free of pain and back at work.[48] Three years later his recovery was startling: previously able to walk only a few yards, he could now hike ten miles over rough terrain.[49]

After five years' experience with the operation, Vineberg was sure of its efficacy. Patients who were least severely disabled – those who experienced angina only during exercise – did particularly well, with 88 per cent returning to work after treatment.[50] But he was well aware that his colleagues would only be satisfied by proof that new and useful blood vessels were being formed on the heart, and devoted considerable effort to proving beyond doubt that this was happening. Controversy raged for several years, with many surgeons unwilling to accept his findings. In 1960 a sensational piece of research was published which did not merely cast doubt on Vineberg's work, but had profound implications for surgery in general.

While Beck and Vineberg persevered with their operations for angina, a few other procedures had become popular with surgeons elsewhere. One of the most successful, pioneered in Italy in the early 1950s, involved placing a ligature around the two internal mammary arteries. Although the results were often excellent, there was a great deal of scepticism about the technique, since there seemed to be no plausible reason why it should work: all it did was impair blood flow to the muscles and bones of the chest. So a group at the University of Washington decided to settle the matter with a double-blind trial, the first time such a thing had ever been used to test the outcomes of internal surgery. It involved seventeen patients with angina, randomly divided into two groups. The first group were given the genuine operation: under local anaesthetic, a surgeon made a skin incision and then tied the mammary arteries. The second went through a sham operation, a procedure in which the surgeon merely opened an incision and then closed it again. Crucially, not even the patient's own doctors knew whether they had received a genuine or a fake operation.

The researchers were stunned to discover that there was no difference between the two groups. Of the nine patients who underwent the sham operation, five noted significant improvement, and two who had been severely disabled before their 'surgery' were once again able to engage in strenuous exercise.[51] The artery-tying operation was obviously worthless. Rarely has there been a more striking demonstration of the placebo effect, whereby the mere expectation of recovery improves a patient's condition. As the heart surgeon Donald Effler put it, 'The patient with coronary artery disease gets initial relief of angina from almost anything: this includes walking into the reception room of the surgeon's office.'[52] It was a dramatic indication that clinicians needed to find physical proof of improvement rather than rely on the patient's impressions.

Fortunately for Vineberg, powerful evidence was not long in coming. Donald Effler was in charge of the cardiothoracic surgery department at the Cleveland Clinic where, in 1958, one of his colleagues, the cardiologist Mason Sones, originated a method of observing blood flowing through the coronary arteries of the living heart, a discovery he made entirely by accident. One morning Sones was performing a procedure known as an aortogram, an X-ray of the aorta. To make the relevant structures visible, a special dye had to be injected into the aortic root via a catheter just before the photograph was taken. Unknown to Sones, the tip of the catheter had slipped from its proper position and the dye was instead delivered straight into the right coronary artery. This was a disaster, since it was generally believed that flooding the coronaries with a foreign substance would cause death. Expecting his patient's heart to stop, Sones leapt up to grab a scalpel so that he could open the chest and perform cardiac massage. There was a brief period of arrest, but a few seconds later the patient was very much alive and having a violent coughing fit, more surprised than hurt.[53] Sones immediately realised that this meant it was safe to inject a small amount of dye directly into the coronaries and thereby make them visible on an X-ray. A high-speed cine camera could then provide moving images of the passage of blood through the vessels, and highlight any areas of blockage.

This technique, selective coronary arteriography, was a giant leap forward which not only enabled precise diagnosis of coronary disease, but allowed Sones and his colleagues to study the results of surgical interventions. In 1962 Donald Effler was considering whether to adopt the Vineberg procedure but remained unconvinced of its worth, so at his request two patients who had undergone the operation several years earlier were sent to the clinic for examination. After studying X-rays of the grafts, Sones found that Vineberg's claims were entirely accurate: the mammary artery implanted into the heart had formed new branches which communicated with the coronaries, providing a new source of blood for the myocardium.[54] Vineberg's operation was widely adopted after this emphatic vindication, and surgeons continued to perform it until the mid-1970s. One patient who underwent the procedure in 1969 survived for twenty-one symptom-free years.[55]

The procedures of Beck, Vineberg and others had succeeded in providing a new blood supply to the myocardium, but left the coronary arteries themselves untouched; surgeons flirted with a great many novel techniques in the 1960s as they attempted to move their focus to the vessels actually affected by the disease. The logical – but hazardous – approach to treating blocked arteries was simply to remove the obstruction. Walton Lillehei had shown that this was possible in experiments on cadavers in 1956, slitting open the affected vessels, removing the plaque and then stitching them back together.[56] Later that year Charles Bailey successfully used this technique – known as coronary endarterectomy – on a patient, inserting a fine cannula through an incision in the artery to remove a 7-millimetre plug of fatty deposit.[57]

Unlike the Vineberg operation, which took months to establish a new circulation, endarterectomy restored blood flow immediately, raising the possibility that it could be used to treat a patient in the immediate aftermath of coronary thrombosis. But scraping the delicate vessels with a metal instrument was likely to damage them, and a less traumatic method of endarterectomy was also developed, using a high-pressure jet of carbon dioxide gas to blast obstructions out of the diseased arteries.[58] Both approaches suffered from the same shortcoming: the coronary arteries tended to become constricted where they had been incised and sutured, once again reducing the diameter of the vessel. There was no point in intervening at all if the condition simply recurred a few months later. Åke Senning found a way round this difficulty, using a strip of artery taken from elsewhere in the body to cover the incision.[59] It was an idea as simple as patching the threadbare elbow of a much-loved coat – but required phenomenal dexterity, since the 'sleeve' in question was only 2 millimetres wide. For the few who could master the technique it was a valuable means of restoring a diseased coronary artery to its natural diameter, once any blockage had been cleared. Though they held a place in the cardiac surgeon's repertoire for several years, endarterectomy and patch-grafting were soon to be superseded by an operation incomparably better.

In 1962 a young Argentinian called René Favaloro joined Effler's department at the Cleveland Clinic from a tiny rural hospital in the Pampas. Born in 1923 in La Plata in eastern Argentina, Favaloro studied medicine at the city's university, intending to become a surgeon, but his early career was blighted by the oppressive political climate of the time. In 1949 he was offered a prestigious training post, on condition that he first signed a piece of paper affirming the policies of President Juan Perón's regime. This he refused to do, choosing instead to live in self-imposed exile in Jacinto Aráuz, a small and impoverished town more than 400 miles away.[60] He was eventually joined there by his brother, and from nothing the two men built up a small but well-equipped hospital with its own laboratory and operating theatre. Favaloro performed thousands of operations, accumulating experience which ranged from childbirth to major abdominal surgery. Despite his isolation he kept abreast of the rapid development of cardiac surgery, and after twelve years decided to move to America to be trained in the new speciality.

When Favaloro arrived in Cleveland he spoke English poorly and knew nobody. Although he was thirty-nine and vastly experienced he was also unlicensed to work as a surgeon, so was obliged to study for the relevant qualifications. But his boss Donald Effler was willing to overlook this detail, allowing him to assist in the operating theatre. In his spare time Favaloro spent hours watching Mason Sones's large archive of X-ray films, learning how to interpret them and trying to identify the recurring features of coronary disease. When he finally began work as a staff surgeon the Vineberg procedure was the operation of choice for most patients, and in 1966 Favaloro introduced a significant improvement. Instead of implanting one internal mammary artery he used both, doubling the area of the myocardium that could receive a new blood supply.[61] But he and his colleagues were still dissatisfied. The Vineberg procedure was slow to have any effect, and endarterectomy was plagued with complications including blood clots. It was time to experiment.

Favaloro was fascinated by the success of the Cleveland Clinic's vascular surgeons, who had been doing innovative work in the reconstruction of diseased blood vessels. They used sections of vein taken from the patient's own leg to replace the arteries supplying the kidneys, or to provide a detour around an obstructed vessel in the limbs. A harvested vein makes an ideal substitute for a diseased artery, though with one caveat: most veins, unlike arteries, contain valves to prevent blood flowing backwards. The surgeon must therefore be careful to attach it the right way round, since blood will only travel in one direction through the vein. Joining two vessels like this is known as 'anastomosis', a Greek word meaning to 'provide a new mouth'.

In early 1967 Favaloro began to think that using a vein graft in this way might be a good method of bringing a new blood supply to the heart muscle.[62] He had also noticed that a substantial number of patients with coronary disease had only a localised blockage near the top of the artery: below this point the vessels were still healthy. A graft attached below the obstruction could theoretically deliver all the blood the myocardium needed.[63] This was not quite a new idea, since a similar scheme had been proposed by Alexis Carrel more than half a century earlier. In a famous paper on experimental heart surgery published in 1910, Carrel wrote: 'In certain cases of angina pectoris, when the mouth of the coronary arteries is calcified, it would be useful to establish a complementary circulation for the useful part of the arteries.' This was prophetic in the extreme, especially if one considers that it was written at a time when many experts believed angina to be a stomach disorder. Carrel even managed to attach a portion of preserved artery between the descending aorta and the left coronary artery of a dog, but the animal died: he had no heart-lung machine, and the operation interrupted the circulation for too long for the heart to recover.[64]

Carrel's visionary genius is underlined by the fact that nobody attempted to repeat his bypass procedure for another forty-three years. In 1953 two surgeons on opposite sides of the world stumbled across similar techniques for attaching a new blood vessel to the coronaries. Vladimir Demikhov, a maverick researcher at the Institute of Surgery in Moscow famous for a series of bizarre experiments in organ transplantation, succeeded in performing bypass operations on a series of dogs, some of which survived for over two years.[65] Unaware of his work, Gordon Murray in Toronto used a piece of preserved carotid artery to bring blood from a dog's aorta into its coronary circulation.[66] He suggested that the technique might be used in humans, but most of his colleagues were incredulous, believing that the 2-millimetre-wide coronary arteries were too small to have anything attached to them. The equipment of the period certainly made such an anastomosis extremely difficult: surgeons only had access to rather unwieldy multifilament thread made from cotton or silk. In the next decade a new generation of polymer suture material would be developed, finer than a human hair and stronger than steel, making it possible to stitch tissue with unprecedented accuracy.

Given surgeons' obsession with priority, it is strange that there is so much disagreement about who was the first person to perform a coronary artery bypass graft (CABG, pronounced 'cabbage'). In the 1960s no fewer than five surgeons independently devised a procedure recognisable as a CABG and applied it to a human patient; and the man generally acknowledged as its inventor, René Favaloro, was the last to do so. This confusion arose because the pioneers of cardiac surgery sometimes worked in isolation, unaware that colleagues elsewhere were doing very similar research; and also because several were not aware of the potential impact of what, to them, seemed a minor innovation.

The first was Robert Goetz, a little-known surgeon in New York, who on 2 May 1960 used a metal ring to attach a patient's internal mammary artery to his right coronary artery. The procedure was a miracle of choreography, with four surgeons all taking a role as the two arteries were stitched together in a breathtaking seventeen seconds. Haste seems to have trumped speed, however, as the anastomosis was accidentally ripped apart in the confusion, and it took a further ninety seconds to repair the damage. The patient survived for a year, but many of Goetz's colleagues were bitterly opposed to what he had done. All trace of the operation mysteriously disappeared from hospital records, and he was never allowed to repeat it.[67] Two years later David Sabiston, a surgeon in North Carolina, used a vein taken from the leg to bypass a blocked coronary artery, but his patient died shortly afterwards from a stroke.[68]

The next in this series of 'firsts' was a thrilling piece of improvisation. In November 1964 Edward Garrett, a junior colleague of Michael DeBakey's in Houston, was operating on a forty-two-year-old truck driver whose coronary arteries were 85 per cent obstructed by fatty deposits. His attempts to scrape them out failed when the vessels disintegrated, and in desperation Garrett decided to employ a technique he had only practised in animals. An incision was hurriedly made in the patient's leg, a portion of the saphenous vein was removed, then used to bypass the coronary blockage. Although this was a notable

surgical achievement, Garrett seems to have overlooked its significance. He did not make any public report of the case until seven years
later, when the patient was still alive and without symptoms.[69]

The work of the Russian Vasilii Kolesov also went unrecognised –
at least in the West – for some years. Kolesov was a military surgeon
amid the horrors of the siege of Leningrad, and continued to operate
in the most basic conditions while German bombs rained down on his
beleaguered hospital.[70] Around a million people died during the siege,
many of them from starvation, and given the terrible deprivation in
wartime Leningrad it is not surprising that many of the survivors
developed severe cardiovascular disease. Kolesov naturally developed
an interest in the subject, and when he became aware of Demikhov's
work he resolved to turn it into a procedure which could be used on
humans. His first bypass graft was performed on 25 February 1964,
using a mammary artery which was sutured to a branch of the left
coronary. The patient did well, and Kolesov continued to perform the
procedure on a regular basis – the only surgeon in the world to do
so for the next three years.[71] But it was not until 1967, when one of
his articles was translated into English and published in an American
journal,[72] that experts outside Russia knew anything of his consistent
success.*

Favaloro's first attempt, on a middle-aged woman, used a slightly
different technique from those tried before. Rather than attach a new
blood supply to the coronaries he simply used a short length of saphenous vein to bypass the obstruction, cutting out the blocked section of
artery and then using the graft to bridge the gap.[73] Though he subsequently used the technique on more than fifty patients, it was fiddly in
the extreme, and he eventually abandoned it. He decided it would be
both easier and more effective to use the graft to divert high-pressure
blood direct from the aorta to the coronaries – the exact method used

---

* Donald Effler is known to have read this article, so it is likely that Favaloro and his
colleagues at the Cleveland Clinic were aware of Kolesov's work when they embarked
on their historic series of operations later that year.

in Houston five years earlier, although Garrett's silence meant that Favaloro had no idea that that operation had even taken place.

One afternoon in the summer of 1967, Eugene Pottenger, a vegetable wholesaler in DeKalb, Illinois, was moving boxes of produce around his warehouse when he felt a strange sensation in his neck. An archetypal small-town entrepreneur, Pottenger had started his business as a market stall during the Depression, and built it into a substantial operation. After the family doctor referred him to a specialist he had a terrible shock: his coronary arteries were found to be dangerously obstructed, and he was told that without surgery he could expect to live for only another three months.[74] When Favaloro offered him the possibility of prolonging his life by undergoing a new operation he did not hesitate, and on 19 October 1967 a vein from Pottenger's upper thigh was extracted and used as a bypass graft from his aorta to the right coronary artery, restoring blood flow to his starved myocardium.[75] Given the state of his arteries before that first operation, it is nothing less than astonishing that he lived for another twenty-six years.[76]

Surgeons have been known to be gung-ho when introducing new operations, trusting to instinct rather than proceeding with careful deliberation. In this instance, Favaloro's enthusiasm was tempered by the calm rationality of Mason Sones, who urged him to withhold judgment until he knew whether the grafts were still functioning months later.[77] The outcomes were excellent, however, and within two years they were able to present the long-term results of their first 100 operations, of more than 300 already performed.[78] In 1970 Favaloro was invited to take part in a conference at the South Bank in London. There was huge interest in his presentation, and when he arrived at the small venue it was already clear that there were more delegates than seats. As the discussion began, the doors gave way with a crash, and an unseemly stampede of middle-aged doctors piled into the already packed room. Chaos was followed by controversy when Favaloro was asked about the mortality rate for his new procedure and revealed that he had already performed it on over 1,000 patients, of whom fewer than 5 per cent had died.[79] This was a staggeringly low figure for a new operation, and the senior cardiologist leading the discussion, Charles Friedberg, voiced his disbelief. Favaloro replied with some heat that anybody who doubted him was welcome to visit his office to check the numbers for themselves.[80] It is not known whether anyone took him up on this offer, but there was nothing dubious about Favaloro's figures; the operation was just as good as his results implied.

Favaloro was not complacent about his success, continuing to look for ways of improving the procedure, and later that year he began to incorporate a modification suggested by the New York surgeon George Green. Originally a head and neck specialist, Green taught himself to sew tiny blood vessels using a microscope, and when a colleague told him about the problem of coronary surgery he realised that the technique should make it possible to suture even arteries as small as 1 millimetre in diameter. While Favaloro was using vein grafts to construct his bypasses, Green turned his attention to the internal mammary artery. His approach, used for the first time on 29 February 1968, entailed attaching the internal mammary to a coronary artery, using a microscope to place the tiny stitches.[81] This only improved the circulation to one side of the heart, however, and he realised that even better results could be achieved if he added a vein graft to the other side.

Favaloro came to similar conclusions, and even before he adopted Green's technique had begun to place more than one graft on different parts of the coronary arteries. Double, triple and even quadruple bypass grafts became commonplace, with even more used for particularly tricky cases. In 2004 the former US president Bill Clinton became the highest-profile quadruple bypass patient, although the bar had already been set higher by his erstwhile Russian counterpart Boris Yeltsin, who eight years earlier received five grafts in an operation supervised by Michael DeBakey. They are mere amateurs, however, compared with the Indian businessman Mithalal Dhoka, who in 2012 became the first person in the world to be given an astonishing twelve bypass grafts, in an operation which lasted more than eleven hours.[82]

*

The rise of the bypass was phenomenal. In 1930 the main cause of heart disease was still rheumatic fever, but twenty years later the illness was in retreat: mutation had apparently rendered it less lethal, and antibiotics offered a cure. But as one threat receded, another loomed. Coronary artery disease was running rampant in developed nations, fuelled by a rise in smoking and the increasing affordability of a high-fat, meat-based diet. The problem was particularly acute in the US, and in 1971 more than 20,000 CABGs were performed there alone. With each procedure costing at least $10,000 (around $60,000 at today's prices) this was a lucrative business – especially in countries where insurance companies, rather than governments, paid the bill. As increasing numbers of surgeons acquired sports cars and second homes, sceptics began to ask whether the operation was more for the benefit of doctor or patient. These included the best known name in heart surgery, Christiaan Barnard, who suggested that if the procedure were made illegal, half of the profession would be put out of business.[83] The same view was articulated in a report published in a major journal in 1977 which speculated that 'self-aggrandizement' and 'personal or institutional expansion' had motivated the adoption of CABG.[84] More seriously, doubts were cast on whether the operation even worked. A major study of the first ten years of results concluded that there was no evidence that it had any long-term effect on angina symptoms, or protected against heart attacks.[85]

Favaloro was exasperated by these findings, because he knew that they were deeply flawed. There was still a vocal group of clinicians who refused to believe that such a simple procedure could improve cardiac function, and their articles on the subject made little attempt to hide their bias. But the main problem was the data itself. Researchers had collected detailed statistics on thousands of people who had undergone bypass surgery, but these numbers were meaningless unless they could be compared with outcomes in patients who had been given some other treatment. Such direct comparison was at that point impossible, since nobody had yet undertaken a clinical study with a proper control group to act as a baseline. What was needed was a randomised controlled trial (RCT), and in 1977 the first of several such studies published its results. These RCTs worked by randomly dividing patients into two groups: one would receive a bypass operation, and the other the best available drug therapy, allowing a straightforward comparison of survival and quality-of-life data. Debate continued to rage for the rest of the decade, though it had little effect on the number of patients willing to undergo the procedure. And then in 1980 a panel commissioned by the US government to examine the results of several new clinical trials came down emphatically on the side of CABG. It reached the conclusion that the operation enhanced quality of life, reduced myocardial ischaemia and improved survival; it was 'a major advance in the treatment of patients with coronary artery disease'.[86]

In the last forty years the basic outlines of the operation have remained much the same, though some details have changed. Many surgeons remained suspicious of George Green's use of the internal mammary artery until research published in 1986 showed that his method was superior to using vein grafts alone.[87] Other vessels have also been used as an alternative to the saphenous vein, including the radial artery from the forearm. Another development was more surprising, and an unusual example of surgeons returning to methods previously rejected as primitive. Many of the first bypass operations took place without the benefit of the heart-lung machine – it was not strictly needed, since the procedure did not entail opening the cardiac chambers. But suturing two blood vessels a millimetre in diameter is little fun if they are dancing in time with the heartbeat, and most surgeons eventually chose to use the pump and operate on a motionless heart. Not all, however. Two surgeons from South America – the Brazilian Enio Buffolo[88] and the Argentinian Federico Benetti[89] – opted to do without whenever possible. Their experience with the technique began in the late 1970s, but it was not until almost two decades later, when they revealed their startlingly good results in thousands of patients, with low mortality and long survival, that the wider surgical community began to take notice. In 1996 Benetti was invited to demonstrate his technique and give a talk at the John Radcliffe Hospital in Oxford. Most of the audience thought his ideas outlandish – until one of the patients who had undergone this major procedure the previous day walked up to the podium to lend his support.[90]

As many soon realised, there were good arguments for the 'off-pump' method. The damaging effects of prolonged cardiopulmonary bypass had been known since the 1980s, and any measure which reduced potential harm to the patient was welcome. Dispensing with the costly heart-lung machine also made it possible for surgeons in poorer parts of the world to perform many more operations – Benetti's method was taken up with particular enthusiasm across Asia, where up to 95 per cent of CABGs now use the off-pump technique.[91] It has not so far achieved the same dominance in Europe and the US, owing to continuing doubts about which method is safer – though one recent study suggests that the off-pump operation is indeed preferable for many patients.[92]

One morning in late 2015 I visited the Bristol operating theatre of Gianni Angelini, a surgeon who has been at the forefront of introducing off-pump coronary artery bypass grafting to the UK. The patient was a man in his eighties with a long list of previous ailments; until recently he would have been regarded as too old and ill to undergo such a procedure. When I arrived, his naked and unconscious body was being shrouded in surgical drapes, leaving just his left leg and the centre of his chest uncovered. While one surgeon began to open his chest, noisily cutting through the breastbone with an electric saw, another made a long incision in his leg and began to dissect the saphenous vein free of surrounding flesh. Much of the next hour was taken up with the tedious task of freeing the left internal mammary artery from the inside of the chest wall: the air filled with the smoky tang of burning flesh as Angelini's first assistant used an electrosurgical scalpel to separate it, millimetre by millimetre, from its bed beneath the ribcage. Every side-branch was carefully closed with a metal clip to prevent bleeding. Eventually a loop of blood vessel about ten centimetres long dangled free from the ribcage; this was cut at its bottom end and clamped, ready to be used as a graft. By this time the vein had also been successfully harvested from the leg and filled with saline to keep it in pristine condition until it was needed.

Only now did Angelini open the pericardium to reveal the heart. This was not the pristine pink muscular organ familiar from illustrations, but a flabby object covered in yellow fat. Its contractions became irregular as it reacted grumpily to the indignity of public exposure. Angelini – known to his colleagues as 'Prof' – examined it closely to identify the parts of the coronary circulation where he intended to attach the three bypass grafts, putting his hand underneath the heart to lift it up a few inches and look at the other side. A special instrument known as a stabiliser was then attached to the table; this device, designed by Angelini, has a metal foot like that of a sewing machine, which gently holds on to the part of the heart where sutures are being placed, keeping it still and minimising the disconcerting effect of the heartbeat. Angelini made a tiny incision in one of the coronary arteries and quickly inserted a short plastic tube into the vessel. This shunt would allow blood to continue flowing while he began to attach the new vessel above it. The first graft was the internal mammary artery, which the surgeon now trimmed to ensure a perfect join. In the earlier stages of the operation the mood had been jovial as the theatre staff swapped hospital gossip, but the room now fell silent as he began the delicate business of the anastomosis – joining the arterial graft to the tiny coronary artery.

Using fine polypropylene thread, Angelini placed stitches around the circumference of the graft to attach it to the wall of the coronary artery over the site of his original incision. At the last minute the plastic shunt was removed from the vessel, the sutures were pulled tight and the anastomosis was complete. Having satisfied himself that the join was perfect and would not leak, he moved on to the second bypass graft. The process was then repeated using a section of the vein harvested earlier from the patient's leg. One end was affixed to the aorta, the other to a different part of the coronary circulation. A third and final graft was similarly attached from the aorta to the back of the heart. After three hours in theatre the heart was festooned with three new loops of blood vessel; Angelini lifted it up once more to check his work, and then placed it gently back in its bed.

Pacing wires were attached to the myocardium to regulate the heartbeat, and thick plastic tubes pushed through the skin to drain any fluid from the chest cavity. The sides of the chest, which had been wrenched apart by retractors to expose the heart, were released to their normal positions, the two halves of the ribcage were reunited with loops of thick wire, and finally the muscle and skin were carefully stitched, leaving only a thin suture line as evidence of the life-saving alterations that had been wrought beneath.

René Favaloro used to emphasise that CABG is only a palliative procedure: there is no surgical cure for coronary disease.[93] There is no medical cure, either, but physicians now have an array of drugs capable of slowing its progress and easing its symptoms so that many patients will never need surgery. By far the most significant development of recent years is the advent of angioplasty and stenting, which allow a blocked coronary to be reopened via a catheter inserted through a blood vessel and without the need for major surgery. These innovations, as we shall see, had such a dramatic impact that for a time they threatened to render bypass surgery redundant. But the procedure pioneered by Favaloro fifty years ago has stood the test of time and remains one of the most successful and frequently performed operations in surgical history.

The story of its creation has a sad end, because a life touched by so much triumph ended in tragedy. On 29 July 2000 René Favaloro shot himself in the heart at his apartment in Buenos Aires. The surgical foundation he had set up on his return to Argentina and into which he had sunk huge amounts of his own money was in deep financial trouble, and the country was in the grip of a recession. In a farewell letter Favaloro expressed frustration at his inability to persuade the government to help him, and despair at the corruption which riddled its institutions. He asked for his ashes to be scattered in the mountains near the town where he had practised as a humble country doctor, and wrote his own poignant epitaph:

> Do not talk of weakness or courage; the surgeon lives with Death, his inseparable companion – I walk hand in hand with him.[94]

8. ONE LIFE, TWO HEARTS

Cape Town, 3 December 1967

As Ann Washkansky drove home one December afternoon after visiting her husband in hospital in Cape Town, she came across the scene of an accident. A large crowd had gathered, and a body lay in the road covered by a blanket. The dead woman's daughter lay prostrate beside her, with paramedics frantically trying to save her life. As police beckoned to Mrs Washkansky, urging her to drive on, she had no inkling that twenty-four hours later the young girl's heart would be beating in her husband's body.

The operation in which this tragic coincidence turned into a surgical miracle is now the most famous in history. In the early hours of 3 December 1967, Christiaan Barnard became the first surgeon to transplant a human heart. Half a century later, few people remember more than this impressive fact. Some may recall that the patient's name was Louis Washkansky and that he lived for a few weeks; or that the world rejoiced and celebrated Barnard, a genius whose feat heralded the era of the heart transplant.

The truth of the matter is more nuanced, and far more interesting. Barnard was an accomplished clinician with undoubted star quality, but he was not even the first surgeon to give a patient a new heart. While he became, overnight, the most famous doctor on the planet, the names of the researchers who had made transplantation a reality remained unknown to the public. It would be natural to assume that the procedure was technically difficult; but, as Åke Senning observed, 'One must merely sew. And when one knows where to sew, there is no problem.'[1] Nor was the achievement universally acclaimed: some physicians felt it happened far too soon, while others had grave reservations about its ethical implications. The ensuing debate lasted several years, and changed the very definition of what it is to be dead or alive.

Like the Moon landing two years later, Barnard's operation was seen as emblematic of the modern age, a triumph of cutting-edge technology over the natural limitations of human life. One commentator heralded 'the opening of a new era in medicine . . . an era as significant as the age of the atom'.[2] But optimism soon gave way to crushing disappointment. Dozens of surgeons began to transplant hearts, but only a handful of their patients survived more than a few weeks. By 1970 most had abandoned an operation that had promised so much and delivered so little. For years afterwards only a handful persevered; the 'new era' did not begin in earnest until the 1980s, when improved knowledge and a novel wonder drug finally made cardiac transplantation a valuable and reliable operation.

In retrospect it is tempting to see the first human heart transplant as the apotheosis of cardiac surgery, the ultimate peak which the profession was trying to scale. In truth, few were interested in attempting this bold step, which was part of a much broader enterprise involving specialists in many different branches of medicine. Their goal was to show that when parts of the body were beyond repair they might be replaced – new organs substituted for old, just as a mechanic replaces a faulty component in a car engine. Attempts to do so date back at least two millennia to ancient India, when Sushruta described the use of skin grafts during rhinoplasty, surgical reconstruction of the nose.[3] In the sixteenth century the Italian surgeon Gaspare Tagliacozzi also became celebrated for his skill in this procedure, using a flap of skin from the upper arm to repair noses mutilated in combat. While the results were often excellent, Tagliacozzi noticed that the operation only worked if the patient's own tissue was employed: a graft taken from a donor soon withered and died. Using somebody else's skin was 'difficult and almost impossible', he wrote; 'The singular character of the individual entirely dissuades us from attempting this work on another person.'[4] He had hit upon the central problem of transplantation: rejection. The body recognises foreign tissue as alien and wages war against it. More than four hundred years later this remains the single most challenging aspect of transplanting organs from one body to another.

With the advent of anaesthetics and aseptic technique in the nineteenth century, surgeons were able to attempt more ambitious reconstructive operations. They achieved wonders in piecing together bodies mutilated by injuries or deformed by tumours, but attempts to replace lost skin with grafts were always unsuccessful. Russian surgeons even tried to use skin taken from dogs, frogs and chickens to repair burns in human patients, with universally disastrous results.[5] In the 1880s the scope of these experiments broadened, as researchers began to investigate the possibility of transplanting endocrine tissue – hormone-producing glands such as the thyroid, testicles and ovaries – from one individual to another in order to treat infertility and cases of thyroid deficiency. But in the closing years of the century, when surgeons discovered a way of suturing blood vessels together, a far more exciting possibility presented itself: transplanting an entire organ and connecting it to the patient's own circulation.

The first to demonstrate that this was not an outlandish dream was the Austrian Emerich Ullmann. In 1902 he transplanted one dog's kidney into the neck of another; since the experiment was merely intended to demonstrate the feasibility of the procedure he left the recipient animal's own kidneys in place. The neck was chosen because its arteries and veins lie close to the skin, considerably simplifying the operation. He attached the donor kidney to these vessels and sutured its outlet duct, the ureter, to the external wound. Urine dripped from the opening, proving that the organ had a good blood supply and was working as usual.

A few months later Ullmann attempted to treat a woman suffering from renal failure by transplanting a pig's kidney into her elbow, but inevitably the operation was a failure. This did not deter others from attempting similar procedures: the Frenchman Mathieu Jaboulay used pig and goat kidneys in humans, while the German Ernst Unger tried those of an ape.[6] In 1906 a surgeon in New York, Robert Tuttle Morris, announced what appeared to be a major breakthrough in transplant surgery. Four years earlier he had replaced the diseased ovaries of a young woman with those of a donor; on 15 March his patient gave birth to a healthy daughter.[7] The implications were immense: if the fertilised egg had come from the new ovaries, the child was biologically the donor's rather than that of the woman who had given birth to her. Most experts today believe that Morris had unwittingly left behind some of the woman's own tissue when removing her ovaries, and that this was the source of the ovum; since DNA testing lay many decades in the future it was impossible to establish who the child's mother really was.[8]

The most thorough of these early transplantation researchers was Alexis Carrel. As the pioneer of blood-vessel surgery he was uniquely well equipped to perform such intricate procedures, and his boundless imagination allowed him to see possibilities that others did not. With his collaborator at the University of Chicago, Charles Guthrie, he succeeded in removing the heart of a small dog and attaching it to the blood vessels in the neck of a larger one. An hour after the operation it began to beat spontaneously, and continued to do so for another two hours. Between 1904 and 1907 Carrel and Guthrie attempted all manner of experiments. They transplanted lungs (both with the heart and without), kidneys, thyroid glands and entire limbs.[9] Most spectacular of all, in 1908 Guthrie created a two-headed dog, transplanting one animal's head on to the neck of another. The grafted head reacted to light and sounds and appeared to be conscious for three hours before it was – mercifully – put to sleep.[10]

While some researchers performed such trials as a way of investigating the function of individual organs, Carrel made clear that he saw transplantation as a serious therapeutic option. He pointed out that contemporary surgery was by and large limited to extirpation – cutting out diseased tissue. 'On the other hand,' he wrote, 'when the extirpation of an organ is necessary the ideal treatment would be the immediate transplantation of a sound organ to take its place.'[11]

This was fantastical stuff, and it reached wider attention in 1907 when Simon Flexner, the director of Carrel's research institute, told a meeting of the American Association for the Advancement of Science that replacing diseased organs would one day be a possibility.[12] The press reacted with astonishment: 'May Transplant the Human Heart', read one headline.[13] The news also inspired what may be the earliest work of fiction about a heart transplant, a short story by the English writer Edgar Jepson. In 'The Rejuvenation of Bellamy Grist', an elderly American poet becomes the first human to undergo the operation, receiving the heart of a chimpanzee called Moko. He is restored to such robust health that other leading citizens sign up for the procedure, their hearts 'worn out by our strenuous American life'. Problems emerge, however, when the austere poet begins to climb trees and produce works with titles such as 'Ode to a Ripe Banana' and 'The Joy of Nuts'.[14] The effect is comical, but Jepson was articulating the fears of many who still believed that the heart was the repository of the soul, and that a patient given a new one would in some way take on the characteristics of the donor.

There was a long pause in attempts to transplant the heart after the work of Carrel and Guthrie, and when work resumed in the 1930s it was not with clinical use in mind. The brain plays an important role in regulating the heart and its reaction to emotion and stress. Signals generated in the medulla, a region of the brain stem, are transmitted to the cardiac muscle via a pair of nerves, modifying functions including the heart rate. A group led by Frank Mann at the Mayo Clinic in Minnesota wanted to find out how the organ would behave if isolated from the central nervous system, and decided that a good way to do so would be to study a transplanted heart. In experiments on dogs in 1933 they took a heart from one animal and implanted it into the neck of another, attaching its major vessels to the carotid artery and jugular vein. It continued to beat but played no part in the circulation of blood, since the recipient animal's own heart had been left in place. Hearts transplanted in this way would function for up to eight days, but generally stopped beating considerably sooner. Mann concluded, rightly, that this was not because of any shortcoming in operative technique, but because of 'some biologic factor', an incompatibility between the donor tissue and the recipient which would have to be overcome in order for transplanted organs to survive for any length of time.[15]

Researchers struggled to understand why tissue transplanted from one body into another was quickly rejected, though as early as 1902 Emerich Ullmann had observed that the appearance in the body of foreign cells 'calls forth ferments into the circulation which destroy the transplanted tissue'.[16] In 1941 a government committee formed to investigate the treatment of war wounds asked the British biologist Peter Medawar to find a way of improving the success of skin grafting, a procedure that was badly needed to treat soldiers with extensive injuries. Although the method had been widely used in the First World War, surgeons could not understand why it was so prone to failure. Medawar performed skin grafts on rabbits, and found that if a first graft failed and the animal was given another from the same donor, the second graft died much more quickly than the first.[17] He quickly realised what was happening: this was a classic adaptive immune response. The body's immune system slowly recognised the first graft as alien tissue, and after a few days lymphocytes, white blood cells, began to attack it. Once the threat had been identified the lymphocytes began to produce antibodies specific to the donor tissue, so that if a second graft were attempted it was quickly recognised and rejected. This insight was crucial, because it suggested a way around the problem: if the immune response could be somehow suppressed, the body might tolerate the transplanted tissue indefinitely. Once effective immunosuppressive drugs had been found, this approach underpinned all subsequent attempts at transplantation.

During the 1940s the most exciting research into the transplantation of organs was taking place in Soviet Russia. This work was almost unknown in the West until twenty years later, when an English translation of a book by Vladimir Demikhov revealed the macabre feats that he and others had achieved. In one operation he cut two dogs in half and created a hybrid animal by joining them in the middle.[18] More than twenty times he succeeded in attaching a puppy's head to the neck of a fully-grown dog, creating a two-headed beast which survived for up to four weeks. The transplanted head reacted to its surroundings, lapped from a saucer of milk and snapped its jaws angrily if provoked.[19]

His longest series of experiments involved giving a dog a second heart, implanted in the thorax, which would play an active part in the circulation. On 31 March 1949 one of these animals was displayed to members of the Academy of Medical Sciences in Moscow. To their amazement he demonstrated that this apparently healthy animal had two heartbeats. The dog was then anaesthetised and its chest opened to show the two hearts beating independently and at different rates.[20] Demikhov also performed no fewer than sixty-seven heart-lung transplants and, on Christmas Day 1951, became the first person to attempt an orthotopic heart transplant. His previous transplants had been heterotopic: that is, the organ had been placed in an abnormal location in the body. In orthotopic transplantation the recipient's own heart is completely excised and replaced by a donor organ, which is sewn into its anatomically normal location. The first operation was a failure, but one later dog survived for thirty-two hours and was well enough to drink and walk around the laboratory.[21] 'These experiments', he wrote, 'have shown beyond doubt that from the point of view of surgical technique, such operations are possible.'[22]

Unaware of Demikhov's work, several American groups had also made progress with orthotopic transplantation, using a newly discovered drug, the steroid cortisone, to suppress the immune system.[23] In 1957 a young surgeon in California entered the fray; though his contribution would later be overshadowed by that of Christiaan Barnard, many still see him as the true father of heart transplantation. Norman Shumway became a doctor – and a transplant surgeon – by accident. Born in Michigan in 1923, he volunteered for military service at the beginning of the war and owing to a shortage of army surgeons was sent to medical school. After qualification he studied in Minnesota, where John Lewis had performed the first open-heart surgery in 1952, and became interested in the use of hypothermia – the focus of his research when he joined Stanford University five years later.

There he was fortunate to meet the ideal collaborator: Richard Lower, six years his junior, whose seventeenth-century namesake had been the first to perform a blood transfusion. In their early experiments Shumway and Lower cooled dogs to well below normal body temperature to investigate the possibilities of hypothermic surgery. This entailed a lot of standing around waiting, and Shumway suggested they spend the time more usefully by removing the heart and then replacing it. It would be good practice for them, but there was also the possibility of conducting 'bench surgery' – repairing cardiac defects while the heart was outside the body. Excising the heart entailed cutting through the major vessels – the aorta, pulmonary artery and both venae cavae – as well as the four smaller pulmonary veins. This was simple enough, but when it came to replacing the organ they found that sewing the severed vessels back together was almost impossible. They realised that it would be simpler if they had an extra margin of tissue to work with; after all, a tailor making a jacket sleeve does not immediately cut it to the desired length, but leaves some extra material and trims it when the sewing has been completed. Lower suggested taking a donor heart from a second dog, leaving a good length of the major vessels attached to the organ. This made the procedure considerably easier, since arteries and veins could now be comfortably sutured into their new location.[24]

Thus did the careers of two of the greatest transplant surgeons begin: through boredom. Finding that the dogs were often well enough to run around after the operation, Shumway and Lower turned their diversion into a major research project. They used the department's new heart-lung machine to support the dog's circulation while its heart was being excised and until the new one was in place, and developed a simplified procedure which removed the need to cut and then suture each of the heart's eight blood vessels. Four of these are the pulmonary veins, the vessels that return freshly oxygenated blood from the lungs to the left atrium. Shumway realised that if they removed the heart by cutting through both atria, he could leave a cuff of tissue containing the ends of these vessels, together with both venae cavae, the veins which enter the right atrium. Instead of suturing six individual vessels, they would only have a single line of tissue to sew, leaving only the pulmonary artery and aorta to be attached. Several researchers elsewhere reached the same conclusion, including Russell Brock in London, who had begun his own animal experiments in 1959.[25]

Shumway and Lower found that the results were surprisingly good. Even without any attempt to prevent rejection, their dogs lived for as long as three weeks. A transplanted heart had no nerves connecting it to the brain, but it appeared this made no difference to its function. The only significant problem was rejection, and they concluded that if they could only prevent the immune system from attacking the new organ, it should continue to work for the normal lifespan of the animal.[26] Their sunny optimism echoed that of Brock, who observed that the heart was, after all, only a pump.[27] This would soon become a familiar refrain, as surgeons tried to convince a sceptical public that they would not lose their soul, or their ability to love, should they undergo the procedure.

Heart transplant researchers were also buoyed by developments elsewhere. Attempts at kidney transplantation had recently intensified, and in 1951 French surgeons performed a number of operations using kidneys taken, controversially, from the bodies of guillotined criminals. These attempts all failed, but in Boston three years later the plastic surgeon Joseph Murray, who had become obsessed with the challenge of human organ transplantation, achieved the first successful kidney transplant. Luckily he did not have to worry about rejection: his patient, Richard Herrick, had an identical twin, Ronald, who was willing to donate one of his own kidneys. Since the brothers were genetically indistinguishable, Richard's immune system did not recognise the new kidney as alien tissue and he made an uneventful recovery.[28] Rejection remained an apparently insuperable problem, but this was an immense achievement nevertheless: Murray succeeded in conquering numerous technical difficulties which had baffled earlier surgeons. Richard Herrick was the first long-term survivor of a transplant operation, living for another eight years. This was well publicised, and rightly so: it was proof that giving a patient a new organ could have dramatic results.*

By 1964 Shumway felt that the surgical elements of the operation had been perfected: cutting out a diseased heart and sewing in a new one was a relatively straightforward technical procedure. Encouragingly, new drugs and radiotherapy had reduced the incidence of rejection in kidney transplantation, developments which led Shumway to conclude that cardiac grafts were 'just around the corner'.[29] Indeed, a team led by James Hardy at the University of Mississippi was already rehearsing for the great moment. The previous summer Hardy had performed the world's first human lung transplant on John Richard Russell, a fifty-eight-year-old convicted murderer suffering from cancer. The new lung (taken from an emergency-room patient who had died from a heart attack earlier that day) worked well, but Russell died eighteen days later from a pre-existing kidney complaint.[30] Hardy had been working on heart transplantation since 1956, and few in the field possessed such wide-ranging expertise. From December 1963 he and his team were on the lookout for a suitable patient: somebody in terminal cardiac failure who could not be helped by any conventional treatment, but who might be saved by a new heart.

---

* Murray shared the 1990 Nobel Prize in Medicine for this achievement.

On 18 January 1964 newspapers worldwide published a sensational story under the headline 'Human Heart is Transplanted':

> A bold attempt to give a man another heart was made by
> Mississippi surgeons Friday. The transplant worked for an
> hour. It was the first known successful human heart trans-
> plant in the world . . . The heart came from a dead man. It
> was revived and transplanted into the chest of a man dying of
> heart failure.[31]

This was complete fiction. A member of the hospital staff had given
the press a tip-off, having discovered that Hardy's team had a patient
and a donor heart and were all set to operate. But the transplant never
took place: when Hardy opened the man's chest he found that a simple
surgical repair would be enough to help the patient.[32] This was all useful experience, however, as the team had gone through every stage of
the transplant protocol except the actual procedure.

Less than a week after this dry run Hardy was able to perform the
operation in earnest. On 17 January, Boyd Rush, aged sixty-eight, had
been admitted to the hospital in a sorry state. After years of high blood
pressure his circulation was so poor that he had developed gangrene
in both legs, which had to be amputated. A cardiologist concluded
that his case was hopeless without a transplant, and on the evening of
23 January his heart started to fail. Hardy had three potential organ
donors lined up, young patients who were dying from brain damage
and being kept alive on ventilators. He realised that if he turned off
one of these machines to obtain an organ he risked prosecution for
murder, and decided that he would only use a heart from a donor who
had died naturally. He knew the chances that this would happen at
just the right moment were minimal; so he had a contingency plan.

A few weeks earlier Hardy had paid a visit to Keith Reemtsma, a
kidney-transplant surgeon in New Orleans. The only patients it was
possible for him to operate on were those with a close relative willing
to donate a kidney, which meant that very few transplants took place.

Reemtsma decided to use kidneys from primates in order to increase the numbers who might benefit from the operation – an easy thing to do, since in the early 1960s the sale of monkeys, chimps and even big cats remained unregulated. It was a controversial procedure, but the results surprised everybody. One patient, a dock worker called Jefferson Davis,[33] lived for two months with the kidneys of a former circus chimpanzee, while others were given organs from baboons and monkeys.[34] Hardy was impressed by what he saw, and it occurred to him that in extremis a primate heart might be an acceptable back-up should a human organ not be available. He bought four large chimps and, to test his hunch, measured the cardiac output of the biggest of them, a hefty specimen of over 100 pounds. At 4 litres per minute it was low by human standards, but he concluded that if it were really necessary it would suffice for a small adult.[35]

As Boyd Rush's heart failed his blood pressure plummeted, and his breathing could only continue with mechanical help. Hardy went to check on the condition of the prospective organ donor, and found that he was unlikely to die imminently – they would not be using his heart that night. Instead the largest chimpanzee was tranquilised and prepared for surgery. Hardy reasoned that his patient had lost both his legs, reducing the volume of blood in his body, so the chimpanzee heart might be just enough to keep him alive. When Rush arrived on the operating table his pulse was irregular and his blood pressure almost non-existent. He was comatose and barely needed anaesthesia. His heart arrested as Hardy was opening his chest – with not a minute to spare they succeeded in attaching him to the heart-lung machine.

With the patient safely on the pump, Hardy summoned his staff to the operating theatre to decide what to do next. They could either turn off the heart-lung machine and let their patient die, or transplant the chimpanzee heart. After a quick discussion the five senior staff took a vote: four were in favour of continuing with the chimp heart, and one abstained.[36] While one team went into the adjoining room to open the animal's chest, Hardy excised Rush's failed and useless organ. He looked down with awe at a sight he was the first to see: a

living patient with a hole where his heart should be.[37] The chimpanzee's heart was handed to him in a metal bowl. It had been rinsed out
with a cold solution and was now being perfused with human blood. It
took forty-five minutes for Hardy to sew it into place. As the new heart
was rewarmed to normal temperature it began to quiver. Hardy gave
it a single shock with the defibrillator, and after a short hiatus it leapt
into a regular and powerful beat. The initial signs were encouraging,
but Hardy soon realised the ape's heart could not cope with the job it
was being asked to do. After watching it struggle for an hour he gave
up hope of seeing his patient regain consciousness.[38] As the chimpanzee heartbeat faded away, so did the life of Boyd Rush, the first human
to receive a new heart.

When Hardy looked up from the table he was surprised to find
the room full of people, many of whom he did not recognise. More
than twenty-five uninvited guests had talked their way in, keen to see
history being made. Realising that the operation would soon be common knowledge, he arranged for the hospital authorities to issue a
brief press release stating that a heart transplant had taken place. No
mention was made of the chimpanzee, leading many in the press to
speculate about the identity of the unnamed donor, and beginning a
long and dishonourable tradition of heart transplant PR disasters. A
second statement was hurriedly published to clarify matters.

Hardy had thought long and hard before proceeding with transplantation, and solicited advice from many of his colleagues. He
was taken aback by the hostility the operation aroused in America,
with surgeons and the public alike uniting in condemnation. In his
memoirs, written twenty years later, Hardy recalled that it was 'as if
there had been a recent bereavement in the family, for the lung and
heart transplants were never mentioned by friends'.[39] It was apparent that he had broken a taboo, and Hardy decided not to involve
another patient unless there should be a palpable change in the public mood. Two thousand miles away in Stanford, Norman Shumway
had followed developments with interest before coming to the same
conclusion.

Though would-be heart transplanters kept a low profile for the next few years, important work was being done behind the scenes. Experimental animals started to live for dramatically longer, thanks to improved management of rejection. Richard Lower discovered that the powerful immunosuppressive drugs often caused dogs to die from infection, and began to use them only if rejection was detected.[40] He and Shumway subsequently kept one animal alive for a year with a new heart.[41] Their collaboration ended in 1965 when Lower moved to Virginia, where he performed a mirror image of James Hardy's feat by transplanting a human heart into a chimpanzee. This may seem a macabre thing to do, and Lower was so worried about adverse publicity that he never reported it, but it was a significant achievement. It was the first time that a beating human heart had been deliberately stopped and removed from a cadaver, sewn into another body and restarted – and it kept the ape alive for several hours afterwards.[42]

Meanwhile a surgeon in Brooklyn, Adrian Kantrowitz, was having notable success in transplanting puppy hearts. Despite the difficulty of working with such tiny organs, most animals survived the procedure. No effort was made to prevent rejection, yet some lived for several months.[43] Kantrowitz believed this was because the puppies' immune systems were still developing, and reacted less aggressively to foreign tissue – which seemed to bode well for the possibility of heart transplants in small babies. By early 1966 he felt that he was ready to operate on an infant. The ethical situation was less fraught than with adults, since the babies who would be candidates for a transplant were those born with major congenital heart defects which were otherwise impossible to treat, and whose life expectancy was measured in weeks or days. As for donors, Kantrowitz chose to use only anencephalic infants, those born with most or all of their brain missing. Since these babies could neither feel pain nor sense their surroundings, and usually died within hours, there were likely to be few moral qualms about their role as organ donors.

Kantrowitz came very close to being the first surgeon to perform a human-to-human heart transplant. In May 1966 he had identified a possible recipient, a baby boy with a catastrophically malformed heart. A few weeks later a hospital in Oregon responded to his plea for donors, and an anencephalic baby was flown all the way to New York. On the morning of 30 June the donor's heart stopped beating, and everything was made ready for surgery – but it had been starved of oxygen for too long to be restarted, and Kantrowitz abandoned the procedure. Although several other donor infants were found, they could never be matched to a suitable patient, and it was not until late the following year that Kantrowitz and his colleagues had a chance to try again.[44]

As 1967 drew to a close three American surgeons were on the brink of making history. Shumway, Lower and Kantrowitz had all performed hundreds of heart transplants on animals, thoroughly investigated the management of rejection and assembled expert teams able to deal with every aspect of the operation and its aftermath. More or less everybody in the medical profession imagined that one of them would be the first to take the momentous step of transplanting a human heart. And then on 4 December came the news that nobody was expecting: a surgeon in faraway South Africa had beaten them to it.

Christiaan Barnard was certainly an outsider in the world of transplantation. Few outside Cape Town knew he was even interested in the subject; he had done little research and published nothing about it. Born in 1923 in the vast open spaces of the Karoo, the desert heartland of South Africa, Barnard was the son of a priest in the Dutch Reformed Church who tended a large congregation drawn from the impoverished Cape Coloured community. Living in relative poverty and surrounded by his father's parishioners, Christiaan grew up without any of the racial prejudice so common among white South Africans at the time – a fact reflected in his later refusal to segregate his surgical wards by race, as the government demanded. After training as a surgeon he performed important research into intestinal atresia, a congenital abnormality in which part of the bowel is narrowed or missing. He proved the cause of this condition by operating on canine foetuses as they lay in the womb,[45] an extraordinary feat which later made possible the entire field of surgery on unborn infants.[46]

Partly on the strength of this work, Barnard won a scholarship to continue his training in Minnesota, where he was given the best possible grounding in open-heart surgery by the pioneer in the field, Walton Lillehei. When he returned home two years later the chief of surgery, Owen Wangensteen, was so impressed with his protégé that he raised funds to buy a heart-lung machine so that Barnard could establish an open-heart programme at Groote Schuur Hospital in Cape Town – the first in Africa.[47] Barnard did not disappoint: with his brother Marius, also a surgeon, he was soon performing some of the most difficult cardiac operations on children, with results as good as any in the world.[48]

Marius worked closely with Christiaan for thirteen years and took part in the famous transplant, yet chose never to assist him at the operating table. He described his first few months working for his brother as 'utter hell', and was appalled by Christiaan's belligerent behaviour towards his staff.[49] He was not alone in his opinion that Christiaan was not a naturally gifted surgeon, even describing him as 'cumbersome' – but any deficit in talent was more than made up for by his unshakeable perfectionism. And he was not short of self-belief: 'I have a tremendous ego, I know that, and I must feed it, or I become miserable and unhappy,' he told one interviewer.[50] Though urbane and charming, he was uncompromisingly, obsessively competitive. When his teenage daughter Deirdre emerged as a talented international water-skier, Barnard brought the same unwavering fanaticism to her coaching. In a revealing passage from his autobiography he recalled his frustration when he realised that she had not inherited this ruthless streak: 'I had failed to transplant into her my own hunger for victory. She was still not going to beat her fists and cry if she lost . . . She would never make it.'[51]

Barnard's interest in the possibilities of transplantation was aroused in 1962, when a South African newspaper reported Demikhov's creation of a two-headed dog. He immediately went to the animal laboratory to repeat the experiment, an exploit that earned him considerable local notoriety. The following year he performed a heart transplant on a dog and predicted in a talk to students at the University of Pretoria that the operation would soon be possible in humans[52] – but made no serious effort to begin a concerted programme of research. That all changed in the summer of 1967, when he travelled to America to visit several transplant specialists and find out what progress was being made. Soon after his return to Cape Town he decided to perform a kidney transplant as preparation for the more technically complex procedure with a heart: it would give him an opportunity to test the anti-rejection protocols he had learned in America. As a dry run it could not have gone better: the patient, a middle-aged woman called Edith Black, made an excellent recovery and lived for another twenty years.

After this success Barnard was buoyant. Colleagues were less enthusiastic about the possibility of a heart transplant, but his enthusiasm brooked no argument. Any initial reluctance was not reflected in the care they paid to the necessary preparations, which were meticulous. Barnard's team included consultants in every relevant specialism, as well as experts in rejection, tissue compatibility, infection, and pre- and post-operative care. There was, however, one curious omission. While Shumway, Lower and Kantrowitz had practised the operation hundreds of times on dogs, Barnard seemed to think such rehearsals unnecessary. Marius did perform a number of canine transplants, but regarded them as personal practice in general cardiac surgery. Christiaan later suggested in self-justification that these experimental operations were a significant part of the hospital's preparations for a human transplant, a claim Marius treated with derision.[53]

In October Barnard decided that his team was ready. After much persuasion the director of the hospital's cardiac clinic, Velva Schrire, agreed to let him know if he came across a suitable candidate for a heart transplant. A month later Schrire summoned Barnard to his office to tell him that he had found one. His name was Louis Washkansky, a fifty-four-year-old grocer with a litany of health problems. Diagnosed with diabetes in 1955, he had since had three heart attacks and been repeatedly hospitalised. He was so ill that the slightest exertion made him breathless; his damaged heart had ballooned to a grotesque size. So poor was his circulation that he had developed severe oedema, swelling caused by fluid retention, which had to be drained using tubes inserted into his legs.[54] When Barnard watched an X-ray film of Washkansky's heart in action he was shocked: two-thirds of the muscle of the left ventricle was dead and useless, and the coronary arteries were almost obliterated.[55] Barnard could barely believe that he was still alive.

Given this bleak outlook, it is hardly surprising that when offered the extraordinary possibility of a new heart he accepted without hesitation. All that remained now was to find a donor organ, and after one false alarm they found one. On the afternoon of 2 December a local family, the Darvalls, went out to visit friends, stopping en route at a bakery to buy a cake. As Mrs Darvall and her twenty-four-year-old daughter Denise crossed the road they were hit by a car. Mrs Darvall was killed instantly, and Denise suffered a terrible head injury. Though an ambulance arrived within minutes, it was soon apparent that nothing could be done for her. At the hospital a few miles away the news was broken to her father, who readily agreed that her organs could be used for transplantation.

Marius Barnard and his wife were at home that evening celebrating their sixteenth wedding anniversary when he received a phone call from his brother summoning him to Groote Schuur. When he arrived at the hospital Denise Darvall had already been seen by a neurosurgeon, who confirmed that she was beyond medical help. With everything in place, Washkansky was taken to the operating theatre at 12.50 a.m. and anaesthetised. In the room next door Denise Darvall lay on the operating table, dead but not-dead, her heart still beating but her brain no longer functioning. Marius took charge of preparing her for the procedure while Christiaan began the transplantation operation on Washkansky, opening his chest and inserting cannulas for the heart-lung machine. By 2.20 a.m. he was ready, and a message was sent next door for Denise Darvall's artificial respirator to be switched off. Twelve minutes later her heart stopped.[56] Immediately her chest was opened and she was connected to the heart-lung machine, which cooled her blood to preserve her organs. Christiaan cut through the major vessels of the heart and placed the precious object in a bowl of cold preserving solution, before carrying it next door, where it was immediately perfused with blood from the pump.

This was the point of no return; but having now seen Washkansky's ruined heart at close quarters Barnard knew that without a transplant he was finished. Bypass was begun, and Washkansky's body cooled to 30°C to protect his brain from damage during the long procedure. After placing a clamp across the aorta to exclude it from the circulation, Barnard cut through the vessel just above the opening of the coronary arteries. The pulmonary artery was also severed, and then Barnard cut away the rest of the heart, leaving a cuff of tissue, the portions of the atria containing the ends of the venae cavae and pulmonary veins, in situ. He placed Denise Darvall's heart into the chest and began to cut into the left and right atria, making holes to match the tissue that he had left behind. Washkansky's diseased organ had been far larger than the new one, so he trimmed the cuff to ensure that it would fit. Then he began to stitch, attaching the left atrium and then the right with two layers of sutures. The pulmonary artery was next to be attached, and finally the aorta was trimmed to length and sutured. When Barnard was satisfied that his stitches were airtight the clamp across the aorta was released, allowing Washkansky's blood to flow into the new heart muscle for the first time.

The transplant was now complete, but the team had to wait for Washkansky's body to be returned to normal temperature before they could find out whether the new heart would work. After a tense half-hour the anaesthetist Joseph Ozinsky finally announced that the temperature in the oesophagus had reached 36°C.[57] Barnard applied the paddles of the defibrillator to the quiescent organ, which jolted as a pulse of electricity passed through it. There was a breathless pause, and then the heart contracted for the first time in its new body. 'Dit werk,' Barnard said quietly in Afrikaans: 'It works.'[58]

It was 5.52 a.m. Barnard and his team had been operating for four and a half hours, but there was much still to do. It took three attempts to wean the patient off the heart-lung machine and demonstrate that the donor heart would support Washkansky's circulation on its own. His chest was closed, and anaesthesia was finally stopped at 8.30 a.m.[59] The patient was now attached to a drip containing powerful steroids which would suppress his immune system, reducing the chances of rejection. When all were satisfied that Washkansky's vital signs were stable he was taken to a room specially prepared for him. Because of the dangers of infection the most stringent precautions had been taken: every object, from the mattress to the walls, had been scrubbed with disinfectant, and any staff who were to come into contact with the patient screened for possible bacterial contamination. This sterile cell would be Louis Washkansky's home for the remaining eighteen days of his life.

An exhausted Barnard had barely returned home before the media frenzy began. It was the biggest news story since the assassination of President Kennedy: within hours the world's media had descended on Cape Town. The operation was meant to be a secret, and it remains a mystery how the press found out: Marius (and many others) suspected Christiaan had tipped them off, but the surgeon always fiercely denied having done so.[60] Louis Washkansky instantly became the world's most famous patient, with constant bulletins on his condition. The early reports were encouraging: within a few days he was sitting up in bed and talking to his nurses, while the symptoms of heart failure had started to subside. The function of his other organs steadily improved, indicating that his circulation was drastically better. When he was well enough Barnard allowed him to give interviews. It was natural that there should be huge interest in his condition, but the hospital allowed access to their patient on a scale which would not be contemplated today: Washkansky was visited by cabinet ministers, photographers, newspaper journalists and representatives of all the major broadcasting organisations.[61] He coped with these invasions with good grace, although he bridled when a BBC interviewer asked how he, as a Jew, felt about receiving the heart of a Gentile.

On 15 December, twelve days after the operation, Washkansky was allowed out of bed, but later that evening came the first signs that all was not well. He started to have difficulty breathing, and an X-ray showed a shadow on his lungs.[62] The diagnosis was pneumonia, and because tests failed to identify any infectious agent Barnard decided this was a sign of rejection – a crucial mistake. In fact Washkansky had an infection which had migrated from a wound in his leg and needed antibiotics; instead he was given a larger dose of anti-rejection drugs, further depressing his immune system at just the moment it was needed to fight the bacterium. Barnard can be forgiven for this error: distinguishing between the symptoms of rejection and infection is still one of the biggest challenges for the transplant surgeon, fifty years later.

By the time Barnard's team realised the true cause of Washkansky's pneumonia it was too late. They threw the pharmacological kitchen sink at the infection, but he continued to deteriorate. On 21 December, eighteen days after the transplant, he finally succumbed. Washkansky's family received condolences from thousands of people who had never laid eyes on this remarkable patient, let alone met him.

Barnard was devastated. He attended the post-mortem, but was overcome with emotion and had to leave the mortuary. Though it felt like a failure, the pathologist's findings showed that the operation had been a success. The cause of death was pneumonia; although there were signs of rejection, these were trivial and had not affected the out-come.[63] If the infection had not supervened, Washkansky apparently might have lived for considerably longer.

While the operation prompted adulation in the media, the reac-tion of most surgeons was bewilderment. In New York, Adrian Kantrowitz learned of it from his daughter, who had heard the news on the radio. He was stunned: Lower or Shumway would have been no surprise, but Barnard was not the name he expected.[64] He had a baby awaiting transplantation in his hospital, and was worried that proceeding with the operation would be seen as rushing to get in on the act. But on 4 December an ideal donor, an anencephalic infant, was transferred to Maimonides Medical Center and he decided to go ahead. Two days later he operated, but his tiny patient, a two-week-old baby boy, lived only a few hours before the transplanted organ failed.[65] In early January a second, adult, patient died just a few hours after the operation.[66] Although Kantrowitz had emulated Barnard's achievement, he was the first of many to discover how elusive ultimate success could be.

Norman Shumway joined the transplant club within days, but his first patient, a fifty-four-year-old man, fared little better than those of Kantrowitz. Remarkably, the operation took place less than twenty-four hours after the patient had been admitted to hospital in terminal cardiac failure. The donor heart came from a forty-three-year-old woman who had suffered a massive stroke. The operation on 6 January went without a hitch, but complications began within hours and never receded. Infections and gastrointestinal bleeding followed, and he died a fortnight later.[67]

In early February Barnard flew to London to take part in a television debate, a special edition of the BBC's science magazine *Tomorrow's World* entitled 'Barnard Faces His Critics'. It was an extraordinary occasion. A large studio audience included many of the most eminent British surgeons and physicians, as well as several outspoken opponents. The questioning was not entirely friendly: five more transplants had been performed since Barnard's first operation, only one patient was still alive, and public opinion was beginning to turn. Some of the most biting criticism came from another transplant surgeon, Roy (later Sir Roy) Calne, who at the age of thirty-seven was widely regarded as Britain's leading expert in the field. As the discoverer of the first effective immunosuppressive agent, azathioprine, he had already begun kidney transplantation and later that year would become the first European to transplant a liver. Although supportive of the decision to perform the operation, he condemned the 'nauseating' publicity that had accompanied it, and attacked the decision to publish photographs of patient and donor. Still more hostile was the writer and broadcaster Malcolm Muggeridge, a devout Catholic whose comments were coloured by his religious convictions. Describing transplantation as 'deeply repugnant', he wondered 'what the fury of Heaven would be at the notion that our bodies are collections of spare parts'.[68]

Such voices were, however, in the minority. Another heart surgeon, Donald Longmore, dismissed the 'phoney' ethical arguments and emphasised the exciting possibilities of the operation. He introduced one of his own patients, a retired milkman called Bill Bradley, who was brought on stage in a wheelchair. The raucous audience fell silent as he explained softly that he had been waiting five years for the possibility of a new heart. 'I will take it tomorrow, given the opportunity,' he said. 'I can become a new man, I can live a life, instead of this.' A sometimes fractious debate ended with a dose of sobering reality.

Nineteen sixty-eight was to become the most tumultuous year in the history of heart surgery. Suddenly everybody was performing cardiac transplants. As Adrian Kantrowitz noted in a special edition of the *American Journal of Cardiology*, 'It is unusual that a new surgical procedure, experimental in nature, has been so quickly taken into clinical practice in so many divergent centres throughout the world.'[69] By the end of October more than sixty operations had taken place, in India, Venezuela and Czechoslovakia as well as leading centres in America and Europe.[70] Many of these should never have gone ahead, performed by surgeons with trivial knowledge of the procedure in hospitals where there was little or no understanding of the complexities of rejection. As one eminent American surgeon, Lyman Brewer, pointed out, the operation had become a status symbol for those seeking the adulation and publicity that came with it.[71]

The most prolific of the early transplanters was Denton Cooley, who candidly admitted that he regretted not having been the first. His reaction to news of Barnard's operation was to send a telegram of congratulation, goading his colleague with the prediction that he would soon be reporting on his first hundred cases.[72] It was not until

May that he performed his first, on a forty-seven-year-old account-ant who did quite well until rejection set in six months later; a repeat transplant also failed, and he died shortly afterwards.[73] Cooley – who prided himself on his speed and accuracy – took a mere three hours to complete an operation that had taken Barnard eight. He was intoxi-cated by the acclaim that followed, admitting to a colleague that he rel-ished the public perception that he was a 'supersurgeon': 'Overnight', he said, 'the surgeon becomes some sort of deity!'[74] By the end of the year Cooley had performed eighteen operations, including one heart-lung transplant on a two-month-old girl.[75] But only six of his patients were still alive, and the longest any of them survived was little more than a year.

If these results were not particularly impressive, the overall pic-ture was hardly more encouraging: a survey compiled in December 1968 found that fewer than half of the sixty-five patients given a new heart in the preceding twelve months were still alive.[76] So poor were the early results that heart transplantation might have been quickly abandoned had it not been for one beacon of hope: Christiaan Barnard's second patient, a retired dentist called Philip Blaiberg, who lived for more than nineteen months. After a long and arduous recovery he became the first transplant patient to leave hospital, but not before he had had the unprecedented experience of holding his own, dead heart. This encounter provided the title for his book, *Looking at My Heart*, in which he recorded his astonishment at becoming an inter-national celebrity; daily bouquets of flowers arrived at his flat and he received endless offers to give talks and appear on TV.[77] As the world gradually became aware that most transplant patients survived for only a few miserable weeks in hospital, pictures of this amiable South African strolling in his rugby-club blazer, and even swimming in the sea, gave a hint that transplantation might one day fulfil the exalted expectations of the public.

With doubts emerging about the worth of the operation, there was also growing disquiet about the ethical questions it raised. Of particu-lar concern was the status of the donor. A heart only remained viable if taken from the body a short time after it stopped beating. Surgeons quickly realised that the ideal donor would be a young person who had suffered a brain injury of some kind. A young body was more likely to have healthy internal organs, and a head injury would often leave the heart unaffected. There was another advantage, too, but one that created an ethical minefield. Modern medical technology such as mechanical ventilation often made it possible to keep the heart beating for some time, even when the brain was catastrophically damaged. A potential donor might therefore be left on life support until surgeons were ready to perform a transplant. But was such a patient alive or dead? By the 1960s, many doctors were satisfied that absence of brain activity was a conclusive sign of death, but among the public it was generally believed that anybody with a beating heart was still alive. Even if it were accepted that a person's brain was dead, it was not clear whether it would be morally defensible to take out a heart that was still beating, or to turn off a ventilator so that it stopped.

Worse, the law had not kept up with recent medical developments. In 1963 a young man from Newcastle was assaulted and suffered fatal head injuries. When he stopped breathing he was put on a ventilator; his wife, when told that his condition was hopeless, gave permission for doctors to switch off life support and remove a kidney for transplantation. The man's assailant was arrested, but attempts to try him for murder failed: the court ruled that the victim had died at the hands of the doctors who turned off his ventilator, so the defendant could only be convicted of common assault.[78]

Similar problems beset Donald Ross when he performed the first heart transplant in Britain – and the tenth anywhere – in May 1968. Press interest was overwhelming, and photographs of Ross and his team standing beaming on the doorstep of the National Heart Hospital were on many front pages. But a note of uncertainty had crept into the coverage. *The Times* printed a sceptical article by its medical correspondent under the headline 'British Heart Transplant May Be Too Early'.[79] The *Guardian* quoted a consultant cardiologist, Donald Scott, who condemned the operation as 'almost amounting to cannibalism'.[80]

The fuss did not appear to bother the patient, forty-five-year-old Frederick West, who cheerfully admitted that he was not interested in the details of the procedure. He made an excellent recovery at first, and was able to drink sherry with his wife three days after receiving his new heart, but died on 18 June after suffering blood clots on the lungs, an avoidable consequence of the technique employed to stitch in the new heart.[81]

Within weeks of the operation Ross and his team were facing calls for their prosecution. The source of the donor heart was Patrick Ryan, a labourer who had been fatally injured when a concrete slab fell on his head. His heart stopped in the ambulance but was restarted, and he was kept on a ventilator until the surgeons were ready to remove his heart. Some questioned whether the doctors had in fact killed him to harvest his organs, and there was considerable media coverage of the ensuing inquest. This was heard in front of a jury and there seemed a genuine prospect that it might give a verdict of unlawful killing. On the stand, one of Ross's colleagues, the surgeon Donald Longmore, produced Ryan's skull from his briefcase, demonstrating that the injury had removed the top half of his brain.[82] The coroner accepted the medics' assertion that Ryan had died in the back of the ambulance, and the jury returned a verdict of accidental death.[83] Ross and his team were off the hook, but the controversy showed no signs of abating. A few months later Ross sent a circular to several hospitals asking staff to notify him if any suitable heart donors were admitted. The head of the intensive care unit at St Thomas' Hospital reacted furiously, denouncing the 'gang of vultures' waiting to snatch out his patients' organs.[84] This echoed the sentiments of the cartoonist Gerald Scarfe, who had depicted Christiaan Barnard as a sharp-beaked vulture ripping the heart from a living patient.

Medics knew they had a problem, and steps were finally taken to ensure that such cases would not arise in future. On 5 August two organisations independently released ethical guidelines intended to clarify the main issues surrounding death. Delegates at the World Medical Assembly in Australia issued a document known as the

Declaration of Sydney, which acknowledged that death was not a clear-cut process: tissues often continued to function for hours after the death of the individual. This was significant, since it gave physicians justification for declaring a patient dead before the heart had stopped beating.[85] Still more important, however, was the report of a committee from Harvard University published the same day. It called for a new definition of death that would be enshrined in law. The key criterion was to be the status of the brain: if the central nervous system was dead, so was the patient. Brain death could be diagnosed if the patient was unresponsive, could not move or breathe, and lacked normal reflexes (for instance, if the pupils no longer reacted to light). Crucially, the committee proposed that a respirator should only be turned off after death had been declared – this would protect doctors from the possibility of legal action.[86]

The Harvard report had profound consequences, particularly in the US, where a new definition of death was eventually enshrined in federal law in 1981.[*] [87] It came too late, however, to prevent one of the most notorious episodes in the history of transplantation. On 8 August 1968 the Japanese surgeon Juro Wada performed his country's first heart transplant, using an organ taken from the body of a boy who had drowned while swimming. It was later alleged that the donor was still breathing when he reached hospital, and that Wada had given him a muscle relaxant to hasten his death. He then declared the boy brain-dead – a gross violation of a principle established elsewhere that the person certifying the death of a donor should not be the surgeon wanting to use their organs.[88] The recipient died three months later, prompting a criminal investigation which eventually saw Wada charged with murder, professional negligence and the illegal disposal of a body.[89] The case failed through lack of evidence, but its effects were chilling. Public trust in the medical profession plunged, and further operations

---

[*] There remains no such definition in English law, though precedent has established brain death as a standard criterion.

in Japan became impossible. It was not until 1999, more than thirty years later, that the next heart transplant took place there.[90]

This was an isolated incident, but enthusiasm was waning elsewhere too. After the peak of 1968, the 'year of the transplant', there was a steep fall in the number attempted. In December 1970 the American Heart Association compiled the results of all 166 reported transplants and found that only 23 patients were still alive. Surgeons were realising that while the procedure itself was technically straightforward, ensuring the patient's survival thereafter was a formidable challenge – one requiring expertise which only specialist centres could offer.

In September 1971 *Life* magazine published an exposé by Thomas Thompson, a journalist who had spent several months in transplant units in Houston. The cover carried the unambiguous headline 'The Tragic Record of Heart Transplants: A New Report on an Era of Medical Failure'. Thompson revealed that in addition to the high mortality of the operation, many survivors experienced dreadful side-effects from their anti-rejection drugs: the powerful steroids caused facial swelling, depression and even psychosis.[91] What had originally seemed the dawning of a new medical age was now widely regarded as a dangerous and failed endeavour.

In the early 1970s transplantation virtually ceased. In some countries efforts simply petered out; in others a formal decision was taken to abandon the operation. In February 1973 the UK's chief medical officer Sir George Godber called a meeting of clinicians to discuss the situation, after which a letter was sent to specialist centres recommending they cease all transplants.[92] This communication was described as 'advisory', but surgeons were in no doubt that it amounted to a prohibition. For the next five years only a handful of brave souls were willing to persist with heart transplants. Shumway and Lower, who had unrivalled expertise in the subtle problems of rejection, were in it for the long haul. Barnard also continued, and his results were better than most: four of his team's first ten patients lived for more than a year. One of them, Dirk van Zyl, returned to his job within months of being given a new heart, and did not miss a day's work until his retirement fifteen years later – an indication that transplantees could not only live for a long time, but with excellent quality of life.[93]

While Shumway and Lower made incremental improvements to their existing techniques, Barnard went in several new directions. In 1974 he began to employ a radical alternative to the conventional transplant method, using two hearts rather than one. The idea came to him after a patient died on the operating table because the new organ could not be started. The man's son asked Barnard why he could not put the diseased heart back, since at least it worked.[94] Barnard realised that this was not as silly as it first appeared. The original heart could be left in place and a donor heart implanted in parallel with it. The new organ would support the old one, possibly allowing it to recover; if rejection set in, the original heart would be able to support the circulation until the episode had been averted. From November 1974 Barnard adopted this approach exclusively; one-year survival improved from 40 to 61 per cent, almost as good as the results achieved by Shumway. Ten of these patients survived even after their donor organs failed, showing that two hearts were indeed sometimes better than one.[95]

Three years later Barnard attempted to use donor organs from non-human species. This approach, known as xenotransplantation, had been employed by James Hardy in the disastrous first human transplant attempt in 1963. Six years later Denton Cooley had attempted to use a ram's heart when no human donor was available, with a similarly dismal outcome: it began to shrivel even as it was being sutured in place, and the patient was dead before Cooley could substitute the pig's heart he had as back-up.[96] In London Donald Ross also attempted xenotransplantation in 1968, in an operation that took place before his first human-to-human transplant. Ross intended to transplant a pig's heart in parallel with the patient's failing organ, anticipating the approach later taken by Barnard. The evening began badly when one of the porcine donors escaped and was recaptured by Donald Longmore after a helter-skelter pursuit through the streets of central London; a senior nurse, woken by the animal's squeals, made a complaint to hospital managers, and was distinctly unamused to discover a plate of pork chops on her front doorstep the following morning.[97] The operation itself was an abject failure: the patient died within an hour. It was an episode that began as farce and ended as tragedy, and unsurprisingly no effort was made to report it to the wider world.

Barnard was no more successful. His first xenotransplant took place in October 1977 when a young woman undergoing routine surgery could not be weaned off the heart-lung machine. He opted to implant a baboon heart as an adjunct to the failing organ; this was a temporary measure, intended to buy a few days until a human donor could be found.[98] The decision prompted a furious row with his brother Marius, who refused to take any part in the operation.[99] Barnard succeeded in restarting both hearts, but the patient died after a few hours. A second operation, this time using a chimpanzee heart, took place shortly afterwards; this time the patient lasted four days.[100]

The final – and most controversial – attempt at cardiac xenotransplantation took place seven years later when a surgeon from California, Leonard Bailey, gave a two-week-old infant the heart of a baboon. Bailey had been investigating the possibilities of xenotransplantation for six years and had succeeded in keeping a goat alive with a sheep's heart for five months. He believed that enough was now known about the immunological problems for transplant surgeons to risk crossing the species barrier. In October 1984 a paediatrician told him that he might have a suitable candidate. Stephanie Fae Beauclair was less than a week old and had been born with hypoplastic left heart syndrome, a congenital condition which at the time was almost universally fatal. Bailey met her parents and explained that although there was an operation which might improve her prospects, its results were so poor that a transplant represented her best hope. They gave their consent, and blood samples were taken to test for compatibility with a donor organ. Surprisingly, tissue from a baboon provoked a less aggressive response from her immune system than samples from her own parents. The decision was taken to go ahead with the xenotransplant.

The operation on 26 October was an intimidating technical challenge. The donor heart was the size of a walnut, and suturing its tiny vessels without leaving any leaks required dexterity of the highest order. When Bailey shocked the new organ and it began to beat once more the surgical team hugged each other with relief. For the next few weeks newspapers carried daily updates on the condition of 'Baby Fae'. At first she did well, and within a week was feeding and being held by her mother. Drugs succeeded in quelling an episode of rejection, but on 9 November there were signs that the new heart was beginning to fail. Despite the team's best efforts she deteriorated steadily and died six days later, having lived for three weeks with the heart of a monkey.[101]

The sorrow that greeted Baby Fae's death was accompanied by mounting criticism. Opposition had begun while she was still in intensive care, when a small group of animal-rights activists picketed the hospital holding placards with the legend 'Ghoulish tinkering is not science'. Anger intensified when it emerged that Bailey had not even attempted to look for a human heart before going ahead; one had in fact become available on the day of the operation.[102] Many surgeons argued that a xenograft was doomed to fail: though baboons and humans are genetically similar, tissue from a foreign species was far more likely to provoke acute rejection. In his report of the operation Bailey tried to defend himself from attacks on his clinical judgment. He argued that a newborn's immune system was poorly developed and therefore more likely to tolerate a xenograft, and pointed to the post-mortem findings, which he said showed no signs of rejection. He suggested that her death was instead attributable to the donor having a different blood type.[103] Few shared his opinion, with one expert publically accusing Bailey of 'wishful thinking'.[104]

The Baby Fae operation brought an end to the first era of xenotransplantation. Medics realised that they had not yet conquered the immunological barrier between humans and other species – moreover, conventional transplantation was suddenly looking a far more hopeful option. A few months before Baby Fae was born, a surgeon in New York, Eric Rose, had performed the first successful paedi-atric transplant on a four-year-old boy, James Lovette. Although he later needed a second new heart, James lived into his twenties.[105] The story with adults was even more encouraging: increasing numbers of patients were surviving for a year or more after transplantation. The first months were always the most dangerous period for a transplant patient, so keeping significant numbers alive for as long as this gave some hint that indefinite survival might soon become possible, or even routine.

What had changed? Many transplant surgeons would say that the crucial breakthrough was the introduction in the early 1980s of a pow-erful new drug, cyclosporine, which drastically reduced the threat of rejection. But this is only part of the story. As early as 1973 Norman Shumway had been able to report that over a third of his patients lived for two years or longer.[106] Much of this success was achieved simply by improving the diagnosis of rejection episodes, and finding a regime of drugs that would treat them. The most important contribution was made by a young surgeon from Northern Ireland, Philip Caves, who joined Shumway's team as a research fellow in 1971. Shumway was at first perplexed by his new recruit, who shunned the operating theatre in favour of a long sojourn in the library. When Caves emerged several weeks later it was soon apparent that his time had not been wasted: he showed Shumway some little-known research by a Japanese sur-geon, Souji Konno, who had devised a method of removing tissue sam-ples from inside a beating heart.[107] Caves realised that the symptoms of rejection appeared some time after the white blood cells began to attack the donor organ. By inspecting sections of cardiac muscle through a microscope, he suggested, it should be possible to detect the process even before the patient became unwell. With the help of a technician he designed and made an instrument called a biop-tome, a tiny pair of pincers attached to a length of piano wire, which could be inserted into a neck vein and passed down inside the heart. Once there it would snip off a tiny portion of the cardiac wall and retain it for microscopic examination. This process, endomyocardial biopsy, was an immense improvement on existing methods of spotting rejection. Transplant patients were given regular biopsies and if necessary received drugs in doses tailored to the severity of the episode.[108] Catching it early meant that most incidents of rejection could be treated without the patient even needing to return to hospital.[109] Survival rates soared, and the proportion of patients living for five years doubled to 40 per cent.[110]

In 1973 Caves received a visit from his friend Terence English. A South African who had nearly abandoned medicine to work as a mining engineer, English was a newly appointed consultant cardiac surgeon at Papworth Hospital in Cambridgeshire. He was surprised to find so many of Shumway's transplant patients looking happy and well, and deeply impressed when Caves showed him his work on endomyocardial biopsy. English had arrived at Stanford without any interest in heart transplantation, but his friend's enthusiasm was so great that he left California intent on establishing a new programme in the UK.[111] It took several years and endless political manoeuvring, but English eventually managed to persuade the authorities that the time was right to resume transplantation.

Britain's first transplant since the moratorium took place at Papworth on 14 January 1979. English began to excise the donor heart while a second team prepared the recipient for surgery. He had just finished when he received a phone call from the anaesthetist in the other operating theatre, who told him that the patient had suffered a heart attack while being put to sleep. Although they had managed to resuscitate him, they could not tell whether there would be any long-term consequences. English decided to go ahead with the operation anyway, and though the new heart worked perfectly the patient had suffered irreversible brain damage and died eighteen days later. In English's words, 'the shit hit the fan,' but he was determined to continue despite any public furore.[112]

His second attempt in August went much better: the recipient, Keith Castle, proved to be the perfect advertisement for transplantation. Waking from the anaesthetic his first question was about the football results; auspiciously, his team Fulham had won their first game of the season 4–3. Later, TV pictures of the cheery south Londoner riding his bike, playing golf and enjoying a pint in his local pub endeared him to the British public and showed how a heart transplant could transform the life of somebody previously unable to walk more than a few steps. Despite failing to heed English's advice to give up smoking, Castle lived for almost six years.

The following year another British surgeon, Magdi Yacoub, began a second transplant programme at Harefield Hospital, and steadily improving survival rates ensured that official approval – and, more importantly, funding – followed. It was only in 1981, after twenty-nine transplants, that English and his team at Papworth started to use the revolutionary new immunosuppressive agent cyclosporine.[113]

The story of this miracle drug began in 1969 when H. P. Frey, an employee of the Swiss pharmaceutical company Sandoz, was on holiday with his family in the mountains of southern Norway. Scientists at the firm were trying to develop new antibiotic agents, and members of staff who travelled abroad were asked to fill a small plastic bag with local soil in case it contained organisms with antimicrobial properties.[114] The sample brought back by Frey included a fungus identified as *Tolypocladium inflatum*, and microbiologists found that it produced a substance that was given the code number 24–556, and later named cyclosporine. They were disappointed to find that it had no antibiotic effects, but tests revealed another interesting property: when administered to animals it impaired their immune systems.

Experiments showed that when rabbits were given the substance after kidney transplants they lived indefinitely, while those that received no immunosuppressive therapy died in less than a month.[115] In Cambridge Roy Calne tested it in heart transplants on pigs, and found that it greatly increased survival times. His assessment was that it was more effective in suppressing rejection than any other drug his team had tried.[116] He began to use it clinically for kidney and liver transplants, but his earliest human patients suffered serious side-effects, including cancer. This problem was eventually solved in

Pittsburgh by Thomas Starzl, who discovered that the toxic effects of cyclosporine were mitigated if it was administered in smaller doses as part of a cocktail of drugs.[117]

Heart surgeons were circumspect about adopting the new drug, waiting until its efficacy had been proved before risking their own patients. The results of clinical trials in the early 1980s were eagerly awaited, and did not disappoint. Cyclosporine was found to be a potent weapon against rejection, significantly improving life expectancy for heart transplant patients: 76 per cent of those given it lived for over a year, compared with 62 per cent of those who were not.[118] Many sceptics were finally convinced, and the number of transplants performed each year soared from 182 in 1982 to more than 4,500 by the end of the decade. It became routine for patients to live long and healthy lives, with average survival today more than a decade.[119] The most spectacular success story was that of John McCafferty, at time of writing the longest-lived heart transplant patient. When Magdi Yacoub performed his transplant in 1982 he was thirty-nine and near death; a year later he walked the sixty miles from his home in Buckinghamshire to Harefield to raise money for the hospital. He ran half-marathons and competed in the British Transplant Games, and lived for thirty-three years with his replacement heart until his death in February 2016.

Norman Shumway described cyclosporine as 'an improvement of [a] magnitude that I think we will never see again'.[120] So it was, but he was also being too modest about his own contribution. More or less overnight, cyclosporine improved one-year survival by around a fifth; but it had *tripled* in the decade before that, a period when Shumway almost single-handedly salvaged heart transplantation from the wreckage of its disastrous early years.

It should be acknowledged that Christiaan Barnard's results were also exceptionally good, with four out of five of his post-1974 patients surviving for over a year. But curiously the pioneer of heart transplantation played only a minor role in its later development. He savoured the fame that his achievements brought him, the endless requests for interviews and the private audiences with President Johnson and the Pope. He became, in the words of a contemporary, 'a bit of a dilettante and one of the world's great womanisers'. The slightly rumpled surgeon was transformed into a nattily dressed socialite who visited nightclubs with Sophia Loren and was invited to spend holidays on Peter Sellers's yacht; his first marriage collapsed after rumours of an affair with the actress Gina Lollobrigida. In the thirteen years that followed the historic first transplant he performed only twenty-one more,[121] and in 1983 gave up surgery for good. His reason for doing so was the rheumatoid arthritis which had afflicted him for twenty years, causing severe pain and hampering his ability to operate. But many of his colleagues suspected him of losing interest in surgery long before he finally put down the scalpel.

In retirement Barnard helped to establish a transplant unit in Oklahoma, but his extracurricular activities did little to enhance his reputation. He lent his name to the 'rejuvenation therapy' of an expensive health spa, and was paid large sums to advertise a face cream – making scientifically dubious claims that outraged many in the medical profession.[122] When he died while on holiday in Cyprus in 2001, the obituaries were fulsome, but paid almost as much attention to the many sexual conquests of the 'playboy king of hearts' as to his surgical achievements.[123] Never has a surgeon's private life been so publicly dissected, or their legacy so hotly debated.

Was Barnard right to perform the first heart transplant? Even among surgeons the point remains moot. Several I spoke to felt that he allowed personal ambition to trump clinical judgment, and that he failed to give Shumway sufficient credit for the years of research that made it all possible. Others pointed out that transplantation was inherently a leap into the unknown, and that no amount of animal experimentation would have been enough to show how the human body would react to being given a new heart. Maybe Barnard was not the person best equipped to transplant a heart in 1967 – but he was the first who had the courage to do so. And where he went, others followed.

So much attention has been paid to Christiaan Barnard and his operation in the half-century since it took place that an intriguing fact has been largely overlooked. In the early 1960s many people doubted that transplantation was really the answer to the failing heart. They believed in an alternative – one which promised to be cheaper, simpler and less fraught with ethical difficulties. Millions of dollars were spent in the quest for a reliable artificial heart, a machine that would act as a permanent replacement for the organ. In an age when two nations were racing to put a man on the Moon, designing a simple hydraulic pump for the human body seemed a realistic technological goal. But this exciting undertaking would soon turn into one of the most rancorous episodes in the history of medicine.

9. CLINICAL TRIAL BY MEDIA

Salt Lake City, 2 December 1982

In 1882 a bored young doctor in colonial India passed the long hours between consultations by writing a ghoulish short story about an artificial heart. Ronald Ross had yearned to be a poet, but his father insisted that he study medicine. It was the right decision, since Ross became the world's leading expert in tropical diseases, later winning a Nobel Prize for his discovery that malaria was transmitted by mosquitoes. Written when Ross was twenty-five but unpublished until long after his death, 'The Vivisector Vivisected' is a chilling tale about a physiologist who seeks to bring the dead back to life. He creates a mechanical heart, a pump which is filled with donkey blood, and successfully uses it to revive a cadaver. In true Gothic tradition the action reaches its macabre climax as a thunderstorm rages outside the dilapidated laboratory: the hapless scientist and his colleague realise that having started to pump they cannot stop without killing their experimental subject, who in a cruel twist turns out to be the physiologist's brother. After hours of frantic pumping they become exhausted and are forced to abandon their hopeless task, as the briefly resuscitated corpse breathes his last for the second time.[1]

Ross's story may not be great literature, but it shows remarkable vision. As a physiologist he understood the inherent difficulties of creating a device to replace the heart, and the contraption he imagined anticipated the work of researchers many decades later. His narrator describes a 'double kind of pump': a pneumatically powered contrivance like two bicycle pumps connected together, each operating at a different pressure to mimic the heart's left and right ventricles, and equipped with valves to ensure the blood flows in one direction. Strangely it was exactly a century later – in December 1982 – that a device strikingly similar in conception, consisting of two plastic pumps powered by air, was implanted into the chest of a retired dentist from Utah – the first time a human had been given a permanent artificial heart. The realisation of Ross's idea was a landmark operation, but deeply controversial; few judged it a success, and relentless press attention ensured that a distasteful melodrama was played out to an audience of millions.

The project to build an artificial heart had begun in a spirit of huge optimism, and was blessed with cutting-edge technology, generous financial support and the keenest scientific minds. In 1968 a government report predicted that within twenty years artificial hearts would become the second largest industry in America, with thousands of patients receiving them each year.[2] It was soon apparent that this forecast was well wide of the mark, and that the difficulties of constructing such a device were greater than anybody had imagined. An endeavour which had begun promisingly descended into acrimony, blighted by accusations of malpractice, industrial espionage and theft. It was not until the 1990s that the 'total artificial heart' became a widely accepted therapy, and although it has scored several notable successes, fewer than 2,000 have ever been fitted.

The artificial heart was originally conceived not as a therapeutic device but as an aid to research. In the nineteenth century many physiologists had used perfusion pumps, crude devices which circulated blood through isolated organs, in order to study how specialised tissues functioned. In 1928 two investigators from London, Henry Hallett Dale and Edgar Schuster, designed something more ambitious: an apparatus capable of 'producing a complete circulation of the heartless animal'.[3] Their device had two pumping chambers, one operating at high pressure to replicate the systemic circulation, and a low-pressure chamber to propel blood through the lungs. Though this was the first attempt to mimic the function of the natural heart, it was only ever intended to enable study on animal cadavers rather than sustain life, and aroused interest only among specialists.

The perfusion pump unveiled in 1935 by two researchers in New York was, if anything, less sophisticated, yet it prompted a storm of publicity. Front-page headlines celebrated the invention of a 'robot heart', and fanciful claims were made about its likely application in humans. Fuelling this press hysteria was the identity of the pump's inventor: Charles Lindbergh, revered for his feat in becoming the first solo pilot to fly the Atlantic nonstop. After the abduction and murder of his young son in 1932, Lindbergh had become a virtual recluse, and his sudden return to the public eye caused a sensation. For several years, it emerged, he had been quietly devoting himself to biological research at the Rockefeller Medical Center, assisting Alexis Carrel in his experiments. Lindbergh first approached Carrel after watching his sister-in-law die from rheumatic heart disease, an experience which made him consider whether a machine could briefly take over the circulation to enable operations to be performed on the heart.[4] What he envisioned was something like the heart-lung machine on which John Gibbon would begin work a few years later; Carrel, however, suggested he channel his energies in another direction. He wanted a pump to perfuse organs outside the body so that they could be studied in the laboratory.

The apparatus designed by Lindbergh consisted of three glass chambers arranged vertically. Rhythmic pulses of gas propelled blood (or an artificial nutrient fluid) from a reservoir in the bottom chamber through the organ under study, which was placed in the upper chamber.[5] After passing through the organ, the blood returned to the reservoir through the middle pressure-regulating chamber. One day, Carrel proposed, a similar device might allow surgeons to remove an organ from a patient's body, operate on it in the laboratory and then return it to its owner.[6] He certainly did not believe that it could be used as a substitute for the human heart. Carrel, though, was a canny operator who understood the value of publicity, so did not object when newspapers portrayed Lindbergh's invention as something it was not. In 1936 he even authorised its use in a horror film, *The Walking Dead*, in which Boris Karloff stars as an innocent man accused of murder and sent to the electric chair. At the film's climax, in a memorable sequence obviously indebted to *Frankenstein*, Karloff's lifeless body is taken to a futuristic laboratory and revived by powerful electric currents. The camera pans across an impressive array of tubes and flasks before settling on the perfusion pump, as one scientist urges another to 'keep that Lindbergh heart pulsating, Nancy – see that it doesn't stop!'[7]

If Lindbergh was not (as has been claimed) the inventor of the artificial heart, it was undoubtedly his involvement that first gave the idea popular currency. And while the version of his device presented by Hollywood was pure science fiction, a researcher in Soviet Russia soon succeeded in making the real thing. As part of his experiments on transplantation in 1937 Vladimir Demikhov constructed a double pump which he used to replace the hearts of dogs. It was small enough to fit inside the chest, and consisted of two chambers with membranes which pulsated to propel blood through the animal's vessels. Power was provided by an electric motor outside the body, with a driveshaft passed through the chest wall. Demikhov managed to keep dogs alive for as long as five and a half hours – the first time anybody had sustained life using an artificial heart. A driveshaft through the chest made this an obviously impracticable long-term measure, and it was not his intention to use the machine for any length of time: he saw it as a sort of storage system, a means of maintaining the circulation for a few hours at most, long enough to preserve organs which might be needed for transplantation.[8]

No other researchers attempted to construct a total artificial heart until the late 1950s; until then all their efforts were directed at assisting, rather than replacing, the organ. One quirky early attempt was made in 1949 by a medical student, William Sewell, while working on his thesis. This was not a high-tech affair: the parts for his device came from a toy shop and cost less than $25. Using an Erector Set (a construction toy similar to Meccano) he assembled a pump powered by compressed air which was used to bypass the right side of a dog's heart, pumping unoxygenated blood from the vena cava through the pulmonary artery and into its lungs. The device was used for as long as eighty-two minutes, with the dogs making a full recovery.[9] Again, this was intended only as an aid to physiological experiments, but offered valuable evidence that a mechanical pump could do the job of an organic one.

The advent of John Gibbon's heart-lung machine in 1953 provided the final proof of this hypothesis, and several investigators were encouraged to explore the possibility of fully implantable devices, influenced by a burgeoning medical interest in the development of artificial organs. This was stimulated by the work of Willem Kolff, whose major contribution to the invention of the artificial heart – like that of Norman Shumway to transplantation – was overshadowed by the headline-grabbing work of others. Kolff was a physician from the Netherlands who had spent the war working in a small hospital in the city of Kampen, where he set up Europe's first blood bank and was involved in the Dutch resistance. In 1943 he constructed an artificial kidney, a device to remove waste products from the blood of patients whose own organs were too diseased to function. The early models were ramshackle affairs, using 50 metres of cellophane tubing (Kolff used sausage skins) wound around a rotating drum immersed in saline.[10] Most of his early patients died, but by the end of the war he had proved the efficacy of artificial dialysis, a technique which has since saved countless lives. In 1950 Kolff emigrated to America, where he continued his work at the Cleveland Clinic, building one of the world's first heart-lung machines. Five years later he became the founding president of a new organisation, the American Society for Artificial Internal Organs, set up to bring together leading researchers in the field.[11]

At the third annual meeting of the ASAIO, Kolff's successor as president, Peter Salisbury, urged his fellow members to devote more attention to permanent organ substitutes rather than temporary devices such as the heart-lung machine. He also presented his own work on a prototype mechanical heart, a hydraulically powered device based on the mechanism of a milking machine. Bizarrely, he suggested that it might be powered by a hand pump operated by the patient, an arrangement which left unanswered the question of how they were expected to sleep.[12] Salisbury's call to arms was effective, however, and in the next few years numerous researchers entered the fray – far more, in fact, than were working on the problems of transplantation. The first to demonstrate a viable device was Kolff, who in 1957 displayed a plastic artificial heart fabricated by his collaborator Tetsuzo Akutsu. To make it as anatomically accurate as possible, Akutsu made a mould of a dog's heart in plaster of Paris, and used this to form a PVC replica. Unlike earlier attempts this mimicked the four-chambered structure of the natural organ, with separate atria and ventricles. It was successfully used to keep a dog alive for ninety minutes,* the first time that this had been done outside the USSR.[13]

Kolff and his colleagues in Cleveland were the early pacesetters, but this soon became a truly international endeavour. A group in Tokyo developed a water-powered heart which kept a dog alive for more than five hours,[14] while another in Argentina achieved thirteen hours.[15] Initially there was little agreement on what an artificial heart should look like, or how it should work. Some imitated the natural ventricles, using plastic sacs which were compressed by fluid or gas to expel the blood. One ingenious design employed a pendulum whose oscillations squeezed each of the two artificial ventricles in turn. Another borrowed the pump used in the heart-lung machine, using rollers mounted on a wheel to push the blood through a plastic tube.

---

* After this ninety-minute period the dog was put down: the purpose of these first experiments was to gather data on how the device worked rather than to achieve long-term survival.

The choice of power source was also critical. At rest, the average human heart pumps around 7,200 litres of blood per day. Moving such large volumes of fluid requires significant amounts of energy, and researchers quickly realised that no conventional power source was small enough to be implanted into the body, making an external power unit inevitable. One option was an electric motor implanted into the thoracic cavity, connected to batteries by wires passed through the skin. Other devices used pneumatic or hydraulic power: the moving parts of the artificial heart were driven by compressed oil, water or gas which had to be pumped from an external unit via tubes passed through the chest wall.

With so many eminent researchers now entering the field, it is surprising that the first patent for an artificial heart was awarded to somebody who lacked even the most basic expertise in medicine or physiology. Paul Winchell was a ventriloquist who had enjoyed national fame as the star of his own TV show in the early 1950s, and later provided the voice for Tigger in Disney's animations of *Winnie the Pooh*. He was also a tireless amateur inventor who registered patents for such indispensable contraptions as a 'non-bulging garter fastener' and an electric flour sieve. His 1963 design for an artificial heart consisted of four polymer sacs, with the 'ventricles' compressed by a pusher plate powered by an electric motor carried in a harness on the outside of the chest.[16] The device, which was never built, was utterly impractical – but Winchell's claim had serious ramifications, since he had established ownership of several design features which others wanted to use in their own devices. When Willem Kolff discovered the patent he was so concerned that he contacted Winchell to negotiate a settlement which allowed him to develop his own heart without infringing any intellectual rights.[17]

While some tried to build a machine that would entirely replace the heart, others took a different approach. In 1957 Bert Kusserow of Yale designed a ventricular assist device (VAD) – a small implantable blood pump intended to augment the output of one of the organ's two pumping chambers.[18] It was not a great success, keeping dogs alive for only ten hours, but the idea was an important one: such a pump could theoretically be used to support a heart that was still viable, but so impaired that it could only function to a fraction of its normal capacity. Much better results were achieved by Adrian Kantrowitz in New York, who used an elegantly simple VAD to augment the output of the left ventricle in dogs, many of which lived for several months with the device implanted.[19] The first application of this technology to humans took place in Houston, where Michael DeBakey began work on circulatory support devices in the late 1950s. In 1961 he employed a young Argentinian, Domingo Liotta, who had constructed several prototype hearts at his base in Cordoba.

DeBakey and Liotta described their first workable VAD as a 'left ventricular bypass pump'. It consisted of a double-walled tube of polyester fabric, with a valve at each end: one end was attached to the left atrium of the heart, and the other to the descending aorta. When air was pumped into the outer tube the inner one collapsed, forcing the blood within it into the aorta. Pulses of air were produced by an external compressor, which was cleverly synchronised with the patient's heartbeat by means of an ECG machine.[20] On 19 July 1963, DeBakey's colleague Stanley Crawford inserted this device into a forty-two-year-old man who had failed to recover after being given a prosthetic aortic valve. The VAD took over much of the work of the patient's diseased left ventricle, pumping as much as 2.5 litres of blood per minute. It worked perfectly, but the patient was already in a dire state when it was switched on, with brain damage and major organ failure, and he died four days later.[21] It was a disappointing outcome, but a moment of real significance: for the first time in history, the human circulation had been sustained by a machine implanted inside the body.

Despite these developments, there was widespread dissatisfaction at the rate of progress. Few institutions had the resources to pay for the necessary equipment, animals and staff; more cash was needed, and lots of it. In 1963 Michael DeBakey appealed to the US government for funds, appearing before the Senate Subcommittee on Health to make his case. He had reason to expect a sympathetic hearing: the committee's chairman, Lister Hill, was the son of Luther Leonidas Hill, the first American surgeon to suture a human heart. DeBakey was duly awarded $4.5 million to continue his research, but two years later the government earmarked the colossal sum of $40 million* for the development of an artificial heart, with the aim of implanting the first device by 1970.[22]

By 1964 DeBakey's team had tried eight different designs of pump, both total artificial hearts and VADs. These included sacs which were placed inside the heart, like an artificial lining to the ventricle. Others were wrapped around the outside of the organ, helping it to contract. But none gave satisfactory results in laboratory tests, and DeBakey realised that the challenges remaining were formidable. The apparent simplicity of the human heart belies its many subtleties, in particular its ability to self-regulate. When the volume of blood returning from the body increases, the heart responds by increasing its output, a relationship named Starling's law after the English physiologist who identified it. Although the two ventricles operate at different pressures, their outputs are finely balanced: in his animal experiments DeBakey found that the dogs usually suffered pulmonary oedema, a build-up of liquid on the lungs caused by unequal stroke volumes between the two ventricles. Though any device needed to be powerful, it also had to be gentle with the delicate red blood cells – otherwise they would rupture, causing serious damage to the patient's kidneys. Another problem lay in the materials at his disposal: the plastics available at the time were not sufficiently durable and had a tendency to cause clots, which could escape into the bloodstream and cause catastrophic blockages in the brain or lungs.[23]

Faced with this succession of obstacles, DeBakey decided to set aside the artificial heart for the time being, and to focus his attention on the development of VADs, which seemed more promising in the short term. Within a couple of years his team had developed a new

---

* This is well over $250 million at today's prices, and represented a far from trivial 0.05 per cent of the entire federal budget for that year.

model powered by carbon dioxide, and tested it on hundreds of calves – some of which lived for as long as three months.[24] More precisely, this was an LVAD (left ventricular assist device), since its purpose was to help the larger and more powerful left ventricle. At a meeting of the New York Heart Association in February 1966, DeBakey gave a talk about his work, suggesting that he would soon be ready to implant the new LVAD in a patient. His remarks caused a frenzy of interest, with one TV company stationing a van outside Methodist Hospital to cover the great moment, whenever it should occur.[25]

They had to wait a while, since the first clinical use of the new LVAD took place more than two months later. On 21 April a sixty-five-year-old retired coal-miner, Marcel DeRudder, was taken into theatre for surgery to replace a diseased aortic valve. When the procedure had been completed, his heart proved unequal to the task of supporting his circulation. Every time the surgical team tried to stop the heart-lung machine his blood pressure fell alarmingly: the cardiac muscle was too damaged to pump enough blood to keep him alive. After a quick discussion, DeBakey decided to use the LVAD, in the hope that its temporary use would allow the weakened myocardium time to recover. One end of the device was attached to the left atrium, the other to the axillary artery, a large vessel in the armpit. The pump itself, which was left outside the body, was a dome-shaped chamber containing a plastic membrane, on one side of which was blood and on the other gas. When carbon dioxide was pumped into the dome the membrane flexed, expelling the blood; when it was sucked out the blood chamber refilled, beginning the cycle once more.[26]

DeRudder never regained consciousness and died five days later, after a massive rupture to his left lung. Although DeBakey had not sought publicity, the resulting blanket media coverage irked his colleagues. One of those who reacted with disapproval was Adrian Kantrowitz, who remarked, 'We don't do things the way Dr DeBakey does – television cameras and all.'[27] He had reason to be irritated, since two and a half months earlier he had performed a similar operation using an LVAD of his own design. This was a simpler device than

DeBakey's, a U-shaped tube of plastic which was fitted across the aortic arch and powered by compressed air. Its other merit was that it had no valves, which meant that it could be used intermittently or switched off entirely without fear of clotting. His first patient died within twenty-four hours but the second, operated on in May, recovered consciousness and seemed to be on the mend until a stroke ended her life a fortnight later.[28]

While treating this woman Kantrowitz was struck by an observation. At one point the pump had been turned off to see if her heart was now strong enough to carry the circulation, and after two hours she was evidently in congestive heart failure, disorientated and having difficulty breathing. When LVAD support was resumed her lung function immediately improved, and she became alert and aware of her surroundings. Kantrowitz became convinced that a less invasive, temporary device for circulatory support would be a valuable way of helping cardiac patients through periods of crisis.[29] He now took a different approach to the problem, one which built on research he had begun more than a decade earlier.

In the early 1950s Kantrowitz was working in the laboratory of Carl Wiggers, a physiologist celebrated for his study of the cardiac cycle, the events which take place during a single heartbeat. He was particularly interested in coronary perfusion, the flow of blood through the arteries that supply the heart muscle. When the heart contracts in systole, the arteries inside the myocardium are twisted and compressed by the high pressure of the ventricles, squeezing blood back towards the aorta. This means that most perfusion takes place during diastole, the pause between contractions, when the vessels are relaxed. To study this sequence in more detail, Kantrowitz enlisted the help of his brother Arthur, a brilliant physicist, and after analysing the complex flow of blood throughout the cardiac cycle they concluded that forcing more blood into the coronaries during the lull of diastole might be a feasible way of improving the condition of patients with heart failure.[30]

Their efforts to exploit this insight came to nothing, but others had more success, notably Dwight Harken, who used an external motor to suck blood from the aorta during systole and pump it back in during diastole.[31] He called this technique counterpulsation, because it created a second pulse in the pause between heartbeats. Although it succeeded in improving coronary perfusion, it had the significant drawback of damaging the red blood cells. Another, more promising, idea involved inserting a catheter into an artery in the neck or chest and threading it downwards towards the heart until its tip lay just above the aortic valve, next to the openings of the coronary arteries. At the end of the catheter was a tiny latex balloon which could be inflated with carbon dioxide.[32] A timing circuit attached to an ECG machine synchronised the inflation of the balloon with diastole, so that blood was propelled into the coronaries.[33] Several people, including Willem Kolff, investigated this approach, but none succeeded in making it work satisfactorily until Adrian Kantrowitz refined it by using helium, which could be pumped more quickly through the narrow catheter than carbon dioxide, and a firmer polyurethane balloon which, unlike latex models, would not stretch and occlude the aorta.[34]

Following successful tests on dogs, Kantrowitz first used this device clinically on 29 June 1967. The patient was a forty-five-year-old diabetic woman who had been admitted early in the morning after suffering a major heart attack. She was ashen-faced, her skin was cold and clammy and her cardiac function was so poor that her pulse was undetectable. After concluding that the prognosis was more or less hopeless, Kantrowitz decided to use the balloon pump. It was inserted through an artery in her thigh and manoeuvred upwards through the aorta until it lay just above the heart. For the next seven hours it pulsated in alternation with the heart, pushing extra blood into the coronaries. Periodically the pump was switched off so that doctors could check the condition of her heart; the first eight times this was tried she seemed to relapse and its use had to be resumed. On the ninth attempt, however, there were unmistakeable signs of improvement. Her blood pressure gradually increased and the colour returned to her face.[35] After three months of convalescence she was well enough to return home from hospital. The only lingering effect of her ordeal was a limp, caused by the incision in her leg, and she remained in good health until her premature death in a road accident eighteen months later.

Although it was slow to catch on, Kantrowitz's balloon pump soon proved its worth, and it still plays an important role today in the management of patients whose hearts cannot sustain the circulation unassisted. When the myocardium is injured the consequence is typically a condition called cardiogenic shock, in which cardiac output is greatly reduced and the major organs no longer receive adequate oxygen. What makes this so dangerous is the body's response, a complex combination of compensatory measures which actually have the effect of exacerbating the original heart failure. Without intervention the patient can rapidly enter a downward spiral, terminating in cardiac arrest and death. The balloon pump is often highly effective at interrupting this vicious circle, increasing cardiac output by as much as 40 per cent and much improving the patient's chances of recovery. But it is an acute measure, useful only for short periods; for chronic conditions a longer-term solution was needed. And this meant either VADs or an artificial heart.

An important milestone was passed in August 1968 when Michael DeBakey used his LVAD to treat a sixteen-year-old Mexican beautician, Esperanza del Valle Vasquez, whose short life had been blighted by rheumatic heart disease. Already in severe heart failure, she was admitted to hospital for replacement of her mitral valve. Surgery presented a grave risk, and DeBakey was not surprised when she could not be weaned off the heart-lung machine. The LVAD was attached, and this was enough to keep her alive for the next four days, until her heart muscle had recovered sufficient function to support her circulation on its own. An extraordinary photograph taken shortly after the operation shows her sitting in bed grinning broadly, with the pump – a plastic object the size of a grapefruit – dangling from tubes implanted in her chest. Esperanza became the first patient to make a complete recovery after the use of an LVAD; it was a promising omen for the greater challenges that lay ahead.[36]

DeBakey's decision to prioritise VADs over the total artificial heart was a pragmatic one, but it did not go down well with some colleagues. Domingo Liotta had joined his laboratory six years earlier hoping that he would soon be able to see one of his prototypes working in a patient, and was upset when his project was effectively sidelined. Late in 1968 he met DeBakey to express his frustration, only to leave his boss's office feeling that he had been brushed off. What he did next might be seen as simply naïve or downright underhand: he arranged a meeting with Denton Cooley.

The relationship between DeBakey and Cooley had never been particularly close, but in the late 1960s it became distinctly chilly. After a decade of collaboration at Methodist Hospital their partnership had ended in 1962 when Cooley moved to St Luke's, a hospital a few hundred yards away – though he remained on the staff of Baylor University College of Medicine, where DeBakey was chairman of the department of surgery. What began as a clash of egos became, with the dawning of the transplant era, a case of mutual antagonism. Cooley was the first Houston surgeon to emulate Christiaan Barnard, performing three transplants in the space of a few days in May 1968. DeBakey, a cautious and methodical man who would only apply a new technique after months of assiduous laboratory work, took the strong view that Cooley had entered the field prematurely and without doing the requisite preparation. By the time he finally chalked up his first transplant in August, Cooley had eleven to his name. Nor can it have helped that the photogenic Cooley suddenly became the best-known face in American surgery, the protégé outshining his mentor.

When Domingo Liotta entered Cooley's basement office in December 1968 he must therefore have understood that his actions would be seen as a betrayal. He told Cooley that he doubted DeBakey's commitment to the artificial heart, and asked whether they could work together with a view to implanting it in a patient. Cooley readily agreed: the thrill of his early transplants had already given way to disenchantment as patient after patient died from rejection, and he saw the device as a promising alternative. Neither felt the need to tell DeBakey about their arrangement, and for the next four months Liotta kept his work with Cooley secret from the man supposedly employing him.

It soon became apparent that Liotta had acted prematurely. The following month DeBakey authorised animal testing of the artificial heart, his interest in the programme evidently very much alive. The results were deeply underwhelming: four of the seven calves died on the operating table, and none of the other three regained consciousness or lived for longer than twelve hours.[37] This only confirmed to DeBakey that months or years of work were still needed before the machine would be ready. On 4 April 1969 he travelled to Washington to attend a meeting of the National Heart Institute, and was just about to go to bed when he received a phone call from a colleague in Houston, who told him that Denton Cooley had performed the first implantation of an artificial heart. DeBakey was dumbfounded: as far as he knew, Cooley had never tried to develop a device, or shown any interest in doing so. The next morning he switched on the television to see Liotta and Cooley being interviewed, showing off a mechanical heart which looked suspiciously like the one from DeBakey's laboratory. When he arrived at his meeting he was surrounded by colleagues anxious to hear further details of the operation; to his intense embarrassment, he was forced to confess he knew as little as they did.[38]

DeBakey flew back to Houston intent on finding out what had happened. He quickly came to the conclusion that Cooley had been determined to be the first to implant an artificial heart, and that Liotta had enabled this by taking DeBakey's prosthesis without permission; in his view it was a straightforward case of theft. Cooley told a different story, claiming that the device was a new model which he and Liotta had developed in secret, and that the operation was not planned in advance but had been a last-ditch effort to save the life of a dying man.

The uncontested facts are these. On 5 March Haskell Karp, a forty-seven-year-old print worker from Illinois, was admitted to Cooley's hospital with advanced coronary artery disease. After two major heart attacks his cardiac muscle was ruined: angiograms showed the left ventricle ballooning with each contraction, indicating that its wall had been terminally weakened by a mass of dead tissue. Cooley recommended a transplant, but Karp was firmly opposed to the idea.[39] Instead he agreed to a less radical operation, myocardial excision with ventriculoplasty, known as the 'wedge procedure'. This entailed cutting out a wedge of dead heart muscle and suturing together the remaining tissue in the hope that it would be enough to keep the organ pumping. Cooley was frank about the risks: Karp stood only a 20 per cent chance of surviving the operation. He offered his patient one glimmer of hope. In the event of failure he could implant a mechanical heart, in the hope that it would keep him alive for long enough to enable a transplant. Karp agreed: if death was otherwise inevitable he would drop his opposition to receiving a new heart.

The operation was scheduled for 4 April, Good Friday. When the anaesthetist, Arthur Keats, went to see Karp at lunchtime that day he found him mottled and blue, struggling for breath; he was so alarmed by his condition that he rushed him straight into theatre. Cooley was quickly summoned, the patient attached to the heart-lung machine, and the operation began. As soon as Cooley opened the pericardium to reveal Karp's heart it became clear why he was at death's door. It was vast, with a grotesque balloon of scar tissue the size of a cantaloupe melon.[40] He excised this useless mass and reconstructed what remained. Attempts to restart the organ were unsuccessful, and – assisted by Liotta – Cooley implanted the prosthesis and switched it on.[41] For the first time in history a human life was being sustained by an artificial heart.

Karp regained consciousness shortly after the chest incision was closed, but could not be moved from the operating theatre since his life depended on a large console pumping compressed gas to the artificial heart through tubes in his chest. How long this machine could keep him alive was anybody's guess, so the race was now on to find a replacement heart. That evening Cooley and Liotta gave a hastily convened press conference at which they described the operation and appealed for a donor organ. Karp's wife Shirley contributed a hand-written note which was widely reproduced in the newspapers:

> Someone, somewhere, please hear my plea. A plea for a heart for my husband. I see him lying there, breathing and knowing that within his chest is a man-made implement where there should be a God-given heart. How long he can survive one can only guess ... Maybe somewhere there is a gift of a heart for my husband. Please ...[42]

A suitable donor was eventually found in Massachusetts, but only arrived after a nerve-wracking delay. The jet carrying the comatose patient developed a mechanical fault in mid-air, and had to make an emergency landing at a military base with its brakes out of action.[43] A replacement plane was quickly dispatched, and the donor was delivered to St Luke's at 5 a.m. the following morning, just as her heart was beginning to fail. The transplant, Cooley's twentieth, was performed quickly and without incident. Cooley was cautiously optimistic about his patient's chances, but his hopes were soon dashed. Within hours, X-rays started to show a worrying shadow on Karp's right lung. It was a fungal infection, and the immunosuppressant drugs Karp was taking left him powerless to fight it. A day later he went into cardiac arrest and died.[44]

While the attempt had been unsuccessful, Cooley's feat prompted reams of adulatory press coverage. But a storm was brewing. DeBakey was not the only one who wanted answers; the National Heart Institute, which had provided generous financial support for DeBakey's research, demanded to know whether the device used by Cooley was that developed in the Baylor College of Medicine laboratories. If so, its use in humans was subject to strict ethical protocols and approval in advance by a special committee – permission which

Cooley had neither sought nor received. Within hours, Baylor initiated the first of several inquiries to investigate the matter. Cooley was defiant, telling journalists immodestly, if accurately, 'I've done more heart surgery than anyone else in the world. I believe I am qualified on what is right and proper to do for my patient. The decisions are made by me with the permission of the patients.'[45]

Cooley claimed, both in public and to the authorities, that he and Liotta had tested no fewer than fifty-seven different configurations of 'their' heart, and that this included implantation in nine calves, of which four had been long-term survivors. But he was unable to provide documentation to prove that any such experiments had taken place, and his story continued to unravel when Liotta admitted that both construction and testing of the device had taken place in the Baylor laboratory, using resources paid for by the government grant.[46] The findings of the various inquiries into Cooley's operation made painful reading for the surgeon, and tarnished his achievement considerably. They found that he had misappropriated a device developed with government funds, and failed to seek ethical approval for an unsuccessful experiment on a human subject.[47] He was also censured for his conduct by the local medical society and by the American College of Surgeons,[48] and subsequently resigned from Baylor. To add to their woes, Cooley and Liotta were then sued for malpractice by the widow of Haskell Karp, who alleged that the surgeons had failed to explain exactly what the operation entailed. The case against them was dismissed, but only after one of the most protracted legal battles in medical history.[49]

The echoes of the Karp affair would reverberate for decades. Cooley soon attempted a reconciliation with DeBakey, but the older surgeon cut all ties with his former collaborator, describing him to friends as a 'non-person'. In a private conversation with a would-be biographer he was still more vicious, accusing Cooley of megalomania, greed and dishonesty. But he saved his harshest words for Liotta, whom he described as 'stupid' and 'unbalanced'.[50] Colleagues in Houston started to refer to the short distance between the offices of DeBakey and Cooley as the 'demilitarized zone', and their falling-out was even the subject of a cover story in *Life* magazine.[51] Although officialdom had painted Cooley as the villain of the piece, public opinion was divided. The influential *New York Post* columnist Max Lerner offered a perceptive assessment of the pair that showed that he well understood the dynamics and egos of the world of heart surgery:

> Neither is wholly right or wrong because both types of men are as necessary and complementary in the progress of the medical arts as the systole and diastole of the heart itself. We need the Cooleys to rush pell-mell along the lines of least resistance in heart transplants and artificial hearts. We need the DeBakeys to make sure that the revolutionary pace proceeds 'with all deliberate speed.' If my older judgment is with Dr DeBakey, my young, temperamental impulses are with Dr Cooley.[52]

This drawn-out soap opera rather overshadowed the important matter of assessing the outcome of the operation, and how the heart had performed. Although it succeeded in keeping Haskell Karp alive for almost three days, there was evidence that the device was highly unsatisfactory in its current form. While it was being used, Karp had suffered serious kidney damage, a complication also noted in the few animal tests which had taken place.[53] Any sober appraisal of the data suggested that the device was far from ready for human use.

The episode dealt a fatal blow to DeBakey's artificial heart programme, although others persevered with their research. Much of the available funding was diverted to a more ambitious aim: the design of a self-contained device which could be fully implanted into the body, rather than remaining tethered to an external power unit. It was hard to imagine anybody attached to such a thing leaving hospital, let alone living a normal life. The main difficulty lay in developing a battery which could provide the power to pump thousands of litres of blood per day while lasting for weeks or months. There was only one energy source with the potential to meet these exacting specifications: nuclear power.

The fascinating but abortive attempt to build a nuclear-powered artificial heart began in the mid-1960s. At about the same time as the US Atomic Energy Authority initiated research into nuclear pace-makers, it received a proposal from a private corporation for a cardiac prosthesis using similar technology. This was a more daunting proposition, since a mechanical pump requires far more energy than a tiny electronic circuit. The project was given the go-ahead, and in 1971 several teams, including one led by Willem Kolff in Utah, undertook the ambitious task of designing a substitute for the human heart, complete with its own miniature atomic power station.[54]

The technology used to power the nuclear heart was an appealing and innovative blend of ancient and modern. A sample of plutonium-238 weighing around 50 grams was enclosed in a hermetically sealed capsule made from tantalum, a hard and chemically inert metal, to minimise the escape of radiation. Through radioactive decay the plutonium heated the walls of the capsule to over 500°C, and this heat was transferred to water vapour which expanded to drive a piston, which in turn provided rotary power to the shaft of the blood pump.[55] The device was, in fact, a tiny steam engine, built on principles which the pioneers of the early nineteenth century would have recognised. Tests showed that the fuel cell would have a minimum lifespan of ten years – more than adequate for the needs of an artificial heart.

Unfortunately the system also had some pretty hefty drawbacks. Scientists asked to assess the device's safety found that it presented a substantial threat to the health not just of the recipient, but of their immediate family. The fuel cell emitted so much radiation that patients were likely to develop leukaemia, and it was virtually certain that they would become sterile – women in as little as a year. Even a spouse sleeping in the same bed as the owner of a nuclear heart was likely to suffer the same fate. The study also suggested that simply coming into contact with a recipient might be enough to cause birth defects.[56] A more outlandish possibility, albeit one taken seriously, was that a recipient might be kidnapped and murdered by hostile agents in order to obtain the plutonium for use in nuclear weapons.[57] But rather than national security concerns, it was the prospect of creating an army of silent killers, capable of giving a stranger cancer merely by standing next to them at a bus stop, that eventually put paid to the nuclear heart: in 1973 funding for the project was withdrawn, and research continued along more conventional lines.[58]

Though largely unheralded outside medical circles, the most encouraging progress was being made by Willem Kolff and his colleagues at the University of Utah. In 1969 his associate Clifford Kwan-Gett made an important breakthrough by designing the first pump that obeyed Starling's law, adjusting its output to compensate for changes in the volume of blood returned to the device.[59] Two years later Kolff asked Robert Jarvik, a twenty-five-year-old medical student, to join the team and help improve the device. This was an inspired move, if a brave one: Jarvik had failed to complete degrees at any of the three institutions he had enrolled at, but what he lacked in application he more than made up for in imagination. He also had a background in engineering, and Kolff immediately recognised his flair for finding mechanical solutions and applying them to the artificial heart. Within a year he had produced the Jarvik-3, which used polyurethane membranes powered by air to pump blood out of the two artificial ventricles.

After more than a decade of research and millions of dollars in funding, the artificial heart could only be seen as a disappointment: nobody had managed to keep an animal alive for longer than three days. But in 1973 this sequence of failures finally came to an end. In Minnesota, Tetsuzo Akutsu's device sustained eight calves for a week, and one for ten days.[60] The following year Kolff and his team surpassed this, using the Jarvik-3 in a calf that lived for eighteen days after implantation.[61] Steady progress was made elsewhere, too: groups in Cleveland and Berlin finally achieved survival times measured in months.[62] Jarvik continued to tweak his device, experimenting with a wide range of materials and designs. In a series of trials which began in 1976, nine calves given a Jarvik heart lived for five months or longer. Among a menagerie of experimental animals which eventually included a sheep called Ted E. Baer and a pair of calves named Charles and Diana,[63] the winner was a Jersey called Alfred, Lord Tennyson, which remained alive and well for 268 days, almost nine months, after implantation.[64]

Most of these devices were designed specifically to replace a cow's heart, but Jarvik also produced a slightly smaller model suitable for humans, which he called the Jarvik-7. Although Kolff had now been working on the problem for over twenty years, he was reluctant to take the momentous step of testing it on a patient. That all changed in 1979, when a young heart surgeon joined his team. William DeVries had worked briefly with Kolff many years before, and when he returned to the university after a break of almost a decade he was astonished by the advances made in his absence. Walking through the building that housed the experimental animals he saw numerous healthy looking cows and sheep with artificial hearts, and was soon convinced that the device was ready for human implantation. It was not easy to per-suade Kolff, who was worried about the implications for his funding should the attempt fail, but after several months of nagging he finally relented.[65]

As it transpired, it was not DeVries but Denton Cooley who implanted the next artificial heart. His second venture with the device in July 1981 was no more successful than the first: the pump caused serious complications in the three days it was in use, and the patient died a week after it was removed and replaced with a donor organ.[66] Cooley again incurred official wrath for his behaviour, earning a rep-rimand from the Food and Drug Administration for using a device which had not been approved for use in humans.

DeVries and Jarvik were attempting something far more ambi-tious, since their device, once inserted, would remain in situ for the rest of the recipient's life. In the autumn of 1982 they finally found a suitable patient. Barney Clark was a local dentist with a chequered medical history stretching back to his thirties, when he had con-tracted hepatitis. A heavy smoker, he later developed emphysema and idiopathic cardiomyopathy, a progressive heart failure of unknown cause.[67] At the age of sixty-one he was almost totally disabled, and drugs had failed to check the degeneration of his cardiac muscle. The amiable Clark was fascinated by medical innovation, so DeVries took him to see his experimental animals with artificial hearts beating in their chests, and invited him to watch as he implanted one in a calf. Clark was at first unenthusiastic, pointing out that the cows were in perfect health when operated on, whereas he was already an invalid.

It did not take long for him to change his mind. At the family Thanksgiving dinner a month later he was so sick that his family were forced to carry him downstairs, and he could eat only a few mouthfuls before returning to bed. He told his wife that he would go through with the operation; not because he thought it would save him, but because he wanted to make a contribution to medical knowledge.[68] When admitted to hospital he was in a pitiable condition, with an enlarged liver and pronounced swelling caused by fluid retention all over his body. To ensure that he could not possibly be accused of any ethical breach, DeVries went through an unusually elaborate consent procedure. Clark was interviewed by a six-strong panel of experts, before being asked to read and sign an eleven-page consent form that listed unambiguously all the many things that might go wrong. He was also shown graphic photographs of Cooley's first operation to leave him under no illusions about what he was about to put himself through. Finally, to guard against any second thoughts, he was made to sign the form again twenty-four hours later.[69] This extraordinary protocol had been the subject of endless discussion by the hospital's ethics committee, and was designed to avoid any repetition of the malpractice allegations that had blighted Cooley's operations.

The regulatory authorities had decreed that DeVries was only permitted to operate if death was imminent; until then he could do nothing but wait for Clark's condition to deteriorate. On the first day of December it started to snow, and when a few flakes turned into a full-blown blizzard DeVries asked his surgical staff to stay on site in case the roads became impassable. That afternoon Clark had an episode of heart arrhythmia which caused him to pass out, and doctors told his family that he was likely to die within hours or days.[70] With a patient who was already comatose and whose blood pressure had plunged to almost nothing, DeVries feared that his experiment was over before it had even begun; but somehow they managed to get him into theatre, open his chest and attach him to the heart-lung machine, and the seven-hour operation was underway.

The procedure had a brutal simplicity to it, and from a technical point of view was not particularly difficult. DeVries began by making two small stab wounds near Clark's navel to accommodate the air tubes which would power the device. Then came the most drastic step: lifting the heart out of the chest cavity, DeVries made an incision which cut it in two, entirely severing the ventricles from the atria. He cut through the aorta and the pulmonary artery, and the redundant portion of the heart – both ventricles, the bulk of the organ – could be discarded. The artificial heart was put in its place, and its Dacron outlet tubes trimmed so that they met the stumps of the major arteries perfectly; if the grafts were left too long they might kink and kill the patient.

The device itself was made of smooth polyurethane, and consisted of two roughly spherical chambers designed to replace the ventricles. Each contained a plastic diaphragm whose pulsations, powered by pressurised air, would propel blood through the body. Their edges were lined with a cuff of Dacron by which each of the two artificial ventricles was carefully sutured to the remaining tissue of the corresponding atrium. It was therefore only the pumping chambers that were new: before entering them, blood would pass through the remnants of Clark's own right and left atria. DeVries attached the drive lines and passed them through a tunnel of muscle so that they emerged through the incisions in the abdomen. The artificial heart was switched on, but was allowed to take over the circulation from the heart-lung machine only when DeVries was satisfied that any air in the blood chambers had been completely evacuated.[71]

It was seven o'clock in the morning when Barney Clark was finally wheeled out of theatre and taken to intensive care. He woke up shortly afterwards and asked for a glass of water, before turning to his wife and saying, 'I want to tell you that even though I have an artificial heart, I still love you.'[72] For his part, DeVries had been working flat-out for twenty-four hours, but knew it would be some time before he would be allowed any rest. Journalists had started to arrive at the hospital while the operation was still in progress, and within days their number had swollen to over 300. Police were summoned to prevent unwanted intruders, and visitors were incessantly questioned for any snippet of news.[73] The hospital administrators had learned the lessons of the transplant era, and regular briefings were organised to satisfy the journalists' insatiable appetite for fresh information.

DeVries found these sessions difficult: he was just thirty-five and had little experience of dealing with the media. What made it all the worse was that he rarely had any good news to pass on. Although Barney Clark regained consciousness within a few hours of the operation, he soon experienced the first in an escalating series of setbacks. On the third day he had to be returned to theatre so that a small lung rupture could be repaired, and this was rapidly followed by kidney failure and mysterious seizures. On 14 December, less than a fortnight after implantation, the artificial heart failed when one of its valves broke, and Clark had to undergo surgery for a third time to replace the entire left ventricle. Further complications followed, but in late February there were finally signs of improvement. Barney was able to talk to his wife, ate normally, and received physical therapy; there was even talk of his discharge from hospital.[74] To give the wider world some evidence of his recovery a short interview was filmed and broadcast on 2 March, though Clark was patently very sick and gave his answers in a monotone while staring into the middle distance. The public reaction to this spectacle was not as positive as DeVries and his colleagues had expected.

Any hope that Clark might ever go home soon vanished. Shortly afterwards he developed pneumonia, and the story thereafter was one of inexorable decline. One by one his organs began to fail, and on 23 March his condition became irretrievable when his lungs and brain stopped functioning. The heart was the last part of his body to keep working, and at 10 p.m., after beating approximately 12 million times, it was finally silenced when DeVries switched it off with the turn of a key. Outside the building it was snowing, as it had been 112 days earlier when Barney Clark became the first person in history to receive a permanent artificial heart.

Clark's survival for more than three months confounded the predictions of the many surgeons who had been pessimistic about his prospects. Surprisingly, even Denton Cooley spoke out against it, suggesting that 'the artificial heart is not ready for elective implantation and cannot even approach the expectation of cardiac transplantation today'.[75] Michael DeBakey criticised Clark's poor post-operative condition and minimal quality of life, while Norman Shumway dismissed the device as a 'clot machine' which was likely to kill patients by giving them strokes.[76] William DeVries had to endure personal as well as professional abuse, receiving threats from anonymous correspondents outraged at his meddling with nature.[77] To cap it all, the medical establishment effectively turned its back on him later that year when the bodies funding research into artificial hearts decided that their resources should instead be concentrated on the simpler and less problematic ventricular assist devices.[78]

DeVries, however, had no intention of giving up. Under the terms of his original agreement with the regulatory authorities he was permitted to perform six more implantations of the Jarvik-7, but the University of Utah raised concerns about the cost. After two years trying to raise funds he admitted defeat and accepted a private healthcare company's offer to fund his work at a hospital in Kentucky.[79] On 25 November 1984 he implanted a second Jarvik heart into Bill Schroeder, a fifty-four-year-old who had been rejected for transplant because of diabetes. By the end of his first week he was walking around his room, but his recovery was marred by a stroke and repeated infections. Nevertheless, three months later he was able to take part in a rehearsal for his son's wedding in the hospital chapel, and was eventually allowed to move to a nearby apartment. His progress was again followed eagerly by the media, and the by-now familiar face of Robert Jarvik made frequent appearances on the news bulletins. With his weakness for garish ties and air of a superannuated rock star he was an arresting figure, and became something of a celebrity. *Playboy* magazine even accorded him the honour of an in-depth profile, an eccentric interview in which he was described sculpting a unicorn-shaped dildo for an unnamed paramour.[80]

In early 1985 DeVries performed two further operations, and for a brief, heady period the hospital housed three patients all living with an artificial heart. The undoubted highlight of Bill Schroeder's recovery came in September, when he was taken on a fishing trip with a portable air pump strapped to the back of his wheelchair. Alas, this was a pleasure which would not be repeated. Shortly before the anniversary of his operation he suffered a major stroke from which he never fully recovered, beginning a slow decline to his death on 6 August 1986.[81]

Bill Schroeder's death was also the end of a chapter for DeVries, signalling the conclusion of his trial of the Jarvik heart. Of his four patients one had died after ten days, but the others were long-term survivors – two for more than a year. These results, he believed, justified his clinical experiments, but he conceded that there were serious problems with the device; in particular, he acknowledged that it had frequently caused strokes, tacitly admitting the truth of Shumway's earlier criticism.[82] Other surgeons in Europe and America used it with some success, however, including Terence English in London. By the time of the last implantation of a Jarvik-7 in 1992, 226 patients in Europe and America had received artificial hearts, most as a bridge to transplantation. Not all of these were Jarviks: ten other models had been used, and often with excellent results. More than a third of patients lived for a year, and two-thirds survived long enough to receive a transplant.[83]

Research into artificial hearts continued, but by the early 1990s many believed that the dream of a permanent substitute for the heart was over. It had been supplanted by the concept of 'bridge to transplant', a compelling new therapy for those with end-stage cardiac failure. The 'bridge' did not have to be a total artificial heart, since VADs had also proved effective at achieving the same goal: in 1984 the Stanford University surgeon Philip Oyer implanted an LVAD into Robert St Laurent, a fifty-one-year-old who was desperately sick after a coronary bypass operation had failed to salvage his diseased myocardium. Developed by the former nuclear physicist Peer Portner, the device was revolutionary in its design, powered by an electric motor rather than compressed air. This removed the need for a bulky external drive unit; instead, a wire passed through the skin was connected to a battery pack which the patient could wear on a belt. A week later the device was removed, and in its place Oyer transplanted the heart of an eighteen-year-old student who had died in a road accident.[84] St Laurent was the first person to successfully receive an LVAD as a bridge to transplant, and lived for another twenty years, in the process also becoming one of the longest-surviving transplant patients.[85]

The first generation of VADs were pulsatile: they pumped blood rhythmically, seventy or so times per minute. This seemed logical, since it simulated the action of the heart. But the late 1980s saw the appearance of a new type of device which drove fluid continuously, like the propeller of a boat. Physiologists had long debated the significance of the pulse, and whether it was an essential feature of the circulation. Some argued that organs had evolved to function with a pulsatile blood supply, and that kidneys, for example, would sustain damage if the blood flow were continuous.[86] Others believed that the pulse was nothing more than 'an expression of the limitations of organic heart design'[87] – a consequence of evolution, but one of no great importance. In 1984 researchers at the Cleveland Clinic put these rival theories to the test by the inventive means of creating a pulseless cow. They took four healthy calves and bypassed

their hearts with a pair of blood pumps – one for each of the ventricles – mounted on the animals' backs. These pumps used rotors to
propel the blood continuously, so for the duration of the experiment
the calves had no heartbeat. All four lived quite happily without a
pulse for a month, suggesting that the same might also be true for
humans.[88]

In April 1988 a pulseless LVAD was implanted in a patient in
Houston by Bud Frazier, a surgeon of immaculate pedigree: after
training with Michael DeBakey he had moved over the road to become
Denton Cooley's right-hand man. He used the Hemopump, a clever
little device which was small enough to be inserted through a blood
vessel. An incision was made in the femoral artery in the groin, and a
catheter containing the pump, just 7 millimetres in diameter, passed
up through the aorta until the device was wedged in the opening of
the aortic valve. Rotors spinning at up to 27,000 rpm propelled blood
from the left ventricle into the aorta, almost entirely taking over the
circulation.[89] The patient, a sixty-one-year-old man suffering an episode of rejection following a heart transplant, was sustained with this
device for two days before making a full recovery. He was eventually
discharged, having briefly become the first human being to live without a pulse.

Like the intra-aortic balloon pump, the Hemopump was intended
only as a short-term measure to help patients through a brief crisis. In
the late 1990s, however, a new generation of continuous-flow LVADs
intended for longer-term use appeared on the scene; the first was
developed by Michael DeBakey, the surgeon responsible for establishing the field more than thirty years earlier. At the age of ninety, and
still as energetic as ever, he supervised clinical trials of a device he had
designed in collaboration with NASA. This partnership was instigated
by a former patient, Dave Saucier, an engineer at the Johnson Space
Center who had received a heart transplant from DeBakey in 1984.
Using NASA's expertise in aerodynamics and technology invented for
the space programme, the team designed a pump the size of an AA battery which resembled a miniature jet engine.[90] The device was placed

inside the chest so that it pumped blood from the left ventricle to the ascending aorta at rates of up to 6 litres per minute.[91]

DeBakey's continuous-flow pump, introduced in 1998, was the first of several second-generation LVADs to be put to clinical use. By the time they appeared on the market, specialists had over a decade's experience with temporary devices, and had noticed that patients often did well even if they failed to receive a transplant within a couple of years; in some cases, the diseased heart even began to recover its function. Clinicians now realised that they might also be useful as 'destination therapy' – a permanent treatment for those patients deemed ineligible for transplant because of age or significant additional health conditions. A major trial was organised involving 129 patients in end-stage heart failure who were not candidates for transplant. They were split into two groups: 68 were given LVADs, and the remaining 61 received the best possible drug therapy. The results of the snappily named Randomized Evaluation of Mechanical Assistance for the Treatment of Congestive Heart Failure trial (REMATCH) were published in 2001, and showed that LVADs reduced the risk of death by almost 50 per cent.[92] American regulators approved one device as destination therapy the following year; NICE, the British equivalent, finally followed suit in 2015.[93]

Today's LVADs are a world away from the bulky, wheezing monsters first used in the 1960s. Easy to implant and almost totally silent, they allow the patient to live a virtually normal life, constrained only by the battery pack that keeps the motor spinning. For many patients unsuitable for transplant they represent the only hope of prolonged survival – and for doctors they represent a real and necessary alternative to giving somebody a new heart. When transplantation began in the 1960s, surgeons could count on a steady stream of organs from young and healthy donors killed in traffic accidents. But in the developed world, at least, roads, and the vehicles we drive on them, are incomparably safer than they were in the 1960s, and the number of donor hearts has fallen correspondingly. Some of those given a VAD as a bridge to transplant will never make it to the top of the waiting list, but if the device keeps them alive and active the result may be almost as good. One surgeon I spoke to told me firmly that trans-plantation will come to be seen as a needlessly crude and expensive aberration: why cut out a patient's heart if you can simply insert a tiny pump?

While VADs have in the last twenty years attracted more atten-tion and funding than the artificial heart, they are not a panacea. Many patients with bilateral heart failure, in which both ventri-cles stop working, will only benefit from a total prosthesis. On 10 September 2011 a 55-year-old Italian, Pietro Zorzetto, was given a transplant after spending 1,374 days – close to 4 years – with a total artificial heart. For much of this time he was in such good health that he was able to go cycling, and asked to be removed from the transplant waiting list.[94] After a quarter of a century of slow improvement, the total artificial heart finally seems to be realising the dreams of its pioneers in the 1950s, becoming a viable means of sustaining the lives of those whose own hearts have long since given up the ghost.

When the pioneers of mechanical circulatory support began their work, they little imagined the decades of controversy, frustration and pain that were to come. But in 2007, the same year that Pietro Zorzetto finally realised their dream by posing for pictures astride his bike, the most bitter and protracted episode of the whole saga finally came to an end when Denton Cooley and Michael DeBakey shook hands for the first time in forty years.

DeBakey was ninety-nine, his former colleague a stripling of eighty-eight. Their reconciliation was engineered by Cooley, who had been reading a book by a former patient, Gene Cernan, the last man to walk on the Moon. Cernan's portrayal of the antagonism between American astronauts and their Soviet counterparts, and how it was transformed into collaboration and finally friendship, moved him, and he decided it was time to seek a truce with his old rival.[95] His initial overtures were rebuffed, but after he wrote a warm letter explaining his motives DeBakey accepted his offer. At a meeting of the Denton A. Cooley Cardiovascular Surgical Society on 27 October 2007, Michael DeBakey was made an honorary member and presented with an award. He was recovering from aortic surgery, and gave a short speech from his mobility scooter.[96]

Both men spoke warmly of each other's surgical achievements, but there were no apologies.

10. FANTASTIC VOYAGE

Lausanne, 12 June 1986

In the 1966 thriller *Fantastic Voyage* a submarine full of scientists is shrunk to microscopic size and injected into the body of a comatose man who has suffered an inoperable brain injury. Over the course of the next hour they navigate his veins and arteries, passing through his heart and locating a blood clot before vaporising it with a laser. It's a fairly silly plot, but the interior of the human body is imaginatively portrayed as a hostile alien landscape, with anatomical details so accurate that the film was once routinely shown to medical students. Though it ends with a tribute to the 'many doctors, technicians and research scientists' who advised the producers, few cinema-goers can have believed that they had just watched a bold vision of the future. Miniaturising a submarine remains beyond our capabilities, but the central premise of *Fantastic Voyage* – that it would one day be possible to operate on the body *from inside* – has since come to pass.

Indeed, another film made the previous year showed that this improbable science-fiction dream was already well on the way to being scientific fact. It was intended only for a small audience of specialists, so the fifteen-minute *Transluminal Angioplasty* can be forgiven its mouthful of a title. It was written, directed and narrated by its star, the Oregon radiologist Charles Dotter, to demonstrate a technique he had invented for removing blockages inside blood vessels. Rather than attack the problem from outside the body, he had hit upon the idea of treating it from within. A flexible catheter was inserted through a small nick in an artery near the skin and gently pushed through the obstruction to create a new channel for the blood. The patient remained awake, and the entire procedure took less than an hour. This was a radical departure from the conventional method of making a large incision under general anaesthetic and opening the artery to clean it. The point is driven home in the film by a montage of gory surgical images – scalpels carving through flesh, needles submerged in bubbling pools of blood – which are then contrasted with the serene and bloodless scene as Dotter gently navigates his catheter towards its unseen destination, exchanging pleasantries with his patient as he does so. In this brief demonstration it is an artery in the leg which is being treated, but Dotter also suggests that the technique might one day be used in the vessels of the heart.[1] Little more than a decade later his prediction would come true, opening a new era in the treatment of cardiac disease.

For decades, doctors concerned with the workings of the heart had been divided into two camps: cardiologists and surgeons. The role of cardiologists was diagnosing cardiac conditions and treating them with drugs; if nothing else was suitable, patients would then be referred for surgical treatment. But in the 1970s something interesting happened: cardiologists began to 'operate' on the heart. This was nothing short of a revolution. Within a few years it became possible to treat coronary artery disease, and to repair congenital defects and even faulty valves, using nothing more than a flexible tube introduced through a tiny needle puncture. This new discipline, interventional cardiology, changed when and how surgery was undertaken, and made some complicated and dangerous operations entirely unnecessary.

The idea of introducing probes into the living heart was not a new one even then. In the nineteenth century several French physiologists did so in order to measure the temperature or pressure of blood within the cardiac chambers, making an incision in the neck of a dog or horse and pushing a tube through the blood vessels until it lay inside the organ. One of them, Claude Bernard, coined the term by which the technique is still known: *cathétérisme* (catheterisation).[2] In choosing this word Bernard was acknowledging the similarity between the method and the ancient practice of inserting a draining tube (catheter) into the bladder to relieve urinary retention. His contemporaries Auguste Chauveau and Étienne-Jules Marey used a catheter to investigate the sounds of the heartbeat, proving that the apex beat, the vibration palpable on the outside of the chest, is simultaneous with the contraction of the ventricles.[3]

Catheterisation provided many important insights to later physiologists, but none was yet brave enough to use it on a human subject. That important step had to wait until the late 1920s, and the work of a young German who was obsessed with the work of Chauveau and Marey. As a student at the University of Berlin, Werner Forssmann came across a picture of Marey holding a catheter which he had just inserted through a horse's jugular vein and into its heart; as he recorded in his autobiography, 'I was so excited by this image that it haunted me day and night.'[4] Forssmann was frustrated by the shortcomings of contemporary methods of cardiac diagnosis, which still relied heavily on the stethoscope; X-rays and the ECG were also in use in larger hospitals, but gave only limited data. He believed that the methods of the French physiologists could be safely adapted for human use, and might provide a wealth of new diagnostic information.

Forssmann was twenty-four, newly qualified and working in a small hospital in the town of Eberswalde when he put his idea into practice. In the summer of 1929 he began by testing the idea on cadavers, and found that a catheter inserted into a vein in the elbow and gently pushed would find its way naturally to the right side of the heart. He then approached his boss, the surgeon Richard Schneider, to explain his plan of doing the same in a living subject. Schneider was sympathetic to his aims, but prohibited him from experimenting on patients. Forssmann offered instead to try the procedure on himself, but this too was forbidden. Schneider, who was friendly with the young man's mother, pointed out that she had lost her husband in the recent war, and he had no desire to tell her that her son had killed himself performing some rash experiment.[5] Forssmann had been expecting this response, and so used all his charm to persuade a theatre nurse, Gerda Ditzen, to help him. When she heard about his idea and was assured that it was entirely safe, she gamely volunteered to be his guinea pig.

One afternoon when most of the staff were taking their siesta, Forssmann and Nurse Ditzen made their way to an empty operating theatre. Forssmann explained that the local anaesthetic he intended to use might make her drowsy, so suggested that she lie on the operating table. This was a ruse; not content with disobeying his boss, Forssmann was also going to trick his accomplice. With ostentatious care he sterilised a patch of her skin with iodine, but out of her sight he had already anaesthetised his own arm. As soon as the skin was numb he made an incision in the crook of his elbow, punctured the vein with a needle and inserted an oiled urinary catheter a short distance. It was then that he admitted his deception: the nurse was furious with him, but agreed to help him complete the procedure. With the catheter tip embedded somewhere near his armpit he walked down several flights of stairs to the basement room where the X-ray equipment was housed. A colleague tried to talk him out of continuing with the experiment, but Forssmann was not to be denied. A strategically placed mirror allowed him to see an X-ray image of his own chest on the fluoroscopy screen, as he carefully fed almost two feet of rubber tubing into his own arm. There was no way of knowing in advance whether this would be painful, but the only sensation Forssmann felt was a slight warmth as the catheter slid along the wall of the vein. Finally the picture showed the catheter tip lodged in the right atrium of his heart, and a photograph was taken as proof of what he had done.[6]

When his superior Dr Schneider heard that his strict instructions had been disobeyed he was incensed, and reprimanded Forssmann for his dishonesty. But his ire was soon spent, and when the young man apologised he was congratulated on his 'great discovery' and invited for a celebratory dinner. Forssmann felt that the cardiac catheter might be a convenient way of introducing drugs directly to the heart, and shortly afterwards used the technique on a desperately ill patient who was suffering from peritonitis, the result of a burst appendix. A cardiac stimulant was injected through the catheter; although the patient appeared to rally briefly, she died shortly afterwards.[7] Encouraged by Schneider, Forssmann wrote an academic paper about his experiences, which was published later that year by one of Germany's most prestigious journals. Forssmann was not prepared for the uproar his work caused: he was accosted by journalists on the street, and his achievement was reported all over the world. One American newspaper remarked that 'other men have performed feats quite as risky, but rarely does anyone try a thing that makes us fidget so much to think about it.'[8]

In the meantime Forssmann had moved to Berlin to continue his training with Ferdinand Sauerbruch, the pre-eminent surgeon of the day. An old-fashioned autocrat, Sauerbruch strongly disapproved of his junior's experiment, and when he learned of it summarily dismissed him.[9] Having endured a torrid couple of months in the Berlin hospital, Forssmann was far from unhappy with this outcome, and returned to Eberswalde to continue his research. He now saw that catheterisation might be a good way to obtain clear images of the heart and major vessels, which give only a faint outline in conventional X-rays. His idea was to inject contrast medium, a liquid opaque to X-rays, directly into the organ so that its structures would be clearly delineated in the resulting photograph. The theory was sound, but the equipment available to him was not terribly sophisticated and the images he obtained were disappointing.[10] Despite the international acclaim that had followed his initial publication, Forssmann struggled to find any in the profession who would support his work, and he eventually gave up his research. Reflecting on the episode almost half a century later, he suggested that the medical establishment of the 1930s still regarded the heart as somehow sacrosanct: 'I had committed the cardinal sin; I had broken into the sanctuary and wantonly destroyed a taboo.'[11]

There was little interest in catheterisation of the heart for the next decade, although a few researchers did try to continue investigations

along similar lines. In 1936 a doctor from Paris, Pierre Ameuille, succeeded where Forssmann had failed, producing the first clear X-ray
images of the structure of the heart.[12] He faced hostility from his cardiologist colleagues, who denounced as 'monstrous' the idea of introducing a tube into the beating organ.[13] But he found a more receptive
audience in a former student, André Cournand, who was visiting
Paris on a break from his job at a hospital in New York. Cournand was
impressed by the images his old teacher showed him, and by his assur-
ances that the procedure was perfectly safe. He also understood that
the technique would be an ideal way of continuing his own research
into the circulation, and when he returned to the United States shortly
afterwards he took a stock of flexible catheters, which at that time
were only manufactured in France.[14]

Cournand's project was a thorough investigation of the cardiopulmonary system, the circulation of blood through the heart and lungs.
He and his colleague Dickinson Richards were particularly interested
in how lung disease affected the flow of blood, and thought that catheterisation would offer a precise method of measuring cardiopulmonary function. They refined their methods through experiments
on dogs and a chimpanzee, and in 1940 they moved to working with
humans.[15] By using the catheter to measure the pressure in the right
atrium, and the oxygen content of the blood before and after it passed
through the lungs, they could calculate cardiac output, the volume of
blood pumped by the heart each minute – a valuable way of assessing
its health. Cournand was able to compare the cardiac outputs of four
patients, one of whom had high blood pressure and heart failure; as
expected, the damaged organ was pumping worryingly small amounts
with each stroke.[16]

The technique was taken up more widely as those who had been
trained by Cournand went to work at other institutions, and many of
them had ideas about new ways in which the procedure could be used.
In 1945 two groups discovered a way of using the catheter to diagnose
congenital heart conditions. Eleanor Baldwin, a physician from New
York, realised that the ability to take samples of blood direct from the

cardiac chambers made it possible to detect cases of ventricular septal defect – until then difficult to diagnose with certainty. If a defect was present, oxygenated blood would be shunted from the left ventricle into the right and mingle with venous blood. Samples taken from the right ventricle via the catheter would therefore show unnaturally high oxygen concentrations when compared with those taken from the right atrium.[17] Similarly, James Warren in Atlanta discovered that the presence of highly oxygenated blood in the right atrium was strong evidence of a hole in the septum between the upper chambers of the heart.[18]

Those outside the US trying to use cardiac catheterisation, however, often faced stubborn opposition. John McMichael, the first to adopt the technique in Britain, began work at a time when Nazi flying bombs were still making daily life in London extremely hazardous. When told that the catheter would cause blood clots and probably kill the patient, he responded by citing the remarkable statistic that in thousands of procedures since Forssmann's first experiment in 1929, not a single death had occurred. He was also able to show that other congenital conditions could be diagnosed by catheterisation, including tetralogy of Fallot and pulmonary stenosis.[19]

McMichael was acutely aware of the debt he owed to the inventor of the method, who had seemingly disappeared from medical life: an article in *The Lancet* published in 1949 noted that 'little is known about the fate of Forssmann'.[20] After much effort McMichael finally tracked him down to a remote village in the Black Forest. The aftermath of the war had been difficult for him: after a spell in a prisoner-of-war camp he had returned home to discover that his house had been flattened in an air raid. He was soon reunited with his family, but his former membership of the Nazi party made it impossible for him to gain a position of any importance, so he settled down to life as a country doctor. He gratefully accepted McMichael's invitation to visit London and talk about his work, finally gaining the recognition denied him almost twenty years earlier. His lasting reputation was assured in 1956, when he shared a Nobel Prize with Cournand and Dickinson Richards 'for their discoveries concerning heart catheterization and pathological changes in the circulatory system'.[21] Although urged to resume the research that had eventually made him famous, Forssmann refused: aware of how much the field had moved on in his absence, he resigned himself to the status of 'living fossil' – as he put it – and spent the rest of his career as a urologist.[22]

Until the late 1940s cardiac catheterisation was performed exclusively on the right side of the heart: this was easily done via a vein, since the catheter would be travelling in the same direction as the blood. Entering the left side meant passing it through an artery and against the flow of blood, which most clinicians thought too difficult and possibly dangerous. A few years earlier a doctor from Cuba, Pedro Fariñas, had shown that this was not the case, pushing a catheter to the base of the aorta in order to obtain beautiful X-ray images of the vessel and its major branches.[23] Sliding it an inch or two further would have taken it through the aortic valve and into the left ventricle of the heart, but he felt that this was too risky to attempt. Henry Zimmerman, a cardiologist working in Cleveland, disagreed. He demonstrated that the procedure was perfectly safe, although it entailed a few difficulties not encountered when investigating the right side of the heart. He used an artery in the forearm to insert a catheter lubricated with olive oil, which then had to be pushed against the direction of the blood flow until it reached the aortic valve. Manipulating it beyond this obstacle was the trickiest step, since the valve is open for just a fifth of a second during each cardiac contraction.[24] The first patient in whom he tried the technique had a leaking aortic valve, and Zimmerman was able to observe how this had affected the blood pressures in the aorta and left ventricle.[25] A few years later a young cardiologist in Maryland, John Ross, devised an ingenious alternative to this technique. He designed a special catheter with a needle at its tip which was inserted through a vein and into the right side of the heart. A small puncture was then made in the septum and the catheter pushed through the hole so that it rested in the left atrium or ventricle.[26] This avoided the difficulty of crossing the aortic valve, and the tiny wound in the cardiac septum was found to heal without complications.

The catheter was not just useful for measuring pressures and taking blood samples. In the early years of heart surgery, surgeons could never be entirely sure what they would find when they opened the patient's chest: a child diagnosed with simple valve disease might turn out to have some exotic congenital problem. The 1950s saw rapid progress in visualising the vessels and interior of the heart, using the catheter to inject contrast medium direct into its chambers. An X-ray taken immediately afterwards would show their structure in far greater detail than had been achieved in earlier decades. The Stockholm-based researcher Gunnar Jönsson found that by precise manipulation of the catheter tip it was possible to choose the part of the circulation highlighted in the resulting X-ray, a technique known as selective angiography.[27] That insight, and Mason Sones's discovery that it was safe to inject the contrast liquid directly into the coronary arteries, were of crucial importance to the rapid evolution of open-heart surgery. An angiogram was a blueprint of the faulty cardiac plumbing which gave the surgeon a clear idea of what to expect and how to fix it.

In June 1963 Charles Dotter was invited to give a lecture to a gathering of radiologists in the spa town of Karlovy Vary in Czechoslovakia. He had been asked to talk about the future of angiography – a young discipline, but one whose role within medicine was well defined. As far as his audience were concerned, their job was to obtain X-ray images of the heart and major vessels in order to reach a diagnosis; surgeons or physicians would then decide on the most appropriate treatment. What they heard in the lecture theatre that day shocked them, for Dotter had far grander ambitions. He told his colleagues that they would soon be not just diagnosing patients, but treating them: 'The angiographic catheter can be more than a tool for passive means for diagnostic observation; used with imagination it can become an important surgical instrument.'[28] This was radical stuff: the idea that the catheter might be an alternative to the scalpel had not even occurred to most of those in the room. Dotter's final words were greeted with a thunderous standing ovation; one of the attendees remembered later that 'It was like a bomb had been dropped.'[29]

Dotter's vision of the future was based on practical experience, not just wishful thinking. A few months earlier he had been performing an aortogram, a routine procedure to obtain X-ray images of a patient's aorta. It entailed inserting a catheter via the femoral artery in the groin and into the abdominal aorta before injecting contrast medium. It was usually straightforward, but this time the femoral artery was obstructed by an atheroma – a fatty deposit caused by atherosclerosis. Dotter found that it took little effort to push the catheter through the obstruction, and without meaning to he provided a new channel for blood to flow through. This was such a simple procedure that he felt sure a catheter could be used routinely to clear a path through obstructed arteries.

Five years earlier a medical student in Cincinnati, Thomas Fogarty, had had a very similar idea. He was still in his early twenties when he invented a new instrument for removing blood clots from inside arteries. He had watched surgeons attempt to do so by making a wide incision through skin and blood vessel before using forceps to scoop up the clot – but this procedure had a disappointingly low success rate, and many patients later had to have a limb amputated. Fogarty constructed a hollow catheter with a tiny latex balloon at its tip; his first prototypes used a finger cut from a surgical glove. The other end of the catheter was connected to a bottle of compressed gas, which could be used to inflate the balloon when required. This device (known ever since as a Fogarty catheter) was placed through an incision in a blood vessel and passed through the clot. The balloon was then inflated and withdrawn, dragging the coagulated blood with it. First used in 1961, the Fogarty catheter was a dramatic improvement on earlier methods of clot removal. It not only reduced mortality, but virtually eliminated emergency amputations. Before its introduction, a fifth of patients lost a limb as a result of failed surgery to remove a clot; afterwards the proportion fell to just 3 per cent.[30] Despite this triumph, Fogarty had immense difficulty in convincing anybody to take his work seriously. When he tried to publish his findings, the first three medical journals he approached declined to print his paper. In 1962 he moved to the University of Oregon to complete his surgical training, and met Charles Dotter – at last, a clinician whose vision matched his own.

Even among friends, Dotter had a reputation as an untamed maverick. A slim athletic man who spent his spare time climbing mountains, he was a restless bundle of energy at work. One Oregon colleague, the surgeon Albert Starr, said of Dotter, 'I never saw him normal; he was always in a hypomanic state.'[31] Although obviously brilliant – he was appointed professor of radiology at the age of thirty-two, the youngest in the US – Dotter was known as 'crazy Charlie', both for his odd manner and his wild ideas. He was evangelical about his work and took his enthusiasm to extremes: on his morning rounds one day in 1961 he gave his students an apparently impromptu talk on the use of the catheter, which he concluded by revealing that he had one in his heart at that very moment, inserted half an hour earlier. To gasps from his audience, he rolled up his sleeve to reveal the end of the instrument, which he then plugged into a monitor in order to demonstrate the pressure readings that could be found in a normal healthy heart.[32]

The new medical era predicted by Charles Dotter finally began on 16 January 1964. Ten days earlier he had met Laura Shaw, an eighty-two-year-old woman who was admitted to hospital with a badly diseased left leg and foot. Three of her toes were gangrenous, and her lower leg was cold and pulseless, indicating that very little blood was reaching it. An angiogram revealed a large area of obstruction in the femoral artery caused by atherosclerosis. The surgeons strongly recommended amputating the diseased foot but she refused, saying that she would prefer to die. With all other options exhausted, Dotter was given the opportunity to try his new technique. He called it transluminal angioplasty – 'angioplasty' meaning the clearing of a blood vessel, and 'transluminal' indicating that the treatment takes place through the lumen, the interior channel, of the vessel.

There were three stages to Dotter's procedure. First a puncture was made in the femoral artery and a guidewire inserted through it, into the vessel and through the area of obstruction. A thin catheter was then slid over the guidewire and also pushed through the atheroma to form a new blood channel. A second, slightly larger, catheter was finally slipped over the first and enlarged the channel still further. This all took a matter of minutes. When Dotter removed the catheter the improvement in his patient's condition was striking: pulses could be felt in her foot, which returned to a normal temperature. Her pain started to disappear, and in the following week the gangrene receded and the leg ulcer healed, signifying an improvement in its blood supply. Three weeks later an angiogram showed that the previously obstructed artery was now completely clear of atheroma.[33] Laura Shaw lived for another three years before dying from unrelated heart disease; until then (as Dotter liked to point out) she stayed on her feet – both of them.

In his first article about transluminal angioplasty, Dotter likened the diseased blood vessels of the leg to a rusty old garden sprinkler. This was in keeping with his therapeutic philosophy; a much-quoted motto of his was 'If a plumber can do it for pipes, we can do it for blood vessels.' He also expressed the sentiment in a pencil drawing which he framed and placed over his desk, showing a monkey wrench and length of pipe crossed like swords in a heraldic badge. Obsessed with machinery since his childhood, Dotter certainly liked to see himself as a sort of medic-cum-mechanic, and he constructed many of his catheters himself using whatever materials he had to hand: guitar strings, speedometer cable, or plastic insulation stripped from an electrical cable.[34]

It is one of medical history's great missed opportunities that Thomas Fogarty and Charles Dotter, the two visionaries of catheter therapy, were not allowed to work together for any length of time. Fogarty was a surgeon, and his superiors were wary of the peculiar radiologist who liked to tease them that the entire discipline of surgery would soon be obsolete. Though discouraged from having much contact with Dotter, Fogarty did collaborate with him on one notable occasion in 1965. In an attempt to improve his angioplasty method, Dotter tried replacing his usual equipment with a balloon catheter made for him by Fogarty, reasoning that what worked for blood clots might also be a good solution for atheroma. This attempt was successful, but Dotter decided the latex balloon was too flimsy for his purposes and did not use it again.[35] Though a one-off, this procedure was of historic significance, the first balloon angioplasty ever attempted. A decade later the technique would become the most powerful weapon in the cardiologist's armoury.

By 1968 Charles Dotter had published seventeen papers on transluminal angioplasty and performed hundreds of successful procedures. He had also gained an international reputation, but strangely he was more famous in the great surgical centres of Europe than he was in his own home town of Portland. American radiologists mostly ignored his work, still regarding the catheter as a diagnostic tool rather than a therapeutic one. But in Germany, Switzerland and the Netherlands, clinicians had taken up transluminal angioplasty with such enthusiasm that they now called it 'dottering'.[36]

In the summer of 1969 Andreas Grüntzig, a thirty-year-old research fellow at the Ratschow Clinic in Darmstadt, had a conversation with a patient that would change the direction of his career. Born in Dresden two months before the outbreak of war, in childhood Grüntzig lost his father – thought to have been murdered by the Nazis – and spent two years living with an uncle in Argentina. He completed his secondary education in Leipzig, but the Communist authorities decreed that he should then begin work as an apprentice stonemason rather than attend university.[37] Determined to become a doctor, Grüntzig fled across the border to West Germany in 1959 and began his medical studies in Heidelberg.[38] Now, a decade later, he had a particular interest in disease of the peripheral arteries, and found himself chatting to a patient with extensive atherosclerosis. The man was worried by the prospect of complex surgery or toxic drugs, and asked the young doctor whether there was any alternative: was it not possible to brush out the deposits from his arteries, as a plumber would grease from a blocked drain? Grüntzig was impressed by this imaginative suggestion, which prompted him to think about arterial disease in an entirely new way. Not long afterwards he went to a lecture given by Eberhard Zeitler, an eminent specialist in vascular medicine and the leading German disciple of Charles Dotter. Grüntzig was fascinated by the idea of 'dottering', and asked his department head for permission to learn more about transluminal angioplasty. The reply was unequivocal: 'I will never allow this kind of technique to be practised at my hospital.'[39]

Grüntzig had to wait another two years before he would be permitted to pursue his ambition. After a move to Zurich, where his new boss was far more sympathetic to the idea of catheter-based therapies, he was allowed to visit Zeitler's clinic to learn the technique. Many of his colleagues remained sceptical, but the unwavering support of one influential member of the surgical department, the pacemaker pioneer Åke Senning, ensured that he was allowed to continue using the Dotter procedure. Over the next couple of years Grüntzig accumulated enough successful cases to show that in the right hands it was a valuable technique. But it was only applicable to a small group of patients, those with accessible lesions in the arteries of the lower extremities, and Grüntzig wanted to treat blockages elsewhere in the body – in particular, those in the coronary arteries. He realised that this would require more sophisticated equipment: the coronary vessels are only a few millimetres in diameter, so simply pushing a probe through the obstruction would not work. Grüntzig knew of Dotter's use of a Fogarty catheter and felt that the approach was promising; the problem was that the balloon was not strong enough to force an occluded vessel open.

What was needed was a less elastic balloon – something like a fire hose, which when not in use is flattened, but when full of water expands to a maximum diameter determined by the stiffness of its material.[40] Armed with a textbook on the chemistry of polymers and a few basic tools, Grüntzig fabricated a series of prototypes at his

kitchen table, helped by his assistant Maria Schlumpf and her husband Walter.[41] PVC proved a suitable material for the balloons, which
were fixed to the catheter with glue, tied with nylon thread, and then
hung out to dry on a washing line.[42] After hundreds of experiments
they found that a sausage-shaped balloon worked best, exerting pressure along its entire length without distortion.

The new catheter was employed clinically for the first time in
February 1974, when Grüntzig used it to clear an obstruction from the
femoral artery of Fritz Ott, a sixty-seven-year-old who was unable to
walk for any distance without debilitating pain. Shortly after treatment his symptoms abated, and he was soon striding long distances
with no discomfort.[43] The balloon used in this procedure was tiny,
measuring just 4 millimetres when inflated, but Grüntzig knew that
to use the same approach on the coronary arteries he would have to
make one even smaller. It took another year of meticulous experimentation until he had a balloon he was happy with. After successful trials
on dogs Grüntzig was eager to move on to patients, but as a matter of
courtesy he first explained his plans to his colleagues in the department of surgery. The coronary arteries were traditionally the preserve
of the surgeon, and he wanted to make sure that they had no objections to a mere cardiologist invading their territory. Senning's jovial
response was the best he could have hoped for: 'Herr Grüntzig, you
will be taking away my patients, but go ahead!'[44]

To minimise the risk to his patients, Grüntzig's first trials took
place in an operating theatre, supervised by a surgeon and using a full
chest incision. If anything went wrong the surgeon could take over
and perform a conventional coronary bypass. The contingency did
not arise, however, and after several successful procedures he decided
that balloon angioplasty was finally a genuine alternative to surgery.
He had to wait several months before a suitable patient was found, but
in September 1977 a thirty-eight-year-old insurance salesman, Dölf
Bachmann, was admitted to hospital in Zurich with severe angina.
X-rays revealed that one of his coronary arteries was blocked a short
distance from its junction with the aorta. Given his age and general

condition a bypass operation would have been straightforward, but after sharing a hospital room with a patient who was recovering from this procedure Bachmann decided that he would rather avoid the trauma of major surgery.[45] He cheerfully accepted the opportunity to be the first to undergo balloon angioplasty. On the afternoon of 16 September Grüntzig himself wheeled his patient into the room where the procedure was to take place – not an operating theatre, but the catheter laboratory, known to its occupants as the 'cath lab'. At this time of day the nearby operating theatre was not in use, and a cardiac surgeon and anaesthetist were present so that they could perform an emergency bypass if it became necessary.

The atmosphere was not that of the typical operating theatre. People were relaxed, coming in and out of the lab as Grüntzig performed the procedure. There was no blood, and the most glaring anomaly was the patient himself, who was wide awake and chatting to the man who was about to clear his blocked artery. The catheter went into the femoral artery without any difficulty and was soon placed into the left coronary. The only moment of real tension arose as Grüntzig pressed a button to inflate the balloon: nobody quite knew what would happen when it briefly obstructed the blood flow to the myocardium. To everybody's surprise the heart carried on beating as normal, and Bachmann did not report any discomfort. To make absolutely sure that the blockage had been cleared, Grüntzig inflated the balloon for a second time. When he measured the pressure in the coronary artery he found that the blood flow was back to normal. 'I started to realise that my dreams had come true,' Grüntzig later recalled.[46] It was a marvellous culmination to a five-year obsession so intense that his daughter Sonja had started referring to the balloon catheter as her 'twin'.[47]

Grüntzig named the new technique percutaneous transluminal coronary angioplasty (PTCA): 'percutaneous' – meaning 'through the skin' – because access to the coronaries is obtained via a needle puncture rather than an open incision. He expected continuing resistance to his ideas, and many experts were unconvinced: after all, placing a balloon inside the coronary artery of a dog was known to *cause* atherosclerosis.[48] Nevertheless, specialists flocked to Zurich to learn the technique – so many of them that they could not be accommodated in the cath lab. Hundreds at a time sat in a large auditorium watching him perform PTCA on a large video screen, the first time that this teaching method (now common practice in medicine) had been used.

Grüntzig's success should have made him the toast of Zurich, but he was becoming increasingly unhappy with the resources at his disposal: the hospital authorities were slow to appreciate the potential of PTCA. American hospitals had embraced the technique with far more enthusiasm, and in 1980 he accepted an invitation to continue his work in Atlanta. The number of centres carrying out the procedure rapidly increased, and his efforts to prove its worth were finally vindicated four years later when a study of more than 2,000 patients found that over two-thirds were free of all symptoms after a year.[49] That was not all: researchers at the University of Göttingen discovered in 1979 that it was possible to use balloon angioplasty to open up the coronary arteries of patients even in the midst of a heart attack.[50] This was something even Grüntzig had been reluctant to try, but it was remarkably successful: a study published five years later found that 90 per cent of patients were long-term survivors.[51]

The explosion in the use of PTCA was truly extraordinary. When Grüntzig left Zurich in 1980 fewer than 900 procedures had been performed worldwide; six years later more than 130,000 had been carried out in the US alone.[52] But it wasn't all good news. As experience accumulated, cardiologists started to notice that many patients suffered relapses. As many as a third of them needed further angioplasty or emergency bypass surgery. Grüntzig was well aware of this problem and worked hard to find a solution. One was eventually found, but he did not live to see it. On 27 October 1985 he was flying back from the Georgia coast with his wife when their plane crashed in a storm, killing them both.[53] His loss was a tragic one, for at forty-six he still had much more to contribute; but he had already changed the face of medicine.

*

A good illustration of the impact of Grüntzig's work is the fate of his first six patients. One died from heart disease shortly after treatment, and another from an unrelated cancer; but the other four were alive and well twenty years later.[54] Dölf Bachmann, the first person to undergo PTCA, was in excellent health and still working in 2015 at the age of seventy-five.[55] While angioplasty almost certainly saved his life, he later suffered a recurrence of his condition which was treated by a revolutionary new device that emerged the year after Grüntzig's death: the stent.

These useful objects are named after Charles Stent, a nineteenth-century dentist who invented a new material for the fabrication of dentures: it was based on gutta-percha, a flexible resin which was also used in golf balls. The word entered surgical parlance when Stent's compound was used by German surgeons in facial reconstruction operations during the First World War; fifty years later it had come to mean a prosthetic tube made of metal or plastic, used to treat obstructions in internal structures such as the urinary tract.[56] Although he did not use the term, Charles Dotter was the first to realise that this concept could also be applied to the blood vessels. In his original description of trans-luminal angioplasty, published in 1964, he floated the idea of a plastic 'splint' which could be inserted into an artery to keep the vessel open.[57] In subsequent experiments he found that plastic exposed to the blood-stream promoted clotting, so instead he designed a metal spring that could be slipped over a catheter and delivered to the site of a previous obstruction. When the catheter was withdrawn, the spring remained in place to keep the vessel open.[58] This technique was successful in dogs, but making a system suitable for use in humans took another decade. By the early 1980s metal stents were finally being used clinically to open up the larger peripheral arteries, such as those in the leg.

The German cardiologist Ulrich Sigwart was unaware of these developments when he had the idea of doing something similar for the coronary arteries. A contemporary and friend of Andreas Grüntzig, he worked a few hours' drive from him in Lausanne and was one of the first to be taught PTCA by him in the late 1970s. His first balloon catheters were a gift from the great man himself, handed to him over dinner one evening. These are disposable items nowadays, but at the time they were so scarce that Sigwart had to sterilise and reuse them.[59] His first intimation of the shortcomings of angioplasty came in 1981, when one of his patients was rushed into surgery for an emergency bypass operation. Ironically, earlier that day Sigwart had submitted the outline of an academic paper in which he boasted that none of his previous hundred patients had suffered any such setback.[60] A number of similar incidents persuaded him of the need to improve the technique.

The problem that he and many others encountered was restenosis – the renewed narrowing of an artery previously opened by the angioplasty balloon. The balloon caused trauma to the wall of the vessel that made its inner layer flake off like badly hung wallpaper. Sigwart hit upon the idea of providing structural support, a sort of internal scaffolding for the vessel. With the help of a local engineer, Hans Wallstén, he developed a prototype. Their first attempt was similar to Dotter's spring, but this design was soon abandoned in favour of one inspired by the children's toy known as a Chinese finger trap.[61] The device was a tiny tube made from stainless-steel mesh, and – most importantly – was self-expanding. When loaded on to the catheter it was long and thin, but when released it would spring back to its usual, larger, diameter. Hospital administrators were unenthusiastic when Sigwart began animal trials, so much so that he was forced to perform the experiments in a wooden hut in the car park.[62] He did not realise at the time that two teams in the US were already working on a similar idea, one of them in collaboration with Andreas Grüntzig.[63] But crucially his was the earliest to be ready for clinical use.

Sigwart had to wait several weeks for his first case, but the definitive proof of its efficacy occurred on 12 June 1986, and in dramatic circumstances.* The hospital in Lausanne was full of distinguished

---

* This was not quite the first use of Sigwart's device. The French cardiologist Jacques Puel had implanted a stent two months earlier, while Sigwart was still trying to obtain authorisation for its use from local health authorities.

cardiologists who had gathered for a course in balloon angioplasty. In the morning they watched, enthralled, as an American specialist, Barry Rutherford, performed a complex procedure on a fifty-six-year-old woman with severe angina. Sigwart was chatting to her afterwards when he noticed her grimace in pain. Instinctively he knew what had happened: the dreaded restenosis. One of the coronary arteries opened by the balloon a short time earlier had collapsed, and little or no blood was passing through it to the myocardium. If she wasn't already in the grip of a heart attack, she soon would be. Sigwart rushed her back into the cath lab and found that the left coronary artery was, as expected, completely blocked. The obvious solution to the problem was a stent.

The metal tube Sigwart intended to implant in her heart was less than 2 centimetres long, with a diameter of 3.5 millimetres. It had to be placed with pinpoint accuracy in a vessel he would never see with the naked eye. First a guidewire was inserted through the femoral artery into the aorta and then the coronary artery. The stent was crimped on to a balloon catheter which was then threaded over the guidewire and gently guided to its destination, with Sigwart intently following its progress on an X-ray screen. When he was sure it was in the right place he inflated the balloon to expand the stent. There was a brief moment of tension while he scanned the screen anxiously to check that it was firmly in place. He was relieved to see that it was, and the effect was instantaneous: blood flow was restored, and the woman's symptoms immediately abated. She was the first patient in such a predicament to avoid emergency bypass surgery.[64]

Sigwart's illustrious visitors were oblivious to this little piece of history: having seen the earlier procedure to its conclusion they had retired to the cafeteria for lunch. A few months later the woman had to return for stenting of the other affected artery, but she was returned to full health. She and Sigwart kept in touch until her death twenty-eight years later.[65] The results of Sigwart's first nineteen cases were published in 1987 to general incredulity.[66] One British cardiologist, Tony Gershlick, recalls his amazement when a colleague returned from a conference and told him that 'they're using watchmaker's springs to keep arteries open'.[67] It was soon clear that stenting was far superior to balloon angioplasty. One in ten patients treated using the older technique later required emergency bypass surgery; stents reduced this rate to virtually nil.[68] In the late 1980s a further refinement appeared on the scene, a tiny catheter-mounted drill with a diamond-encrusted bit which could be slipped into the coronaries to pulverise the atherosclerotic plaque before the insertion of a stent.[69]

As ever, the early models were far from perfect. One cardiologist described using them as 'bungee jumping without checking the knots': stents fell off the catheter, were swept into the bloodstream, and had to be retrieved from remote parts of the body by an exasperated surgeon. Better designs eliminated this technical fault, but a more serious one remained: a significant proportion of implanted stents quickly became obstructed.[70] Researchers found that bare metal caused scar tissue to form on the inside of the vessel, provoking an inflammatory response.

Drugs were the obvious way to prevent this scarring, known as intimal hyperplasia – but how could they be delivered to the coronary arteries? Several possible methods were investigated, but in the early 1990s a number of investigators settled on the same solution: putting them in the stent itself.[71] The first drug used for this purpose was sirolimus, derived from a bacterium identified in a soil sample taken from Easter Island twenty years earlier.[72] Stents coated with this compound would release it slowly into the bloodstream for a few months, long enough to guard against restenosis. After the disappointments of the previous two decades physicians wanted to be absolutely sure that these devices, known as drug-eluting stents, were really an improvement on what they already had, so they were subjected to numerous clinical trials. The results were strikingly good, with one study finding that they reduced the rate of clinically significant restenosis to zero.[73]

The invention of the drug-eluting stent has been called the 'third revolution' in interventional cardiology – the first two being balloon angioplasty and the stent itself.[74] Its success resulted in a long debate – as yet unresolved – about whether it or coronary bypass surgery offer the better long-term results; but for suitable patients stenting is a quick, painless and life-saving treatment which can be performed even in the middle of a heart attack. In the last few years cardiologists have begun to investigate a new type of stent made from magnesium or a special soluble polymer. These devices are bioabsorbable, meaning that in time they dissolve, leaving no trace but a pristine and fully opened vessel.[75]

What makes this such a momentous development is the sheer scale on which it is used. Percutaneous coronary intervention (PCI) has become a crucial weapon in the battle against heart disease, which remains the leading cause of death in the world. Over a million PCIs are performed in Europe every year,[76] around 100,000 of them in the UK,[77] making it one of the most frequently used hospital treatments for any condition. But this is not the only way in which interventional cardiology has, to paraphrase Åke Senning, stolen patients from the surgeons.

Andreas Grüntzig's idea of reaming out blocked coronary arteries with a miniature pipe cleaner was certainly bold, but while he was developing his technique other specialists were working on an even more startling use for the catheter. They hoped to repair hearts distorted by congenital disease, remodelling their internal tissues and removing the need for elaborate surgery. In 1964 William Rashkind, a cardiologist from Philadelphia, proposed a new treatment for cyanotic heart defects, a group of conditions in which a cardiac abnormality results in imperfectly oxygenated blood being circulated throughout the body. His idea was to create an artificial septal defect, a hole between the left and right sides of the heart. This would allow blue, badly oxygenated blood to travel back into the pulmonary circulation, giving it a second opportunity to pass through the lungs before being pumped to the rest of the body. Conceptually this was similar to the Blalock–Taussig shunt, invented two decades earlier to alleviate tetralogy of Fallot, and when Rashkind outlined his idea at a conference one of the first to appreciate its merits was one of the pioneers after whom the operation was named. Helen Taussig wrote to him afterwards, saying: 'It would be wonderful if we can do some of the simpler operations without opening up the chest. I think that is a real advance and a real look into the future.'[78]

Rashkind entered this brave new world two years later, when he treated a newborn infant with transposition of the great arteries (TGA), in which the positions of the aorta and pulmonary artery are swapped. This creates two independent circulations, one pumping blood endlessly through the lungs, while the body receives only useless deoxygenated blood. Babies born with the condition are cyanotic from lack of oxygen, and unless there is some way for blood to find its way from the systemic circuit into the pulmonary one they rapidly die. Rashkind's patient was only hours old when he inserted a catheter into the right side of its heart and manipulated it into the foramen ovale, the small window between the two atria which usually closes shortly after birth. He then inflated a balloon at the catheter tip and withdrew it sharply to tear a larger, permanent hole in the septum.[79] This was not a cure, but like the Blalock–Taussig operation it was an effective, life-saving measure which hugely improved the patient's condition. A journalist from *Time* magazine was allowed to watch one of these early procedures being performed on Bobby Weiner, a sixteen-day-old with TGA, and noted the remarkable change in his skin colour from slate-grey to pink when the balloon was withdrawn. The baby required only a local anaesthetic and sucked on a dummy as the operation took place.[80]

Rashkind continued to investigate other ways of treating congenital disease, and in the late 1970s he developed an alternative method of creating a septal defect. Instead of a balloon, the catheter contained a tiny blade just 12 millimetres long and 1 millimetre wide. As it passed through the blood vessels the blade was retracted, like that of a folded penknife; but when it reached the inside of the heart the operator could turn a lever to expose it, and make an opening between the left and right atria.[81]

Of course, a hole in the heart is only desirable for those with other rare defects; for most people born with otherwise normal cardiac anatomy they can be inconvenient or even life-threatening. Devices for closing atrial or ventricular septal defects via the catheter also started to appear, the first invented by Terry King, a cardiologist from New Orleans. When as a young man he first suggested repairing holes in the heart without surgery, the idea seemed so outlandish that one colleague told him to see a psychiatrist.[82] Brushing off this helpful advice, he and a colleague, the surgeon Noel Mills, spent several years designing a catheter system containing two tiny umbrellas. These were furled as the catheter entered the heart chambers, but when it had passed through the defect they were opened, one on each side of the hole. The two umbrellas then snapped together, forming an artificial barrier over which new tissue would grow.[83] Their first patient, seventeen-year-old Suzette Creppel, received umbrella closure of an ASD in April 1975, made a full recovery and is still alive today.

The scope of catheter interventions to operate inside the heart widened still further in 1981, when Jean Kan, a successor of Helen Taussig as head of paediatric cardiology at Johns Hopkins Hospital in Baltimore, developed a successful method of treating narrowed valves.* Inspired by a talk given by the visiting Andreas Grüntzig, she decided that inflating a balloon inside the valve could be a means of

---

* This breakthrough was anticipated almost thirty years earlier by the remarkable work of a Mexican surgeon, Victor Rubio-Alvarez, who in 1952 used a catheter with a sharp wire at its tip to slice through the fused leaflets of stenotic valves. His technique did not catch on, but it is arguable that the few procedures Rubio-Alvarez performed represent the dawn of interventional cardiology.

correcting pulmonary stenosis.[84] After two years of animal experimentation she performed the first successful procedure on Sharon
Owens, aged eight; in her patient's honour, Kan called the device
the Owens Pulmonary Valvuloplasty Balloon, the name by which it
was known for some years afterwards.[85] Variations of the Owens balloon were subsequently used to treat the other valves of the heart,
beginning with mitral stenosis in 1984.[86]

By the end of the decade, cardiologists had a formidable array
of techniques at their disposal to tackle complex congenital conditions without once picking up a scalpel. Many of these patients were
children, and in addition to avoiding the trauma and long recovery associated with an operation, catheter treatment spared them
the disfiguring scar which is a permanent reminder of open-chest
surgery.

Better still, the catheter provided a treatment for an entire
class of illnesses that were almost impossible to treat surgically.
Arrhythmias, disorders of the heart rhythm, had long been among
the most difficult conditions for physicians to treat, because the
mechanisms behind them are so complex. When a surgeon repairs
a damaged valve or corrects a congenital malformation, the cause
of the problem is usually visible to the naked eye, and fixing it is a
matter of cutting or stitching the structures concerned. The causes
of many arrhythmias, on the other hand, are invisible even when
the organ has been cut open: the heart of a seriously ill patient may
look completely normal. That is because the nature of the problem is
electrical, and the faulty structures are the microscopic conduction
pathways that carry electrical impulses from one part of the heart
muscle to another.

On 19 October 2003 the British prime minister Tony Blair was
spending the weekend at his official country residence, Chequers,
when his heart began to race for no apparent reason. This was not
the first time he had experienced the phenomenon, which he had
previously attributed to drinking too much coffee. When the palpitations failed to subside he went to the local hospital, where he was

told he needed urgent treatment from a specialist in London.[87] News that the premier had been rushed to a cardiac unit caused some panic, but the condition was easily treated. At the Hammersmith Hospital he was diagnosed with supraventricular tachycardia, an arrhythmia which causes the heart rate to increase to over 180 beats per minute. Episodes of SVT are uncomfortable but rarely life-threatening, although over a long period they can cause serious complications. The cause of the palpitations was an abnormal conduction pathway inside the heart, so that parts of the myocardium were receiving an electrical stimulus far more frequently than they should. After a recurrence of his symptoms the following year, Blair returned to hospital for a brief procedure which banished his symptoms for good. Known as radiofrequency ablation, it uses a catheter with a special tip to destroy the tissue responsible for the aberrant electrical signals. Had any of his predecessors been hospitalised with SVT, it is doubtful whether they could have stayed in office: although drugs can sometimes control the condition, it remained incurable until the late 1980s.

The technique of radiofrequency ablation was an innovation that came out of one of the younger branches of medicine: cardiac electrophysiology, the study of the electrical activity of the heart. The discipline was established in the 1960s, as researchers started to unravel the mechanisms responsible for the many different types of arrhythmia, identifying and mapping the specific electrical pathways that caused the organ to misfire. One of the leading lights of this new field was the Dutch cardiologist Hein Wellens – later known as the 'giant of Maastricht' for the importance of his contribution[88] – who decided to study Wolff–Parkinson–White syndrome, a condition which causes an abnormally fast heartbeat. Colleagues of Wellens in Amsterdam had recently discovered that the hearts of patients with WPW syndrome contain an extra conduction route between the atria and ventricles: impulses passing through this so-called accessory pathway can cause the ventricles to contract prematurely, resulting in tachycardia.

Wellens showed that it was possible to deliberately induce and then terminate episodes of arrhythmia by passing an electrode mounted on a catheter into the heart chambers and stimulating the areas responsible with an electrical current.[89] This led to the first surgical treatment for the condition the following year, when surgeons at Duke Hospital in North Carolina operated on a thirty-two-year-old fisherman who had suffered attacks of tachycardia since the age of four, leading eventually to heart failure. After using ECG electrodes to pin down the exact location of the accessory pathway, surgeons opened the heart and made a 6-centimetre incision in the interior wall of the right atrium, severing the connection and curing his condition permanently.[90]

In the following decade this procedure was used to treat a variety of life-threatening arrhythmias, sometimes using cryoablation (extreme cold) to freeze the rogue pathways until they stopped working. But cutting open an otherwise healthy heart to do so seemed an unnecessarily invasive procedure, and using the catheter instead was one obvious way to avoid opening the chest. In the late 1970s a cardiologist in San Francisco, Melvin Scheinman, began a series of animal experiments using high-voltage electricity to burn (ablate) areas of tissue inside the cardiac chambers. The method he eventually adopted used a powerful DC current generated by a defibrillator and passed down a wire inside a catheter into the heart.[91]

While he had some success employing this approach on patients, there were major problems with the technique: it was safer than surgery, but the risks were terrifying. When an ablation went wrong it could make the arrhythmia worse, damage the coronary arteries or even perforate the heart.[92] The answer was not some dramatic technological breakthrough, but a piece of equipment that had been in operating theatres for over sixty years. In 1925 an eccentric plant physiologist in Boston, William Bovie, became interested in the idea of using electricity to perform surgery. He invented an apparatus that produced a precisely modulated current which, when passed through a needle-like electrode, would cut through flesh as easily as a scalpel. By changing the nature of the current it was also possible to dehydrate the tissue, or to arrest bleeding by coagulating the blood. The secret of this versatile device was that it used a particular type of high-frequency alternating current (AC). Most domestic mains power is AC, and typically the current flips direction fifty or sixty times per second. Bovie's equipment produced an electric current that alternated as many as three million times per second, the frequency of radio waves.[93] He demonstrated his invention to the brain surgeon Harvey Cushing, who was so impressed that he used it to operate on a number of patients with tumours he had previously thought inoperable. The results were stunning: as a contemporary press report noted, 'In several of the operations . . . the patients were insane before they went under the electric knife, and came out sane again.'[94]

Bovie's 'electric scalpel' – commonly but inaccurately known as the diathermy knife* – became a staple of the surgeon's toolbox, and in 1987 the German cardiologist Thomas Budde introduced the device to the cath lab when he treated a forty-nine-year-old woman with persistent tachycardia.† Drugs and two previous ablations using DC current had proved totally ineffective in controlling the condition, and the patient was prone to regular fainting fits. A catheter was manipulated into her right atrium, and five pulses of radiofrequency current passed through the electrode at its tip, finally liberating her from the palpitations which had caused her so much discomfort and left her at risk of a stroke and other serious complications.[95]

Radiofrequency ablation was far superior to anything before it: it allowed cardiologists to zap the tiny region that was causing an arrhythmia without doing any damage to surrounding structures. Occasionally the burnt tissue would heal, causing a recurrence of

---

* 'Diathermy' properly refers to heating an object from a distance, as microwaves do food in a microwave oven. The origin of this surgical misnomer is obscure. In America it is commonly known as a 'Bovie'.
† Melvin Scheinman had in fact tested radiofrequency ablation in the late 1970s, but abandoned it when it caused complications in his laboratory animals.

symptoms and necessitating a repeat procedure, but this was rare: in one study, researchers found that 98 per cent of patients were cured at the first attempt.[96] In the early years of the procedure, when it was difficult to pinpoint the area causing a problem, ablation often resulted in the total destruction of the heart's conduction system, so that patients needed a pacemaker to maintain a normal heartbeat. Today's technology is far more sophisticated, often allowing cardiologists to make a precision strike on any unwanted conduction pathways while leaving the rest untouched. While pacemakers remain the usual treatment for most bradycardias (abnormally slow heartbeats), ablation can now be used to treat a wide range of tachycardias, including atrial fibrillation.

In some ways, ablation is the most remarkable of all the many victories won against disease of the heart. Here's a sobering fact: in over a century of evolution, heart surgery has rarely cured a patient. The majority of procedures documented in this book, from the Blue Baby operation to transplantation, valve replacement to stenting, are merely palliative. They may offer relief from symptoms, but they do not cure the underlying condition. Radiofrequency ablation offers a definitive cure for an entire class of patients whose condition was previously beyond the capabilities of medicine. Andrew Grace, an electrophysiologist at Papworth Hospital, was one of the first British specialists to adopt the technique. He recalls the dreadful outlook for patients with serious arrhythmias when he was a newly qualified doctor in the early 1980s: 'I used to think that Wolff–Parkinson–White syndrome was one of the worst things that could happen to a young person. I remember these patients aged eighteen who were on three different anti-arrhythmic drugs surrounded by men much older than them having heart attacks. It was as bad as having cystic fibrosis or something, and now—' he clicks his fingers '—we can fix them in an hour.'[97]

It is more than half a century since Charles Dotter told an incredulous audience that the humble catheter would one day become 'an important surgical instrument'. Subsequent developments have surely exceeded even his expectations: while we haven't quite reached the world of *Fantastic Voyage*, with microscopic submarines navigating the blood vessels, interventional cardiologists now routinely repair congenital abnormalities, treat heart attacks and cure life-threatening arrhythmias – all without lifting a scalpel. The rise of the discipline was so meteoric that some cardiac surgeons began to fear that their own skills would soon become obsolete. That's one prediction that hasn't (yet) come true, but interventional cardiology continues to innovate at a pace not seen in heart surgery since its heyday in the 1960s. And as we'll see in the next chapter, the latest developments have seen surgeons and interventional cardiologists working together more closely than ever before.

11. I, ROBOT (SURGEON)

Boston, 7 November 2005

On a cold, bright January morning I am walking south across Westminster Bridge to St Thomas' Hospital, an institution founded by Augustinian monks in the twelfth century. Today it occupies a white-tiled modernist complex memorably described in Pevsner's *The Buildings of England* as 'monster cubes'.[1] Pevsner rather liked the bold development, but when it appeared on the Thames skyline in the 1970s some of the neighbours were less keen. MPs and peers in the Palace of Westminster, whose agreeable river terrace overlooks the hospital, vented their indignation in Parliament, describing it variously as an 'icebox', a 'monstrosity', and a 'travesty of architecture'. Whatever its aesthetic merits, St Thomas' has a proud tradition of innovation: I am there to observe a procedure generally regarded as the greatest advance in cardiac surgery since the turn of the millennium – and one that can be performed without a surgeon.

The patient is a man in his eighties with aortic stenosis, a narrowed valve which is restricting outflow from the left ventricle into the aorta. His heart struggles to pump sufficient blood through the reduced aperture, and the muscle of the affected ventricle has thickened as the organ tries to compensate. If left unchecked, this will eventually lead to heart failure. For a healthier patient the solution would be simple: an operation to remove the diseased valve and replace it with a prosthesis. But the man's age and a long list of other medical conditions make open-heart surgery out of the question. Happily, for the last few years another option has been available for such high-risk patients: transcatheter aortic valve implantation, known as TAVI for short.

When I arrive in the cath lab, wearing a heavy lead gown to protect me from X-rays, the patient is already lying on the table. He will remain awake throughout the procedure, receiving only a sedative and a powerful analgesic to render it painless. I am shown the valve to be implanted, three leaflets fashioned from bovine pericardium fixed inside a collapsible metal stent. After being soaked in saline it is crimped on to a balloon catheter, squeezing it from the size and shape of a tube of lipstick to a long, thin object like a pencil.

The consultant cardiologist, Bernard Prendergast, has already threaded a guidewire through an incision in the patient's groin, entering the femoral artery and then the aorta, until the tip of the wire has arrived at the diseased aortic valve. The catheter, with its precious cargo, is then placed over the guidewire and pushed gently up the aorta. When it reaches the upper part of the vessel we can track its progress on one of the large X-ray screens above the table. We watch intently as the metal stent describes a slow curve around the aortic arch before coming to rest just above the heart. There is a pause as the team checks everything is ready, while on the screen the silhouette of the furled valve oscillates gently as it is buffeted by pulses of high-pressure arterial blood. When Dr Prendergast is satisfied that the catheter is precisely aligned with the aortic valve he presses a button to inflate the tiny balloon. As it expands it forces the metal stent outwards and back to its normal diameter, and on the X-ray monitor it suddenly snaps into position, firmly anchored at the top of the ventricle. For a second or two the patient becomes agitated as the balloon obstructs the aorta and stops the flow of blood to his brain; but as soon as it is deflated he becomes calm again.

Dr Prendergast and his colleagues peer at the monitors to check the positioning of the device. In a conventional operation the diseased valve would be excised before the prosthesis is sewn in; during a TAVI procedure the old valve is left untouched and the new one simply placed inside it. This makes correct placement vital, since unless the device fits snugly in the annulus there may be a leak around its edge. The X-ray picture shows that the new valve is securely anchored and moving in unison with the heart. Satisfied that everything has gone according to plan, Dr Prendergast removes the catheter and announces the good news in a voice that is probably audible on the other side of the river. Just minutes after being given a new heart valve, the patient raises an arm from under the drapes and shakes the cardiologist's hand warmly. The entire procedure has taken less than an hour.

TAVI is the latest example of the interventional cardiologist's encroachment on the surgeon's territory – and, according to many experts, this is what the future will look like. Though available for little more than a decade, it is already having a dramatic impact on surgical practice: in Germany the majority of aortic valve replacements, more than 10,000 a year, are now performed using the catheter rather than the scalpel.[2] In the UK the figure is much lower, since the procedure is still significantly more expensive than surgery; this is largely down to the cost of the valve itself, which can be as much as £20,000 for a single device. But as the manufacturers recoup their initial outlay on research and development it is likely to become more affordable – and its advantages are numerous. Early results suggest that it is every bit as effective as open-heart surgery, without many of surgery's undesirable aspects: the large chest incision, the heart-lung machine, the long post-operative recovery.

While it has only recently become a clinical reality, the essential idea of TAVI was first suggested more than half a century ago. In 1965 Hywel Davies, a cardiologist at Guy's Hospital in London, was mulling over the problem of aortic regurgitation, in which blood flows backwards from the aorta into the heart. He was looking for a short-term therapy for patients too sick for immediate surgery – something which would allow them to recover for a few days or weeks, until they were strong enough to undergo an operation. He hit upon the idea of a temporary device which could be inserted through a blood vessel, and designed a simple artificial valve resembling a conical parachute. Because it was made from fabric it could be collapsed and mounted on to a catheter; in experiments on dogs Davies showed that it was easy to introduce it via the femoral artery and lodge it in the descending aorta. It was inserted with the top of the 'parachute' uppermost, so that any backwards flow would be caught by its inside surface like air hitting the underside of a real parachute canopy. As the fabric filled with blood it would balloon outwards, sealing the vessel and stopping most of the anomalous blood flow.[3]

This was a truly imaginative suggestion, made at a time when catheter therapies had barely been conceived of, let alone tested. But Davies found that his prototype tended to provoke blood clots, and he was never able to use it on a patient. The idea was forgotten, and another two decades passed before anybody considered anything similar. That moment came in 1988 when a trainee cardiologist from Denmark, Henning Rud Andersen, was at a conference in Arizona attending a lecture about coronary artery stenting. It was the first he had heard of the technique, which at the time had been used in only a few dozen patients, and as he sat in the auditorium he had a thought which at first he dismissed as ridiculous: why not make a bigger stent, put a valve in the middle of it, and implant it into the heart via a catheter? On reflection he realised that this was not such an absurd idea, and when he returned home to Aarhus he visited a local butcher to buy a supply of pig hearts. Working in a poky room in the basement of his hospital with basic tools obtained from a local DIY warehouse, Andersen constructed his first experimental prototypes. He began by cutting out the aortic valves from the pig hearts, mounted each inside a home-made metal lattice, then compressed the whole contraption around a balloon.[4]

Within a few months Andersen was ready to test the device in animals, and on 1 May 1989 he implanted the first in a pig.[5] It thrived
with its prosthesis, and Andersen assumed that his colleagues would
be excited by his work's obvious clinical potential. But nobody was
prepared to take the concept seriously – folding up a valve and then
unfurling it inside the heart seemed wilfully eccentric – and it took
him several years to find a journal willing to publish his research.
When one finally did in 1992 his paper was largely ignored, and crucially none of the major biotechnology firms showed any interest in
developing the device. Andersen's 'crazy' idea worked; but it still sank
without trace.

Thinking that nothing would ever come of it, Andersen sold the
patent for his device and moved on to other projects. And then at
the turn of the century there was a sudden explosion of interest in
the idea of transcatheter valve implantation. In 2000 an interventional cardiologist in London, Philipp Bonhoeffer, replaced the diseased pulmonary valve of a twelve-year-old boy using a valve taken
from a cow's jugular vein which had been mounted in a stent and
put in position using a balloon catheter.[6] In his report, Bonhoeffer
suggested that the technique might be used to replace other cardiac
valves – and in France another cardiologist was indeed already working on doing the same for the aortic valve. Alain Cribier had been
developing novel catheter therapies for years; it was his company
that bought Andersen's patent in 1995, and he had persisted with the
idea even after one potential investor told him that TAVI was 'the
most stupid project ever heard of'.[7] Eventually he managed to raise
the necessary funds for development and long-term testing, and by
2000 had a working prototype. Rather than use an entire valve cut
from a dead heart, as Andersen had, Cribier employed a bioprosthetic
one: three leaflets made from glutaraldehyde-treated bovine pericardium, mounted in a collapsible stainless-steel stent. Prototypes were
implanted in sheep to test their durability: after two and a half years,
during which they opened and closed more than 100 million times,
the valves still worked perfectly.[8]

Cribier was ready to test the device in humans, but his first patient could not be anybody eligible for conventional surgical valve replacement, which is safe and highly effective: to test an unproven new procedure on such a patient would be to expose them to unnecessary risk. In early 2002 he was introduced to a fifty-seven-year-old man who was, in surgical terms, a hopeless case. He had catastrophic aortic stenosis which had so weakened his heart that with each stroke it could pump less than a quarter of the normal volume of blood; in addition, the blood vessels of his extremities were ravaged by atherosclerosis, and he had chronic pancreatitis and lung cancer. Several surgeons had declined to operate on him, and his referral to Cribier's clinic in Rouen was a final roll of the dice. An initial attempt to open the stenotic valve using a simple balloon catheter failed, and a week after this treatment Cribier recorded in his notes that his patient was near death, with his heart barely functioning. The man's family agreed that an experimental treatment was preferable to none at all, and on 16 April he became the first person to receive a new aortic valve without open-heart surgery.

Over the next couple of days the patient's condition improved dramatically: he was able to get out of bed, and the signs of heart failure began to retreat. But shortly afterwards complications arose, most seriously a deterioration in the condition of the blood vessels in his right leg, which had to be amputated ten weeks later. Infection set in, and four months after the operation he died.[9] He had not lived long – nobody expected him to – but the episode had proved the feasibility of the approach, with clear short-term benefit to the patient. Andersen's animal experiments thirteen years earlier had been received with indifference; when Cribier presented a video of the operation to colleagues they sat in stupefied silence, realising that they were watching something that would change the nature of heart surgery.[10]

At first Cribier was only permitted to perform TAVI on desperately sick patients who were too great a risk for surgery. Predictably, many died within weeks, but there were also some astonishing successes: a handful of patients lived for more than five years after being declared untreatable. These results attracted the interest of the large medical device companies, and huge amounts of money were poured into improving the technology. Clinical trials were set up to investigate whether the procedure was as good as its proponents claimed, and in 2010 a large international study concluded that for those too sick for open-heart surgery,* TAVI was far superior to any other treatment.[11] Better still, even if a patient *was* well enough to go under the knife, it made no difference to their survival prospects if they opted for TAVI instead.[12]

When surgeons and cardiologists overcame their initial scepticism about TAVI they quickly realised that it opened up a vista of exciting new surgical possibilities. In 2012 Lars Søndergaard, a medic from Copenhagen, became the first to apply the transcatheter approach to the mitral valve, implanting a prosthesis in an eighty-six-year-old patient.[13] As well as replacing diseased valves it is now also possible to repair them, using clever imitations of the techniques used by surgeons. If the leaflets no longer close properly, a cardiologist can pin them together with tiny plastic clips,[14] or remodel the entire valve by implanting a stiff piece of plastic around its circumference.[15] The technology is still in its infancy, but many experts believe that this will eventually become the default option for valvular disease, making surgery increasingly rare.

While TAVI is impressive, there is one even more spectacular example of the capabilities of the catheter. Paediatric cardiologists at a few specialist centres have recently started using it to break the last taboo of heart surgery – operating on an unborn child. Little more than a century ago most surgeons believed that the adult heart was out of bounds; the notion of foetal cardiac surgery would have been inconceivable, since it is only in the last thirty years that specialists have been able to diagnose foetal heart conditions with any degree of

---

* It remains to be seen whether TAVI is as good as surgery in the long term: clinicians will need years more follow-up data before they can reach any conclusions.

confidence. Although antenatal scans using ultrasound became commonplace in the 1970s, doctors had no idea how to interpret the grainy
black-and-white images of the tiny beating heart. It was 'like trying to
read a foreign language without a dictionary',[16] in the words of Lindsey
Allan, a paediatric cardiologist who in the early 1980s was working at
Guy's Hospital in London. Despite this, she not only devised a method
of visualising the most important features of the foetal heart,[17] but
also showed that it was possible to differentiate between normal and
abnormal anatomy, and to identify specific congenital malformations
well before birth.[18]

Allan was also involved in the first attempts to correct congenital
abnormalities in an unborn child. Her team at Guy's treated a series
of babies with aortic stenosis: shortly after birth they inflated a balloon catheter inside the valve, in the hope that slightly widening it
would improve the blood flow and alleviate the condition. Sadly all
died, having already sustained irreversible damage to the heart muscle while in the womb. Reasoning that the only hope was to intervene
earlier, Allan and her colleagues decided in 1989 to try the procedure
in utero. Under local anaesthetic, a stiff hollow needle was passed
through the mother's abdominal wall, into the uterus and through the
chest of the foetus, directly into the left ventricle of its heart. This terrifying undertaking would have been inconceivable only twenty years
earlier, but ultrasound images allowed the doctors to see the structures through which they were passing the needle. Once the needle
was in the left ventricle a guidewire was passed through it and across
the narrowed aortic valve; the needle was withdrawn, and a balloon
catheter threaded on to the wire and into the heart. During the first
procedure the valve could not be reached, and the foetus died the
next day. The second attempt was more successful: the balloon was
inflated inside the valve, dilating it as intended. The pregnancy continued to term, and a repeat procedure was performed after birth, but
the child's heart muscle was already compromised and it died after
five weeks.[19] These first attempts ended in failure – but later technical improvements made it a viable method of treating valve problems

in pregnancy, successfully extending the lives of babies with the condition. Then, around the turn of the millennium, doctors started to
apply the technique to an altogether more formidable problem.

Nowhere is the progress of cardiac surgery more stunning than in
the field of congenital heart disease. Malformations of the heart are
the most common form of birth defect, with as many as 5 per cent of all
babies born with some sort of cardiac anomaly – though most of these
will cause no serious, lasting problems.[20] The organ is especially prone
to abnormal development in the womb, with a myriad of possible ways
in which its structures can be distorted or transposed. Some we have
already encountered, but there are dozens of others, some vanishingly
rare. Over several decades, specialists have managed to find ways of
taming most; but one which remains a significant challenge to even
the best surgeon is hypoplastic left heart syndrome (HLHS), in which
the entire left side of the heart fails to develop properly. The ventricle and aorta are much smaller than they should be, and the mitral
valve is either absent or undersized. Until the early 1980s this was a
lethal defect which inevitably killed babies within days of birth, but a
sequence of complex palliative operations now makes it possible for
many to live into adulthood.*

Because the left ventricle is incapable of propelling oxygenated
blood into the body, babies born with HLHS can only survive if there
is some communication between the pulmonary and systemic circulations, allowing the right ventricle to pump blood both to the lungs and
to the rest of the body. Until they close a few days after birth, the ductus
arteriosus (between the aorta and pulmonary artery) and the foramen
ovale (between the left and right atria) provide routes for oxygenated
blood to travel back into the pulmonary circulation. Some children
with HLHS also have an atrial septal defect, a persistent hole in the
tissue between the atria of the heart which improves their chances of

---

* Typically a baby with HLHS will undergo three operations, each named after the
surgeon who invented it: the Norwood Procedure a couple of weeks after birth; the
Glenn Shunt a few months later; and the Fontan Procedure a year or two after that.

survival by increasing the amount of oxygenated blood which reaches the sole functioning pumping chamber. When surgeons realised that an ASD conferred a survival benefit, they began to create one artificially in babies born with an intact septum, usually a few hours after birth. But it was already too late: elevated blood pressure was causing permanent damage to the delicate vessels of the lung while the child was still in the womb.

The logical – albeit risky – response was to intervene even earlier. So in 2000 a team at Boston Children's Hospital adopted a new procedure to create an artificial septal defect during the final trimester of pregnancy: they would deliberately create one heart defect in order to treat another. A needle was passed through the wall of the uterus and into the baby's heart, and a balloon catheter used to create a hole between the left and right atria.[21] This reduced the pressures in the pulmonary circulation and hence limited the damage to the lungs; but the tissues of a growing foetus have a remarkable ability to repair themselves, and the artificially created hole would often heal within a few weeks. Cardiologists needed to find a way of keeping it open until birth, when surgeons would be able to perform a more comprehensive repair.

In September 2005 a couple from Virginia, Angela and Jay VanDerwerken, visited their local hospital for a routine antenatal scan. They were devastated to learn that their unborn child had hypoplastic left heart syndrome, and the prognosis was poor. The ultrasound pictures revealed an intact septum, making it likely that even before birth her lungs would be damaged beyond repair. They were told that they could either terminate the pregnancy or accept that their daughter would have to undergo open-heart surgery within hours of her birth, with only a 20 per cent chance that she would survive. Dismayed by this gloomy outlook, the VanDerwerkens returned home, where Angela researched the condition online. Although few hospitals offered any treatment for HLHS, she found several references to the Boston Fetal Cardiac Intervention Program, the team of doctors who had pioneered the use of the balloon catheter during pregnancy.

They arranged an appointment with Wayne Tworetzky, the director of foetal cardiology at Boston Children's Hospital, who performed a scan and confirmed that the condition was treatable. A greying, softly spoken South African, Tworetzky explained that his team had recently developed a new procedure, but that it had never been tested on a patient. It would mean not just making a hole in the septum, but also inserting a device to prevent it from closing. The VanDerwerkens had few qualms about accepting the opportunity: the alternatives gave their daughter a negligible chance of life.[22]

The procedure took place at Brigham and Women's Hospital on 7 November 2005, thirty weeks into the pregnancy, in a crowded operating theatre. Sixteen doctors took part, with expertise drawn from a range of specialisms: cardiologists, surgeons, and no fewer than four anaesthetists – two to look after the mother, and two for her unborn child. Mother and child needed to be completely immobilised during a delicate procedure lasting several hours, so both were given a general anaesthetic. The team watched on the screen of an ultrasound scanner as a thin needle was guided through the wall of the uterus, then the foetus's chest and finally into her heart – an object the size of a grape. A guidewire was placed in the cardiac chambers, and then a tiny balloon catheter was inserted and used to create an opening in the atrial septum. This had all been done before on other patients; but now the cardiologists added a refinement. The balloon was withdrawn, then returned to the heart, this time loaded with a 2.5 millimetre stent which was set in the opening between the left and right atria.[23] There was a charged silence as the balloon was inflated to expand the stent; then, as the team saw on the monitor that blood was flowing freely through the aperture, the room erupted in cheers.

Grace VanDerwerken was born in early January after a normal labour, and shortly afterwards underwent open-heart surgery, the first of three operations she would need in infancy. After a fortnight she was allowed home, her healthy pink complexion proving that the interventions had succeeded in producing a functional circulation. But just when she seemed to be out of danger, Grace died suddenly at the age of thirty-six days – not as a consequence of the surgery, but from a rare arrhythmia, a complication of HLHS that occurs in just 5 per cent of cases. This was the cruellest luck, when she had seemingly overcome the grim odds against her. Her death was a tragic loss, but her parents' courage had brought about a new era in foetal surgery. Grace was the first child to have a device implanted in her heart while still in the womb – a landmark procedure which has since been performed successfully on many other foetuses diagnosed with HLHS.

Grace's story is a dispatch from a new frontier of medicine, a world of microscopic precision and miraculous engineering in which life-threatening heart conditions are treated without recourse to the scalpel. But this is not the only novel method of eradicating the trauma of open-heart surgery. In 1983 the French surgeon Alain Carpentier made a whimsical attempt to imagine the operating theatre of the future. It reads like something out of *Buck Rogers*, complete with lasers to open the patient's chest and a mysterious electrical device which renders patients unconscious without any need for anaesthetics. In Carpentier's mega-hospital of the year 2050, automation has done away with the large surgical teams of the twentieth century. A single surgeon performs a valve repair assisted only by a machine, a robot which fetches instruments and helps with the simpler parts of the procedure.[24] Nothing dates faster than a vision of the future, however, and several of Carpentier's ideas already look like relics of the 1980s. But he did correctly anticipate the use of email to share scans and medical records, and made one other prediction that was surprisingly accurate: fifteen years later he himself performed open-heart surgery assisted by a robot.

If you're now picturing a chrome-plated android endowed with artificial intelligence, superhuman dexterity and impeccable clinical judgment, you may be disappointed. Surgical robots are not the autonomous machines of science fiction: they cannot think for themselves, but are passive devices which can only carry out instructions given by a human. Instruments held by the robot are controlled by a surgeon sitting at a console a short distance from the operating table – the device is, in effect, an extension of the surgeon's own hands. The rationale for creating such a machine was not to automate the process of surgery, but to make it possible to operate accurately through an incision too small to admit the human hand.

Surgical robotics is the natural evolution of an idea born in the late nineteenth century, but which began to have a significant clinical impact only thirty years ago. In the 1890s the German surgeon Georg Kelling became preoccupied with the dangers of abdominal surgery. He wanted to find a way of treating patients without making a large and risky incision, and at a medical conference in 1901 demonstrated a new technique which he called 'koelioscopie'. He made two tiny holes in the abdominal wall of a live dog, through one of which he inserted a cystoscope, a magnifying instrument like a small telescope. Air was then pumped through the second incision to inflate the cavity, giving a clear view of the abdominal organs and creating enough space to manipulate surgical instruments.[25] This was the first demonstration of laparoscopic or 'keyhole' surgery, a technique which only became common practice many decades later when technological developments – notably the invention of flexible optical fibres – made it a genuine alternative to conventional surgery. The advantages of laparoscopy were soon apparent: in the hands of a competent surgeon the smaller incisions reduced operative risk, allowed the patient to recover more quickly and reduced post-operative pain. In the 1980s there was a great deal of interest in these minimally invasive techniques, and it was not long before surgeons began to ponder their application in operations on the heart and lungs.

The principal aim in using such an approach was to avoid sternotomy, the usual method of opening the chest for open-heart procedures. This entails cutting through the skin and the tissue underneath it before splitting the breastbone with a pneumatic saw; metal retractors are then used to pull the ribcage apart and give the surgeon a good view of the heart and surrounding vessels. Although most people recover from a sternotomy without significant pain, it leaves an unsightly scar down the centre of the chest; the incision may take months to heal; and it can be risky to repeat the procedure in the event that further surgery is needed. There were good reasons for looking for an alternative.

In 1996 two surgeons from the Cleveland Clinic, Delos Cosgrove and José Navia, performed a series of mitral valve repairs using a simple, minimally invasive, technique: rather than opening the chest, they tilted their patient slightly and made an incision between two ribs on his right side. This small aperture allowed just enough space to admit instruments and allow them to open the heart chambers.[26] Others adopted the approach, often using a video camera to provide a better view of what they were doing inside the heart. Though the method reduced pain and bleeding, the limitations of working through such small incisions were clear. The instruments were unwieldy – typically twice as long as normal – and even the best high-definition camera gave only a flat two-dimensional image of the complex 3D structures they were trying to cut and sew.

The fundamental challenge – that of performing intricate manipulations in a restricted space – was hardly new. Industry had been using robotics since the 1970s to assemble complex electronics or handle dangerous chemicals, applications where a high degree of precision was required. Smaller desktop robots subsequently became a familiar sight in medical laboratories, so it required little imagination to realise that the technology might be adapted for the operating theatre.[27] In 1988 a robot was used for the first time to assist with a prostate operation, and other applications followed, but only a decade later was one used in cardiac surgery.

On 7 May 1998 Alain Carpentier performed the first robotic heart operation, using a prototype machine with two arms designed to replicate the full range of motion of the human hand. The procedure began with a small incision on the right side of the patient's chest, creating an aperture just 6 by 4 centimetres. Cardiopulmonary bypass was initiated, and once the heart had been taken out of the circulation the right atrium was opened. The camera and robotic instruments were then lowered into the cardiac chambers and Carpentier sat down at a computer console a few feet away from the table. The patient had a large atrial septal defect and an associated aneurysm of the septum; as a 3D image of these features appeared on the video screen, Carpentier had the eerie sense that he was actually inside the organ and inspecting it at close quarters. He slipped his fingers into the motion-sensitive rings controlling the instruments. One of the robotic 'hands' held forceps, the other a pair of scissors, a needle or a device for tying knots, as required. As he worked, a computer continuously analysed his movements and eradicated any tremor: even the best surgeon's hands tremble from time to time. In a procedure lasting several hours, Carpentier was able to cut out the aneurysm and place a patch of pericardium across the septal defect to repair it. The operation was completed without a hitch.[28]

A few weeks later, Carpentier's friend and collaborator Friedrich-Wilhelm Mohr applied the technology to mitral valve surgery, performing complex repairs through three small incisions (known as 'ports') made between his patients' ribs. Mohr used a voice-activated robot capable of responding to simple verbal commands; it could also memorise the structures of the heart and move to particular positions automatically. The system proved so effective that he was able to complete the entire operation with only the assistance of a single scrub nurse – fulfilling the prophecy made by Carpentier more than a decade earlier.[29] But the new surgical tool passed its most exacting test later in the year, when both Mohr[30] and Carpentier[31] showed that it was possible to perform even coronary artery bypass grafting – a notoriously fiddly procedure – using a robotic assistant.

Although the early results of robotic CABG were excellent, doubts were soon raised about a machine's ability to suture the tiny coronary arteries with as much accuracy as the human hand. Devices have now been developed to speed up this process: instead of sutures, tiny metal clips like staples are punched through the edges of the blood vessels.[32] This is still a new procedure, but current research suggests that – in the short to medium term, at least – the outcome of robotic surgery is just as good as that of the old hand-sewn method.[33] Similarly, after thousands of operations on mitral valve repair the results are no worse than would be expected from a human surgeon. Patients undergoing robotic surgery tend to have a shorter stay in hospital, return to work earlier and experience less pain.[34]

So is the robot the future of heart surgery? Alas, probably not. When surgeons adopt a new procedure, one question matters above all others: will this save more lives than existing techniques? Robotic surgery may allow patients to spend less time in a hospital bed, but it is no better at keeping them alive than an old-fashioned surgeon. And there are other barriers to its general adoption: robots are hugely expensive to buy and maintain; surgeons require extra training and experience before they become adept in their use; and operations take longer when a robot is involved. One surgeon put it like this: 'Cardiologists have used innovation to make their jobs easier. We're managing to make our jobs more difficult.' The robotic surgeon will supplant its human counterpart only if and when it can do a better job.

The desire to reduce the effects of surgery by using minimally invasive methods has led some surgeons to explore another, rather disconcerting, possibility. In October 1998 surgeons at Guven Hospital in the Turkish capital Ankara began to perform heart surgery on patients who remained wide awake. Instead of a general anaesthetic they were given a spinal injection to numb the entire chest area while the surgeons completed a coronary artery bypass graft on the beating heart. The rationale behind this strange regression to an earlier medical age is twofold: to eliminate the risks inherent to anaesthesia, and to enable constant assessment of the patient's neurological condition, a useful indicator of rare but dangerous complications.

Today, perhaps the most adventurous pioneer of conscious cardiac surgery is Vivek Jawali, from the Wockhardt Heart Institute in Bangalore, who in 2004 began performing a range of procedures, including CABG, valve replacement and even open-heart repair of congenital defects, without general anaesthetic or mechanical ventilation. In several of his patients a phenomenon previously unknown to medicine was observed: after being attached to the heart-lung machine they spontaneously – and for unknown reasons – stopped breathing. In normal circumstances this would have been an emergency, but because their blood was being oxygenated mechanically there was no cause for alarm.[35]

Conscious cardiac surgery must count among the most surreal experiences anybody has ever had at the hands of the medical profession – so, just for a moment, imagine it from the patient's point of view. You're lying on an operating table, wide awake. Your breastbone has been sawn through to reveal your internal organs – though somebody has considerately hung a surgical drape in front of your face so that you can't catch a glance of your own heart and lungs. A surgeon has not only stopped your heart but cut it open, and at this very moment is rummaging inside it with a forceps and a needle. Weirdest of all, although you can reply to the anaesthetist's questions you haven't needed to breathe for the last hour; the sensation is strangely liberating, like a dream in which the action takes place underwater yet inexplicably you don't drown. You may find the idea distasteful, even repellent, but most patients who have been through the experience report no discomfort or unpleasant memories of the procedure.

Conscious heart surgery is an intriguing idea which has been taken up with enthusiasm in a few centres in India, China and Japan, but is only ever likely to be useful for a small subset of patients for whom a general anaesthetic is clinically undesirable. Like keyhole surgery and robotics, it amounts to an eye-catching innovation rather than a revolution. Indeed, most recent developments in cardiac surgery fall into this category, with little sense of anything radically new on the horizon, of any breakthrough to compare with TAVI. When interventional cardiologists and surgeons reflect on the future of their field the contrast between their responses is surprising. The cardiologists brim with enthusiasm, and cannot wait to explain how catheter interventions might develop in the coming years. Surgeons have less to say, and say it without any great excitement: many agree that there is little remaining scope for innovation. They now have a tried and tested repertoire of operations to treat all the commonly encountered heart conditions. Most are so effective that there is little need to develop new ones; instead, efforts are concentrated on refining existing methods, reducing mortality and the incidence of complications.

Professional sportspeople like to talk about the 'aggregation of marginal gains', the insight that achieving tiny improvements in many different areas will eventually add up to a substantial competitive advantage. The philosophy was pioneered and popularised by Dave Brailsford, the coach under whose guidance the British track cycling team dominated successive Olympics from 2008 onwards. In his determination to improve performance Brailsford studied every conceivable aspect of his cyclists' lives, from the aerodynamics of their riding positions to the bedding they slept on – even bringing in a surgeon to teach them to wash their hands properly as a safeguard against illness. Cardiac surgery is now following a similar path, looking at how outcomes can be improved by comparatively minor changes to operative technique, anaesthesia, medication and follow-up care. Fifty years ago a typical research paper might describe a novel operation, including pictures and a case report or two. Today it's more likely to read like an actuarial report, with reams of data subjected to rigorous statistical analysis. This is important work, but it does not exactly quicken the pulse.

It would be wrong, however, to imply that innovation has ground to a halt. Much of the most exciting contemporary research focuses on the greatest, most fundamental cardiac question of all: what can the surgeon do about the failing heart? Christiaan Barnard believed he had the answer, and half a century later transplantation remains the gold standard of care for patients in irreversible heart failure once drugs have ceased to be effective. It's an excellent operation, too, with patients surviving an average of fifteen years. But it will never be the panacea that many predicted, because there just aren't enough donor hearts to go round. In 2007 there were 88 people on the UK waiting list for a heart transplant; by 2016 there were 249, even though the number of operations performed rose sharply.[36] Fewer than half of patients on the waiting list live long enough to receive a new organ, and some spend a year or more in intensive care before finally undergoing surgery. The lack of available hearts is critical, and there is little that can be done about it: fewer healthy young people die than they used to, a development which is hardly to be regretted.

With nowhere near enough organs available, surgeons have had to think laterally. One new strategy is the use of organs from so-called 'marginal' donors: those aged over fifty or who show some signs of disease. In the 1970s most hearts came from accident victims in their teens or early twenties; at one major European transplant centre the average age of a donor organ now stands at fifty-five, and surgeons routinely transplant hearts taken from donors in their sixties.[37] Another solution is the use of technology to preserve donor hearts, enabling them to be transported long distances. Conventionally, the organ is packed in ice within minutes of its ceasing to contract, a measure that preserves its tissues for up to four hours. In 2006 a new medical device called the TransMedics Organ Care System appeared on the market, a portable pump-oxygenator the size of a small suitcase which circulates warm blood through the heart while it is in transit. Nicknamed the 'heart in a box', it was adopted by Harefield Hospital in 2011 to enable the retrieval of geographically distant donor organs, since it allows a heart to be kept beating and perfused with blood for more than eight hours – long enough to get between any two points in the British Isles.[38]

Desperation has also led surgeons to challenge one of the oldest orthodoxies about transplantation. For many years the only suitable donor was believed to be a brain-dead patient whose heart was still beating; if its contractions had ceased, ischaemia (interruption of the blood supply) would cause permanent damage to its tissues within minutes of death. This remained the accepted wisdom until 2006, when Stephen Large, a transplant surgeon at Papworth Hospital, proved that a stopped heart could in fact be restarted, and continue to function, up to forty minutes after the death of the patient.[39] The discovery suggested an entirely new source of donor organs, although it also raised complex new ethical questions: what criteria should be used to determine death? How soon after the heart had stopped beating was it acceptable to remove it? And how would consent be obtained from family members during the brief window when the organ remained viable? Only after these had been discussed and new protocols agreed was the approach put into clinical practice.

The first modern transplant from a non-beating-heart donor was performed in mid-2014 by surgeons at St Vincent's Hospital in Sydney, Australia.* The organ came from a donor whose life support was withdrawn at the behest of the family. Half an hour after it had stopped contracting it was withdrawn and attached to the Organ Care System. Fresh blood was now pumped through the organ and as oxygen reached the myocardium it began to beat once more – and continued to do so for four hours as it was transported to Sydney by road.[40] There it was implanted into the chest of Michelle Gribilar, a fifty-seven-year-old who had been desperately ill with congenital heart failure. Less than a month later she was well enough to go home, and was soon able to walk long distances without fatigue.

This method was used to perform several transplants, but it had significant drawbacks, in particular the fact that the donor's own blood was used to perfuse the heart while in the Organ Care device – an unsatisfactory arrangement, since at the point of death the blood is full of toxic chemicals produced as a response to stress and injury, which may harm the organ.[41] To get around this problem Stephen Large and his team modified the procedure for Europe's first non-beating-heart transplant, which took place at Papworth in February 2015. When the donor had been declared dead the heart was restarted while still in the body, with the brain deliberately excluded from the circulation to avoid catecholamine storm – the dramatic release of hormones such as adrenaline which would otherwise flood the body during brain death. Once the heart had been assessed and stabilised it

---

* Not the very first, since Christiaan Barnard's early transplants, performed before a consensus had been reached on the definition of brain death, used non-beating-heart donors.

was stopped again, removed from the body and attached to the Organ Care System ready for transplant. The first recipient, a sixty-year-old former boxer called Huseyin Ulucan, did well, but the second was an even more spectacular success. The patient was a man who at twenty-three was dying from heart failure and had spent two months in the hospital's critical care unit. Eight weeks after his transplant his doctors were taken aback when they received a video of him 'recuperating'. Stephen Large was astonished: 'I remember seeing this guy in intensive care [and] thinking, when's it going to happen, the cardiac arrest? Two, three weeks? And now here he is, doing motocross and water-skiing on one leg.'[42]

By returning to non-beating-heart donation it is estimated that it may be possible to increase the number of available organs by as much as 20 per cent.[43] But this will only help in the short term, and I was surprised to find some transplant surgeons yearning for the demise of their own speciality. One said, 'I want to see the end of heart transplantation, or transplantation in general. Relying on the organs of somebody who's died is a strange position to be in. We find ourselves complaining that there isn't enough death!' André Simon, the surgeon in charge of the heart transplant programme at Harefield Hospital, suggests that transplantation will continue to play a role, but only for a small number of carefully selected patients. VADs are now improving at such a rate, he believes, that they will eventually be the answer in most cases, and we may one day even have a reliable and permanent artificial heart.[44]

Indeed, a new generation of total artificial hearts is now in development. For decades the only models available were pneumatically powered, a cumbersome arrangement which left patients permanently tethered to an air pump. The development of VADs with tiny rotary electrical motors provided another option, and several companies are now working on artificial hearts based on the same technology. In addition to being much smaller and more efficient than the pneumatic pumps, these devices are far more durable, since the rotors that impel the blood are suspended magnetically and are not subject to the wear and tear caused by friction.[45] Animal trials have shown promising results, but none has yet been implanted in a patient.

Another type of total artificial heart has, however, recently been tested in humans. Alain Carpentier, who in his ninth decade continues to innovate, has collaborated with engineers from the French aeronautical firm Airbus to design a pulsatile, hydraulically powered device whose unique feature is the use of bioprosthetic materials similar to those used in replacement valves. Unlike earlier artificial hearts, its design mimics the shape of the natural organ; the internal surfaces are lined with preserved bovine pericardial tissue, a biological surface far kinder to the red blood cells than the polymers previously used. The blood is propelled by membranes, which pulsate back and forth under alternating pressure from silicone oil pumped by an electric motor. The device is also the first to regulate its own rate automatically, detecting whether the patient is at rest or exercising. Since the motor is housed inside the body, the patient merely needs to wear a battery on a belt rather than carry a bulky drive unit.[46] Carpentier's artificial heart was first implanted in December 2013; although the first four patients have since died – two following component failures – the results were encouraging, and a larger clinical trial is now underway.[47]

One drawback to the artificial heart still leads many surgeons to dismiss the entire concept out of hand: the price tag. These high-precision devices cost in excess of £100,000 each, and no healthcare service in the world, publicly or privately funded, could afford to provide them to everybody in need of one. Where else to look, then? Some believe that the cure for heart failure will not be provided by a machine, but by a farmyard animal. Researchers realised decades ago that the supply of transplant donors was never likely to meet demand, and began to look for an alternative source of organs. In the 1960s the American surgeon Keith Reemtsma had had some success transplanting chimpanzee kidneys into patients, and although the first attempts by James Hardy and Christiaan Barnard to use non-human hearts all ended in failure the idea seemed credible. If the difficulties could be overcome, xenotransplantation – the transplantation of organs from another species – had one huge advantage: in theory, donor animals could be farmed to produce an almost unlimited supply of organs.

Unfortunately the task proved far more challenging than anybody had imagined. The main obstacle is a phenomenon known as hyperacute rejection. In the 1960s the British surgeon Roy Calne began a series of animal experiments in which he transplanted goat kidneys into dogs. He found that within a matter of minutes the organs died, 'turning port red, maroon, purple, and then black before my eyes'.[48] The immune system quickly recognises cells from another individual as alien, and begins to attack them – but when the tissue comes from a different species the assault is far more aggressive. In the 1980s, when research into xenotransplantation began to gather pace, many investigators believed that hyperacute rejection could be mitigated if the donor organs came from animals closely related to humans, since the immune system reacts more violently to tissues which are genetically dissimilar. Baboons and chimpanzees were the obvious candidates, but these animals take a decade to reach maturity, which makes breeding impractical. Moreover, the heart of even the largest chimp is too small to sustain the average human's circulation. In the mid-1980s David Cooper, a British surgeon then working in Oklahoma, became interested in the possibilities of xenotransplantation. Having abandoned the idea of using primate organs he turned his attention to pigs. Unlikely as it may seem, pigs have hearts very similar to ours; they are also easy to breed, and take only a year to reach full size.

Unfortunately, pig hearts also present a far greater immunological challenge. In his early experiments Cooper found that when a monkey heart was transplanted into a baboon it might function for a few days or weeks before rejection set in. When a pig's organ was used instead, it would last only a few minutes before being destroyed by the baboon's immune system. It transpired that primates, including humans, produce antibodies against pig tissue – an immune response that is not innate, but which develops in the first months of life. Why we should acquire immunity against pigs was mysterious, since antibodies are usually produced against pathogens that the body has recognised as a threat. Why should babies' immune systems learn to attack pig tissue months before they are able to eat solids, let alone pork?

After many months, Cooper's research group discovered that this immune response is not directed specifically at pig tissue, but at a molecule found on the surface of porcine cells. Galactose-α-1,3-galactose is a sugar that plays a role in the biochemistry of all mammals, with the notable exception of primates such as humans. It is also present in the cell membranes of the microbes which colonise our gut shortly after birth, a fact that explains why the human immune system produces antibodies against it. In the first few months of life the body learns to recognise the sugar as a feature of non-human cells, and will attack any structure containing it.[49]

Efforts to get rid of these antibodies stalled until 1992, when a small biotechnology firm in Cambridge, Imutran, unveiled a major breakthrough. Her name was Astrid, and she was a genetically modified, or transgenic, sow. Her DNA had been altered so that her cells produced human decay-accelerating factor (hDAF), a protein specific to human tissues.[50] It was hoped that this would fool the immune system into recognising porcine organs as human, and thus prevent rejection; indeed, in 1995 Imutran announced that surgeons at Papworth intended to perform the first pig-to-human heart transplants the following year. The era of xenotransplantation seemed to be just months away.[51]

The prediction turned out to be horribly premature. Researchers soon found that the immunological barriers were even more complex than they at first appeared. And then experts in another field, microbiology, broached a subject which cast doubt on the entire enterprise: trans-species infection. Transplanting a pig organ into a human might also risk introducing pig viruses into the patient's bloodstream, with unknown consequences. Many diseases we now think of as human – including HIV, Ebola and measles – originated in animals before crossing the species barrier, so there appeared to be a genuine danger of creating new types of infection. Most concerning of all were a group of organisms called porcine endogenous retroviruses (PERVs), viruses which seemed impossible to eliminate, since they are actually part of the pig's genome. Laboratory research published in 1997 showed that PERVs were capable of infecting human cells – in a test tube, at any rate.[52] Nobody knew whether this would also happen in a living body, or what the consequences would be; such setbacks caused many to lose faith in a project which only recently had looked so promising.*

Several companies withdrew their funding for xenotransplantation, and the media lost interest. Ironically, though, it was only after their work had fallen out of the public eye that researchers started to make significant progress with the problem of rejection. In February 1997 a team at the Roslin Institute in Edinburgh introduced the world to Dolly, an eight-month-old sheep who instantly became the most famous ungulate on the planet. She had been cloned from a mammary gland cell taken from another sheep – the first time that specialised adult cells had been used to clone a mammal. Her birth was a watershed in genetic engineering, since it demonstrated that scientists had attained a new degree of sophistication in manipulating DNA. One way of making pig tissue compatible with the human body is to alter its biochemistry – and the best way of doing that is to tinker with the pig's genome. Dolly's creation told researchers that such a thing might be possible.

On Christmas Day 2001, five healthy piglets were born at a research facility in Blacksburg, Virginia. They looked perfectly normal, but in one respect they were profoundly unlike any pig that had lived before. Their cells lacked a molecule called α1,3-galactosyltransferase, an enzyme responsible for the synthesis of the galactose sugar which

---

* Some still have serious concerns about PERVs, though there is no evidence that they cause harm to humans. A team at Harvard recently succeeded in eliminating the genes responsible for the viruses from the pig genome, which may offer a definitive solution to the problem.

provokes hyperacute rejection when detected by the human immune system. Scientists from the University of Pittsburgh had succeeded in 'knocking out' the gene that triggers the production of the enzyme, so that the pigs' cells were incapable of manufacturing the sugar.[53] Creating these so-called 'Gal knockout' pigs was an important step towards a rejection-free xenograft, and David Cooper's team in Boston subsequently transplanted several Gal knockout pig hearts into baboons. Two were given normal pig hearts, and hyperacute rejection killed them both within twenty minutes. But the Gal knockout organs caused no such reaction, and one animal lived for six months with its new heart – a dramatic improvement on previous attempts at xenotransplantation.[54]

This was only the first piece in a complicated jigsaw, however: the animals eventually succumbed to rejection, indicating that there remained other biochemical processes to be mastered. Research established that other parts of the immune system were also implicated, and that the blood coagulation systems of pigs and primates are fundamentally incompatible.[55] In 2009 a group in Germany bred triple-transgenic pigs to overcome several rejection mechanisms simultaneously, a development which produced the best results so far.[56] One baboon lived for a year with a porcine heart implanted in parallel with its own – the experiment was testing for rejection rather than assessing whether the transplanted organ could sustain the circulation on its own.[57]

Research is still identifying further immunological mechanisms which need to be overcome before xenotransplantation can be applied to humans. The transgenic pigs currently being used have as many as six genetic manipulations to alter their biochemistry, and more may be necessary. When baboons are given porcine organs they require immunosuppressive drugs, as do patients who receive a conventional transplant, but the ultimate goal is to produce a pig heart that the human body cannot distinguish from its own tissue. Clinical trials may finally be on the horizon, although they will not be given the go-ahead until researchers can demonstrate consistent long-term survival in primates with a xenograft which actually sustains the circulation.[58]

Research into xenotransplantation – not just for hearts, but kidneys, pancreatic cells and livers – is now going on in several countries including China, South Korea and the US. David Cooper, who has worked in the field for over thirty years, believes that it will not be long before we can reap the benefits: 'You're not going to have to get up in the middle of the night to fly somewhere to get a heart; it won't come from somebody who's brain-dead; you'll be able to do the transplant the next morning on the routine operating list. The patient won't be in an intensive-care unit for three months waiting for a donor – we'll be able to say, we'll transplant him tomorrow.'[59] It's an enticing prospect, but there aren't many surgeons who share his optimism. Several cite Norman Shumway, the father of transplantation, who used to joke that 'Xenografting is the future of transplantation, and always will be.'[60] In addition to the practical difficulties, there are significant ethical and psychological questions which still need to be answered. Many patients may have religious or moral objections to receiving a heart from a pig, or even see it as a threat to their humanity. And so far, with clinical use still some way off, doctors have barely attempted to gauge public opinion on the subject.[61]

Surveying the landscape of possible treatments, there is surprisingly little consensus on the most promising option for heart failure: some proponents of VADs are dismissive of the total artificial heart, while transplant enthusiasts suggest that mechanical devices will always remain too expensive for general use. And there is one still more tantalising notion: that we will one day be able to engineer spare parts for the heart, or even an entire organ, in the laboratory.

Growing tissues outside the body was first proposed in 1897 by Leo Loeb, a German pathologist working in Chicago. While investigating wound healing in the skin of guinea pigs, he succeeded in transplanting cells extracted from a guinea pig foetus and then embedded in a nutrient medium, a mixture of agar and blood serum.[62] Finding that they continued to grow while isolated from the blood and neighbouring tissue, Loeb suggested that by using similar methods it might be possible to cultivate tissues outside their usual biological environment. By the end of the next decade growing cells *in vitro* (from the Latin, 'in glass') had become an indispensable laboratory technique, but it was not until much later that anybody contemplated using it to build specific structures to repair the body. In the 1980s surgeons began to fabricate artificial skin for burns patients, seeding sheets of collagen or polymer with specialised cells in the hope that they would multiply and form a skin-like protective layer.[63] But researchers had loftier ambitions, and a new field – tissue engineering – began to emerge. In an influential article published in 1993, two of its pioneers, Joseph Vacanti and Robert Langer, defined this nascent discipline as applying 'the principles of biology and engineering to the development of functional substitutes for damaged tissue'.[64]

High on the list of priorities for tissue engineers was the creation of artificial blood vessels, which would have applications across the full range of surgical specialisms. In 1999 surgeons in Tokyo performed a remarkable operation in which they gave a four-year-old girl a new artery grown from cells taken from elsewhere in her body. She had been born with a rare congenital defect which had completely obliterated the right branch of her pulmonary artery, the vessel conveying blood to the right lung. A short section of vein was excised from her leg, and cells from its inside wall were removed in the laboratory. They were then left to multiply in a bioreactor, a vessel which bathed them in a warm nutrient broth, simulating conditions inside the body. After eight weeks they had increased in number to more than 12 million, and were used to seed the inside of a polymer tube which functioned as a scaffold for the new vessel. The tissue was allowed to continue growing for ten days, and then the graft was transplanted. During a straightforward procedure the blocked artery was removed, and the tissue-engineered vessel sutured in its place. Two months later the polymer scaffold around the tissue, designed to break down inside the body, had completely dissolved, leaving only new tissue which would – it was hoped – grow with the patient.[65]

The limitation of this technique was that the tissue used to engineer the new artery could only come from another blood vessel, since the cells which make up the lining of these vessels – the endothelium – are highly specialised. But at the turn of the millennium a new world of possibility opened up when researchers gained a powerful new tool: stem cell technology. In contrast to the endothelial cells in the blood vessels (for instance), stem cells are not specialised to one function but have the potential to develop into many different tissue types. One type of stem cell is found in growing embryos, and another in parts of the adult body, including the bone marrow (where they generate the cells of the blood and immune system) and skin. In 1998 James Thomson, a biologist at the University of Wisconsin, succeeded in isolating stem cells from human embryos and growing them in the laboratory,[66] resulting in a wealth of new research into how cells differentiate and possible new therapies. But an arguably even more important breakthrough came nine years later. Shinya Yamanaka, a researcher at Kyoto University, showed that it was possible to genetically 'reprogram' skin cells and convert them into stem cells.[67] The implications were enormous. In theory it would now be possible to harvest mature, specialised cells from a patient, reprogram them as stem cells, then choose which type of tissue they would become.

One possible application of this discovery is in the treatment of heart attacks. When the cardiac muscle is damaged by an interruption in its blood supply the body does little to repair it: scar tissue forms, but few new muscle cells, or myocytes, appear. Existing methods of treatment – whether drugs, CABG or stenting – do nothing to restore the tissue which has been injured, so an effective means of replacing lost myocardium would be a major therapeutic breakthrough. To encourage the growth of new muscle, scientists first tried extracting adult stem cells from the patient's bone marrow and injecting them into the coronary arteries, in the hope that some would adhere to the myocardium and convert into myocytes – but the results were disappointing.*

Rather than engineer new tissue in situ, Sanjay Sinha, a cardiologist at the University of Cambridge, is attempting to grow a 'patch' of artificial myocardium in the laboratory for later implantation in the operating theatre. His technique starts with undifferentiated stem cells, which are then encouraged to develop into several types of specialised cell: not just myocytes, but also smooth muscle tissue and vascular cells. These are then seeded on to a scaffold made from collagen, a tough protein found in connective tissue. The presence of several different cell types means that when they have had time to proliferate, the new tissue will develop its own blood supply. Clinical trials are still some years away, but Sinha hopes that one day it will be possible to repair a damaged heart by sewing one of these myocardial patches over areas of muscle scarred by a heart attack.[68]

Using advanced tissue-engineering techniques, researchers have already succeeded in replicating structures more complex than myocardium, including the creation of replacement valves from the patient's own tissue. This can be done by harvesting cells from elsewhere in the body (usually the blood vessels) and breeding them in a bioreactor, before seeding them on to a biodegradable polymer scaffold designed in the shape of a valve. Once the cells are in place they are allowed to proliferate before implantation, after which the scaffold melts away, leaving nothing but new tissue.[69] The one major disadvantage of this approach is that each valve has to be tailor-made for a specific patient, a process which takes weeks. In the last couple of years a group in Berlin has refined the process by tissue-engineering a valve and then stripping it of cellular material, leaving behind just the extracellular matrix, the structure which holds the cells in position.

---

* A more promising approach, recently pioneered by a group in San Francisco, attempts to convert the scar tissue into new muscle cells in situ. A genetically engineered virus is used to introduce new DNA into the affected cells, reprogramming them into myocytes.

The end result is therefore not quite a valve, but a skeleton on which the body lays down new tissue.[70] Valves manufactured in this way can be implanted, via catheter, in anybody; moreover, unlike conventional prosthetic devices, if the recipient is a child the new valve should grow with them.[71]

If it is possible to tissue-engineer a valve, then why not an entire heart? For many researchers this has come to be the ultimate prize, and the idea is not necessarily as fanciful as it first appears. In 2008 a team led by Doris Taylor, a scientist at the University of Minnesota, announced the creation of the world's first bioartificial heart. They began by pumping detergents through hearts excised from rats. This removed all the cellular tissue from them, leaving a ghostly heart-shaped skeleton of extracellular matrix and connective fibre, which was used as a scaffold on to which cardiac or blood-vessel cells were seeded. The organ was then cultured in a bioreactor to encourage cell multiplication, with blood constantly perfused through the coronary arteries. After four days it was possible to see the new tissue contracting, and after a week the heart was even capable of pumping blood – though only 2 per cent of its normal volume.[72]

This was a brilliant achievement, but scaling the procedure up to generate a human-sized heart is made far more difficult by the much greater number of cells required. Surgeons in Heidelberg have since applied similar techniques to generate a human-sized cardiac scaffold covered in living tissue. The original heart came from a pig, and after it had been decellularised it was populated with human vascular cells and cardiac cells harvested from a newborn rat.* After ten days the walls of the organ had become lined with new myocardium which even showed signs of electrical activity.[73] As a proof of concept the experiment was a success, though after three weeks of culture the organ could neither contract nor pump blood.

---

* While human vascular tissue is easily harvested, for ethical and practical reasons human cardiac tissue is more problematic, hence the use of rat cells.

Growing tissues and organs in a bioreactor is a laborious business, but recent improvements in 3D printing offer the tantalising possibility of manufacturing a new heart rapidly and to order. 3D printers work by breaking down a three-dimensional object into a series of thin two-dimensional 'slices', which are laid down one on top of another. The technology has already been employed to manufacture complex engineering components out of metal or plastic, but it is now being used to generate tissues in the laboratory. The process is a bit like making a three-dimensional colour photocopy, as the finished item is an exact replica of an original. To make an aortic valve, for instance, researchers at Cornell University took a pig's valve and X-rayed it in a high-resolution CT scanner. This gave them a precise map of its internal structure which could be used as a template. Using the data from the scan, the printer extruded thin jets of a hydrogel, a water-absorbent polymer which mimics natural tissue, gradually building up a duplicate of the pig valve layer by layer. This scaffold could then be seeded with living cells and incubated in the normal way.[74]

Pushing the technology further, Adam Feinberg, a materials scientist at Carnegie Mellon University in Pittsburgh, recently succeeded in fabricating the first anatomically accurate 3D-printed heart. He used the heart of a chick embryo, chosen because its complex internal anatomy made it particularly difficult to replicate. The tiny organ, just 2.5 millimetres in diameter, was mapped microscopically to provide a template for the printer, which was set up so that it produced a replica ten times life size. This facsimile was made of hydrogel and contained no tissue, but it did show a remarkable fidelity to the original organ.[75] Since then, Feinberg has used natural proteins such as fibrin and collagen to 3D-print hearts; his group is now aiming to include living cardiac cells in the hydrogels extruded by the device so that it is able to print living tissue and so construct a viable organ.[76] For many researchers in this field a fully tissue-engineered heart is the ultimate prize, but even those involved acknowledge that their goal is a long way off. When I asked one whether he could see it being a realistic alternative to transplantation, he laughed before suggesting that it would take another forty years to perfect.

We are, therefore, left with several competing visions of the future. Within a few decades it is possible that we will be breeding transgenic pigs in vast sterile farms and harvesting their hearts to implant in sick patients. Or that new organs will be 3D-printed to order in factories, before being dispatched in drones to wherever they are needed. Or maybe an unexpected breakthrough in energy technology will make it possible to develop a fully implantable, permanent mechanical heart. More mundanely, it's also conceivable that advances in drug therapy and preventative care will render such dramatic interventions largely unnecessary. A few retired medics can still recall wards full of patients suffering from polio, tuberculosis or scarlet fever; perhaps heart disease will go the same way as these illnesses, which have now virtually disappeared in the West.

Most cardiac surgeons are too cautious to forecast which, if any, of these scenarios is most likely to come to pass. Perhaps they realise that, as a breed, when they do venture to make predictions they often turn out not to be very good at it. In 1910 Harry Sherman, one of the first surgeons to suture a beating heart, gave a talk at a meeting of the Medical Society of the State of California. He told his colleagues: 'I do not see how the majority of heart conditions which come to the physician can look to surgery for relief. A too large heart cannot be shaved down to a proper size, nor can a new heart muscle be made.'[77] If he was being unduly pessimistic, a report published in 2004 by the World Health Organisation went to the other extreme, predicting implausibly that by 2020 'nanosurgeons', microscopic robots, would be able to crawl through arteries to scrape away fatty deposits and make minor repairs.[78]

Whatever the future holds, it is worth reflecting on how much has been achieved in so little time. Speaking in 1902, six years after Ludwig Rehn became the first person to perform cardiac surgery, Harry Sherman remarked that 'The road to the heart is only two or three centimetres in a direct line, but it has taken surgery nearly 2,400

years to travel it.'[79] Overcoming centuries of cultural and medical prejudice required a degree of courage and vision still difficult to appreciate today. Even after that first step had been taken, another fifty years
elapsed before surgeons began to make any real progress; and then
in a dizzying period of three decades they learned how to open the
heart, repair and even replace it. In most fields, an era of such fundamental discoveries happens only once – if at all – and it is unlikely
that cardiac surgeons will ever again captivate the world as Christiaan
Barnard and his colleagues did in 1967. But the history of heart surgery is littered with breakthroughs nobody saw coming, and as long as
there are surgeons of talent and imagination, and a determination to
do better for their patients, there is every chance that they will continue to surprise us.

ACKNOWLEDGEMENTS

Thanks are first due to the Royal Society of Literature and the Jerwood Charitable Foundation, whose non-fiction award immeasurably benefited the book by allowing me to research more deeply without worrying about whether I'd be able to finish the job.

Writing this book would not have been possible without the generous assistance of numerous surgeons, cardiologists, physicians, clinical researchers and others. They invited me into their operating theatres, gave up their meal breaks to talk to me, offered introductions and tips, and lent me books and journal articles. In particular I wish to thank the following, who went out of their way to help in one way or another: Gianni Angelini, Nick Cheshire, Horatio Clare, David Cooper, Martin Elliott, Sir Terence English, Tony Gershlick, Andrew Grace, Marjan Jahangiri, Stephen Large, Marc de Leval, Duncan Macrae, Gavin Murphy, Papworth Hospital NHS Foundation Trust, John Pepper, Bernard Prendergast, Simon Redwood, Benny Rousso, Royal Brompton & Harefield NHS Foundation Trust, Babulal Sethia, Ulrich Sigwart, André Simon, Sanjay Sinha, David Taggart, Angela and Jay VanDerwerken, Francis Wells and Stephen Westaby.

I am also indebted to the staff of the Wellcome Library, my 'office' for much of the last two years, to the National Library of Medicine, and to Oregon Health and Science University Historical Collections and Archives for their assistance in tracking down several elusive documents.

Thanks also to my agent Patrick Walsh for his enthusiasm and advice, and to Stuart Williams and Anna-Sophia Watts at The Bodley Head, whose perceptive editorial suggestions made a huge difference to the final form of the text. To my family, for their advice and peerless grammar pedantry, and finally to my partner Jenny, for her unstinting support as well as tolerance for my endless boring medical questions (and even more boring surgical anecdotes).

LIST OF ILLUSTRATIONS

Quonset hut/Dwight Harken operation site. (*Photo by Thomas Morris*).

'Blue baby' surgery at the Johns Hopkins Hospital, February 1947. *Courtesy of the Alan Mason Chesney Medical Archives of the Johns Hopkins Medical Institutions.*

Michael Schirmer and Anna the Dog, March 1948. (*Photo by Fritz Goro/The LIFE Picture Collection/Getty Images*).

Heart of King George II, from *Observations concerning the Body of His Late Majesty, October 26, 1760*, by Frank Nicholls, M. D., F. R. S. Physician to His Late Majesty. Phil. Trans., published 1 January 1761. Downloaded from http://rstl.royalsocietypublishing.org/ on 24 March 2017.

Michael DeBakey in surgical scrubs at Methodist Hospital, operating room in background, 1978. *U. S. National Library of Medicine. Reproduced with permission of the Baylor College of Medicine Archives.*

A view of a cross-circulation operation performed by Lillehei, August 1954. (*Photo by Al Fenn/The LIFE Picture Collection/Getty Images*).

Hypothermic heart surgery, NIH 1955. Photo by Roy Perry. *U. S. National Library of Medicine.*

John Gibbon with heart-lung machine. *U. S. National Library of Medicine.*

Philip Amundson holding an artificial mitral valve, 13 October 1960. Photo by University of Oregon Medical School. *Courtesy of OHSU Historical Collections & Archives.*

First Pacemaker: Senning and Elmqvist's first pacemaker, 4 October 1978, Stockholm, Sweden. *(Photo by Bettmann/Getty Images).*

Pacemaker Anniversary: Senning, Elmqvist and their first patient, Arne Larsson, holding the first pacemaker, October 1978. *(Photo by Keystone/Hulton Archive/Getty Images).*

First Human Heart Transplant Recipient: Christiaan Barnard and Louis Washkansky, Cape Town, South Africa, December 1967. *(Photo by Rolls Press/Popperfoto/Getty Images).*

Christiaan Barnard, South Africa, 1968. *(Photo by Wieczorek/ullstein bild via Getty Images).*

Cartoon of Christiaan Barnard as a vulture, Gerald Scarfe, 1969. *Courtesy of Gerald Scarfe.*

Overhead view of open heart surgery at Houston Methodist Hospital, 21 April 1966. *(Photo by Bettmann/Getty Images).*

Haskell Karp in Surgery Recovery Room, Houston, Texas, 1969. *(Photo by Bettmann/Getty Images).*

Barney Clark being visited by his wife Una Loy, December 1982. *(Photo by Bettmann/Getty Images).*

Early Artificial Heart, Houston, Texas, April 1969. *(Photo by Bettmann/Getty Images).*

Heart specialist Andreas Grüntzig holding a balloon catheter, 1981. *(Photo by Ted Thai/The LIFE Picture Collection/Getty Images).*

Robotic surgery at Jewish General Hospital, Canada. *(Photo by Felipe Argaez, MedPhoto, JGH).*

FURTHER READING

This is a small and personal selection of the available literature, for the most part written for those without prior medical knowledge. A more extensive bibliography can be found in the notes for each chapter.

Historical Surveys

Cooper, David, *Open Heart: The Radical Surgeons Who Revolutionized Medicine* (Kaplan Publishing, 2010)
> Concentrating on the 'golden age' of heart surgery in the 1950s and 1960s, this lively book by a former colleague of Christiaan Barnard includes many vivid anecdotes from the surgeons themselves.

Friedman, Steven G., *A History of Vascular Surgery* (Blackwell Futura, 2005)
> An accessible introduction to cardiac surgery's sister discipline, including biographical portraits of some of its leading figures.

Richardson, Robert, *Heart and Scalpel: A History of Cardiac Surgery* (Quiller Press, 2001)
> Originally published in 1969, an engagingly written book which provides a detailed account of developments up to and including Barnard's first transplant.

Shumacker, Harris B., *The Evolution of Cardiac Surgery* (Indiana University Press, 1992)
> The most scholarly history of the discipline, written by a surgeon who himself made several important contributions. Comprehensive but aimed at the specialist, and often dauntingly technical.

Stoney, William S. (ed.), *Pioneers of Cardiac Surgery* (Vanderbilt University Press, 2008)
> A valuable collection of interviews with dozens of the most influential surgeons active between the 1940s and the 1980s.

Westaby, Stephen, and Cecil Bosher, *Landmarks in Cardiac Surgery* (ISIS Medical Media, 1997)

> The bulk of this weighty volume consists of facsimiles of original surgical articles reporting some of the major breakthroughs of the first century of cardiac surgery. These are, however, preceded by a readable and lavishly illustrated historical narrative.

Topics in Cardiac Surgery

Cooper, David, and Robert Lanza, *Xeno: The Promise of Transplanting Animal Organs into Humans* (Oxford University Press, 2000)

> Research has moved on considerably since it was first published, but this book by the leading expert in the field is still worth reading for its lucid explanation of the challenges of xenotransplantation.

DeBakey, Michael E., and Antonio M. Gotto, *The New Living Heart* (Adams Media Corp, 1997)

> A beginner's guide to the organ and its diseases, co-written by one of the giants of twentieth-century surgery. A wonderfully clear explanation of how the heart works and what can go wrong with it, although some of the clinical information is now out of date.

Fox, Renée C., and Judith P. Swazey, *The Courage to Fail: A Social View of Organ Transplants and Dialysis* (University of Chicago Press, 1974)
————, *Spare Parts: Organ Replacement in American Society* (Oxford University Press, 1992)

> A pair of influential books by two sociologists who studied the implications of organ transplantation and the artificial heart. They spent considerable time in the hospitals concerned and interviewed many of those involved – and not just the surgeons. *The Courage to Fail* includes a detailed and even-handed assessment of Denton Cooley's controversial 1969 artificial heart operation and its consequences.

Jeffrey, Kirk, *Machines in Our Hearts: The Cardiac Pacemaker, the Implantable Defibrillator, and American Health Care* (Johns Hopkins University Press, 2001)

> An impressively thorough history of both devices which concentrates on the technological rather than medical aspects of the subject.

Nathoo, Ayesha, *Hearts Exposed: Transplants and the Media in 1960s Britain* (Palgrave Macmillan, 2009)

> A fascinating analysis of the controversy caused by the first human transplants, exploring how they altered the relationship between the British media and the medical profession.

Wright, Thomas, *Circulation: William Harvey's Revolutionary Idea* (Chatto & Windus, 2012)

> An engrossing and much-admired account of William Harvey's discovery of the circulation of the blood.

Biography and Memoir

A number of surgeons have written entertaining and revealing (if occasionally partial) accounts of their own work. Barnard's memoirs are particularly worth reading, and he is often surprisingly frank about his own failings. Bigelow's two books are clearly written and modestly put his own considerable achievements into context. Thomas Thompson's *Hearts*, a bestselling double profile of Cooley and DeBakey written at the height of their feud, is a fine piece of reportage by a writer who spent many months in the company of both men. Wertenbaker's *To Mend the Heart* concentrates on the work of Dwight Harken and paints a vivid portrait of the man who launched the modern era of cardiac surgery.

Barnard, Christiaan, *The Second Life: Memoirs* (Vlaeberg, 1993)

Barnard, Christiaan, and Curtis B. Pepper, *Christiaan Barnard: One Life* (Howard Timmins, 1969)

Barnard, Marius, and Simon Norval, *Defining Moments: An Autobiography* (Zebra Press, 2011)

Bigelow, Wilfred G., *Cold Hearts: The Story of Hypothermia and the Pacemaker in Heart Surgery* (McClelland and Stewart, 1984)

———, *Mysterious Heparin: The Key to Open Heart Surgery* (McGraw-Hill Ryerson, 1990)

Cooley, Denton A., *100,000 Hearts: A Surgeon's Memoir* (Dolph Briscoe Center for American History, University of Texas at Austin, 2012)

Cooper, David, *Chris Barnard: By Those Who Knew Him* (Vlaeberg, 1992)

Edwards, W. Sterling, *Alexis Carrel: Visionary Surgeon* (Thomas, 1974)

English, Terence, *Follow Your Star: From Mining to Heart Transplants – a Surgeon's Story* (AuthorHouse, 2011)

Favaloro, René G., *The Challenging Dream of Heart Surgery: From the Pampas to Cleveland* (Little, Brown, 1994)

Forssmann, Werner, *Experiments on Myself: Memoirs of a Surgeon in Germany* (St Martin's Press, 1974)

Longmire, William P., *Alfred Blalock: His Life and Times* (unknown publisher, 1991)

Malinin, Theodore I., *Surgery and Life: The Extraordinary Career of Alexis Carrel* (Harcourt Brace Jovanovich, 1979)

Murray, Gordon, *Medicine in the Making* (The Ryerson Press, 1960)

Romaine-Davis, Ada, *John Gibbon and his Heart-Lung Machine* (University of Pennsylvania Press, 1991)

Shumacker, Harris B., *The Life of John H. Gibbon, Jr., Father of the Heart-Lung Machine* (Fithian Press, 1999)

Thomas, Vivien T., *Pioneering Research in Surgical Shock and Cardiovascular Surgery: Vivien Thomas and his Work with Alfred Blalock. An Autobiography* (University of Pennsylvania Press, 1985)

Thompson, Thomas, *Hearts: DeBakey and Cooley, Surgeons Extraordinary* (Pan Books, 1974)

Wertenbaker, Lael, *To Mend the Heart* (Viking Press, 1980)

NOTES

ABBREVIATIONS

BMJ   *British Medical Journal*
JAMA   *Journal of the American Medical Association*

INTRODUCTION

1. J. Pegrum and O. Pearce, 'A stressful job: are surgeons psychopaths?' *Bulletin of the Royal College of Surgeons of England* 97, no. 8 (2015), 331–4

2. R. Chelliah, R. Showkathali, B. Brickham et al, 'Multi-disciplinary clinic: next step in "heart team" approach for TAVI', *International Journal of Cardiology* 174, no. 2 (2014), 453–5

1. BULLET TO THE HEART

1. Dwight E. Harken, 'Administrative and basic clinical considerations in the European theater of operations', *Surgery in World War II: Thoracic Surgery* (ed. John B. Coates; Washington: Office of the Surgeon General Dept. of the Army, 1963), 113–60

2. D. E. Harken, 'Foreign bodies in, and in relation to, the thoracic blood vessels and heart: Techniques for approaching and removing foreign bodies from the chambers of the heart', *Surgery, Gynecology and Obstetrics* 83 (1946), 117–25

3. William S. Stoney, 'Interview with Alden H. Harken': www.mc.vanderbilt.edu/diglib/ sc_diglib/cardiac_surgery/harken.html

4. Harken, 'Administrative and basic … ', Coates (ed.), op. cit.

5. Lael Wertenbaker, *To Mend the Heart* (New York: Viking Press, 1980), 41

6. Nicholas L. Tilney, *Invasion of the Body: Revolutions in Surgery* (Cambridge, MA: Harvard University Press, 2011), 165

7. Stoney, op. cit.

8. Stephen L. Johnson, *The History of Cardiac Surgery, 1896–1955* (Baltimore, London: Johns Hopkins Press, 1970), 12

9. Sir Gordon Gordon-Taylor (ed.), *The British Journal of Surgery: War Surgery Supplement no. 3: War Injuries of the Chest and Abdomen* (Bristol: John Wright & Sons, 1952), 399

10. Stephen Paget, *The Surgery of the Chest* (Bristol: Wright & Co, 1896), 121

11. B. M. Ricketts, *The Surgery of the Heart and Lungs* (New York: The Grafton Press, 1904), 146

12. J. W. Haward, *A Treatise on Orthopaedic Surgery* (London: Longmans, Green, 1881)

13. James E. Garretson, *A System of Oral Surgery* (London: J. B. Lippincott, 1884)

14. H. Macnaughton-Jones, *A Treatise on Aural Surgery* (London: J. & A. Churchill, 1881)

15. Robert B. Carter and William A. Frost, *Ophthalmic Surgery* (London: Cassell, 1889)

16. Henry Morris, *Surgical Diseases of the Kidney* (London, 1885)

17. Henry Savage, *The Surgery, Surgical Pathology and Surgical Anatomy of the Female Pelvic Organs* (London: J. & A. Churchill, 1882)

18. Reginald Harrison, *On Some Points in the Surgery of the Urinary Organs* (London: J. & A. Churchill, 1888)

19. Nicholas Senn, *Intestinal Surgery* (Chicago: W. T. Keener, 1889)

20. Henry Smith, *The Surgery of the Rectum* (London: J. & A. Churchill, 1882)

21. D. B. Kirkpatrick, 'The first primary brain-tumor operation', *Journal of Neurosurgery* 61, no. 5 (1984), 809–13

22. Ambroise Paré, *The Workes of that Famous Chirurgion A. Parey: Translated by Thomas Johnson* (London, 1649)

23. R. K. French, 'The thorax in history: 1. From ancient times to Aristotle', *Thorax* 33, no. 1 (1978), 10–18

24. Pliny, John Bostock, and H. T. Riley, *The Natural History of Pliny* (London: Henry G. Bohn, 1855), 3

25. Galenus, Friedrich W. Assmann and Carl G. Kühn, *Opera Omnia* (20 vols; Hildesheim: Olms, 1965), 8: 304–05

26. Francis Adams, *The Medical Works of Paulus Ægineta* (London, 1834), 2: 418–21

27. Alexander Read, *A Treatise of the First Part of Chirurgerie* (London: Francis Constable, 1628)

28. Paré, op. cit., 296

29. Barthélémy Cabrol, *Alphabet Anatomic, auquel est contenue l'explication exacte des parties du corps humain, et reduites en tables selon l'ordre de dissection ordinaire: Avec l'ostéologie, et plusieurs observations particulières* (Tournon: C. Michel & G. Linocier, 1594)

30. Johann Dolaeus and William Salmon, *Systema Medicinale: A Compleat System of Physick, Theoretical and Practical* (London: T. Passinger, 1686)

31. William Babington, *Medical Records and Researches: Selected from the Papers of a Private Medical Association* (London: T. Cox, 1798), 1

32. 'Extensive wound of the heart, in which the patient survived one hour and a quarter', *London Medical Gazette* 3, no. 72 (1829), 653–54

33. John H. Fuge, 'Case of gunshot wound of the heart', *Edinburgh Medical and Surgical Journal* 14, no. 1 (1818), 129–31

34. 'Case of wound of the heart, in which the patient survived the accident nearly ten days', *London Medical Gazette* 2, no. 49 (1828), 729

35. Baron Dupuytren, 'Clinical observations on wounds of the heart', *London Medical Gazette* 13, no. 322 (1834), 661

36. Rudolph Matas, 'Surgery of the vascular system', *Surgery: Its Principles and Practice* (ed. William W. Keen; 7 vols 5; Philadelphia: W. B. Saunders Co, 1909), 17–350

37. 'Extensive wound of the heart …' op. cit.

38. Dupuytren, op. cit.

39. 'Extensive wound of the heart …' op. cit.

40. 'Case of wound of the heart', *The Lancet* 32, no. 829 (1839), 605–06

41. Samuel S. Purple, 'Observations on wounds of the heart and their relation to forensic medicine', *New York Journal of Medicine* 14 (1855), 411–34

42. George W. Callender, 'Removal of a needle from the heart; recovery of the patient', *Medico-Chirurgical Transactions* 56 (1873), 203–12

43. Lew A. Hochberg, *Thoracic Surgery Before the 20th Century* (1st ed.; New York: Vantage Press, 1960), 545–6

44. William Harvey and Robert Willis, *The Works of William Harvey* (London: Sydenham Society, 1847), 382–3

45. John B. Roberts, 'The Surgery of the Pericardium', *Annals of Anatomy and Surgery* 4 (1881), 247–52

46. DaCosta, John Chalmers, *Modern Surgery, General and Operative* (3rd ed.; Philadelphia and London: W. B. Saunders Co, 1900), 303

47. L. Birkbeck, G. Lorimer and H. Gray, 'Removal of a bullet from the right ventricle of the heart under local anaesthesia', *BMJ* 2 (1915), 561

48. H. C. Dalton III. 'Report of a case of stab-wound of the pericardium, terminating in recovery after resection of a rib and suture of the pericardium', *Annals of Surgery* 21, no. 2 (1895), 147–52

49. DaCosta, John Chalmers, op. cit.

50. George T. Vaughan, 'Suture of wounds of the heart', *JAMA* 52, no. 6 (1909), 429

51. Charles Ballance, 'Examples of the resources of surgery in certain emergencies', *The Lancet* 179, no. 4612 (1912), 139–44

52. Charles A. Elsberg, 'An experimental investigation of the treatment of the wounds of the heart by means of suture of the heart muscle', *Journal of Experimental Medicine* 4, 5–6 (1899), 479–520

53. Adolfo Crotto and Luigi Lucatello, *Atti dell'XI Congresso Medico Internazionale, Roma, 1894* (Rome: Ripamonti e Colombo, 1895), 4

54. Axel Cappelen, 'Vulnus cordis. Sutur af hjertet', *Norsk Magazin for Laegevidesnsk* 6 (1896), 285–8

55. John Bland-Sutton, 'A clinical lecture on the treatment of injuries of the heart', *BMJ* 1, no. 2578 (1910), 1273–6

56. 'Cardiac surgery', *JAMA* 26, no. 24 (1896), 1183–4

57. Frederick A. Willius et al., *Classics of Cardiology* (1983), 2: 42–3

58. 'Operation on a human heart', *North Otago Times* XXVI, no. 8943, 16 July 1897

59. 'Novel or strange', *Cornishman*, 6 May 1897

60. G. S. Brock, 'Penetrating wound of the pericardium and left ventricle; suture; recovery', *The Lancet* 150, no.3857 (1897), 260–1

61. L. L. Hill, 'A report of a case of successful suturing of the heart, and table of thirty-seven other cases of suturing by different operators with various terminations, and the conclusions drawn', *Medical Records and Researches: selected from the papers of a private medical association* 62 (1902), 846–8

62. Willius et al., op. cit.

63. Rudolph Matas, 'Surgical treatment of perforating and bleeding wounds of the chest', *JAMA* 32, no. 13 (1899), 687–92

64. M. Launay, 'Plaie double du coeur par balle (ventricule gauche), suture, guerison', *Bulletin de l'Académie Nationale de Médecine* 48 (1902), 185–8

65. 'Extracted bullet from heart', *Los Angeles Herald* 31, no. 39, 9 November 1903

66. Werner von Manteuffel, 'Schussverletzung des Herzens.: Naht. Extraktion der Kugel aus der hinteren Wand. Heilung.,' *Zentralblatt für Chirurgie* 41 (1905), 1096–7

67. Eugene H. Pool, 'Treatment of heart wounds: report of successful cardiorrhaphy and tabulation of cases', *Annals of Surgery* 55, no. 4 (1912), 485–512

68. George Benet and Charles G. Spivey, 'Suture of stab wound of the heart', *JAMA* 104, no. 22 (1935), 1979

69. G. W. Brewster and Samuel Robinson, 'Operative treatment of wounds of the heart: With report of a recent case of bullet wound of the heart, lung, and liver', *Annals of Surgery* 53, no. 3 (1911)

70. Charles A. Ballance, *The Bradshaw Lecture on the Surgery of the Heart* (London: Macmillan & Co, 1920), 68–71

71. Birkbeck, Lorimer and Gray, 'Removal of a bullet ...', op. cit.

72. Rudolph Matas, 'Military surgery of the vascular system', *Surgery: Its Principles and Practice* (vol. 7, ed. William W. Keen; Philadelphia, London: W. B. Saunders Co, 1921), 713–819

73. A. L. d'Abreu, 'War wounds of the chest', *British Journal of Surgery: War Surgery Supplement no. 3: War Injuries of the Chest and Abdomen* (ed. Sir Gordon Gordon-Taylor; Bristol: John Wright & Sons, 1952)

74. Matas, op. cit., 728–9

75. William W. Davey and Geoffrey E. Parker, 'The surgical pursuit and removal of a metallic foreign body from the systemic venous circulation', *British Journal of Surgery* 34, no. 136 (1947), 392–5

76. Matas, op. cit., 713

77. Wertenbaker, op. cit.

2. BLUE BABIES

1. Timothy G. Buchman, 'Shock: Blalock and Cannon', *Archives of Surgery* 145, no. 4 (2010), 393–4

2. William P. Longmire, *Alfred Blalock: His Life and Times* (unknown publisher, 1991), 97–8

3. Robert M. Freedom, *The Natural and Modified History of Congenital Heart Disease* (Oxford: Blackwell, 2004), 190

4. 'Kirkcaldy Has a Blue Baby', *Dundee Courier*, 12 November 1947

5. 'Interview with William Longmire', in *Pioneers of Cardiac Surgery* (ed. William S. Stoney; Nashville, TN: Vanderbilt University Press, 2008)

6. Longmire, op. cit., 101–04

7. Vivien T. Thomas, *Pioneering Research in Surgical Shock and Cardiovascular Surgery: Vivien Thomas and his Work with Alfred Blalock. An Autobiography* (Philadelphia: University of Pennsylvania Press, 1985), 44

8. Joyce Baldwin, *To Heal the Heart of a Child: Helen Taussig, M.D.* (New York: Walker, 1992), 39–40

9. 'Interview with Denton A. Cooley', in Stoney (ed.), op. cit.

10. Thomas, op. cit., 92–3

11. 'Interview with William Longmire', in Stoney (ed.), op. cit., 68–70

12. Longmire, op. cit., 104

13. Helen B. Taussig, 'Personal memories of surgery of tetralogy', *History and Perspectives of Cardiology* (ed. H. A. Snellen, A. J. Dunning and A. C. Arntzenius; Leiden University Press, 1981), 159–72

14. Alfred Blalock and Helen B. Taussig, 'The surgical treatment of malformations of the heart: in which there is pulmonary stenosis or pulmonary atresia', *JAMA* 128, no. 3 (1945), 189–202

15. Price Day, 'Taussig-Blalock and Blue Babies', *Baltimore Sun*, 3 February 1946

16. Blalock and Taussig, op. cit.

17. ibid.

18. Helen B. Taussig, 'On the evolution of our knowledge of congenital malformations of the heart. The T. Duckett Jones Memorial Lecture', *Circulation* 31, no. 5 (1965), 768–77

19. Renée Matthews, obituary, *Cardiology News* 6, no. 3 (2008), 39

20. Blalock and Taussig, op. cit.

21. 'Interview with William Longmire', in Stoney (ed.), op. cit., 70–71

22. Freedom, op. cit., 186

23. Thomas, op. cit., 101

24. Alfred Blalock and Michael Ravitch, *The Papers of Alfred Blalock* (Baltimore: Johns Hopkins Press, 1966), xliii

25. Longmire, op. cit., 153–4

26. 'Roger, the "Blue Boy", will live', *Sevenoaks Chronicle and Kentish Advertiser*, 12 December 1947

27. 'New heart for Christmas', *Daily Mail*, 27 December 1947

28. Blalock and Ravitch, *The Papers of Alfred Blalock*, xlviii

29. 'London notes', *Yorkshire Post and Leeds Intelligencer*, 22 March 1948

30. Longmire, op. cit., 156–7

31. 'Gift of health fills the stocking of boy who was doomed to die', *New York Times*, 13 December 1948

32. Thomas, op. cit., 153–4

33. B. M. Ricketts, *The Surgery of the Heart and Lungs* (New York: The Grafton Press, 1904), 247–71

34. 'The antivivisection bill', *JAMA* 28, no. 4 (1897), 177–8

35. Alfred Blalock, 'The technique of creation of an artificial ductus arteriosus in the treatment of pulmonic stenosis', *Journal of Thoracic Surgery* 16 (1947), 244–57

36. James M. Mason, 'Observations on surgery of the colon. Indications for primary resection and anastomosis and for exteriorization procedures', *Transactions of the Southern Surgical Association* 62 (1950), 152

37. Sherwin B. Nuland, 'Man vs Dog: a bioethical trade-off; animal research reflects our regard for human life', *Los Angeles Times*, 5 September 1989

38. 'Blue Baby research', *Life*, 14 March 1949

39. 'McKeldin's official majority 92,998; Miller by 8,910', *Star-Democrat* (Easton, Maryland), 24 November 1950

40. Chris Smith, 'Information on Anna', cited 10 June 2015: www.hopkinsmedicine.org/mcp/Front_page/anna/

41. C. W. Lillehei et al., 'Direct vision intracardiac surgical correction of the tetralogy of Fallot, pentalogy of Fallot, and pulmonary atresia defects: report of first ten cases', *Annals of Surgery* 142, no. 3 (1955), 418–42

42. James Mackenzie, *Diseases of the Heart* (London: Henry Frowde, 1908)

43. F. J. Poynton, 'A lecture on congenital heart disease', *BMJ*, no. 1 (1906), 1458

44. William J. Rashkind (ed.), *Congenital Heart Disease* (Benchmark papers in human physiology 16; Stroudsburg, PA: Hutchinson Ross, 1982), 91

45. Robert Boyle, 'An account of a very odd monstrous calf', *Philosophical Transactions* 1, 1–22 (1665), 10

46. Thomas Bartholinus, *Thomæ Bartholini Acta Medica et Philosophica Hafniensia. ann. 1671* (1673), 5

47. Richard van Praagh, 'The First Stella van Praagh Memorial Lecture: the history and anatomy of tetralogy of Fallot', *Seminars in Thoracic and Cardiovascular Surgery. Pediatric Cardiac Surgery Annual* (2009), 19–38

48. Bartholinus, op. cit.

49. Étienne-Louis Arthur Fallot, 'Contribution à l'anatomie pathologique de la maladie bleue (cyanose cardiaque)', *Marseille Médical* 25 (1888), 77–93

50. Douglas Waugh, *Maudie of McGill: Dr Maude Abbott and the Foundations of Heart Surgery* (Toronto: Hannah Institute & Dundurn Press, 1992), 42–4

51. E. Braunwald, 'Nina Starr Braunwald: some reflections on the first woman heart surgeon', *Annals of Thoracic Surgery* 71, 2 Suppl (2001), 7

52. K. Smith, 'Maude Abbott: pathologist and historian', *Canadian Medical Association Journal* 127, no. 8 (1982), 774–6

53. Baldwin, op. cit., 50

54. Charles Harris, *The Heart and the Vascular System in Ancient Greek Medicine: From Alcmaeon to Galen* (Oxford: Clarendon Press, 1973), 294–5

55. Nathaniel Highmore, *Corporis Humani Disquisitio Anatomica* (The Hague: Samuel Brown, 1651): 194–5

56. C. N. LeCat, 'Concerning the foramen ovale being found open in the hearts of adults', *Philosophical Transactions* 9 (1747), 134–5

57. Rashkind (ed.), op. cit., 173–4

58. Traver J. Wright and Randall W. Davis, 'Myoglobin oxygen affinity in aquatic and terrestrial birds and mammals', *Journal of Experimental Biology* 218 (2015), 2180–89

59. George A. Gibson, *Diseases of the Heart and Aorta* (Edinburgh: Young J. Pentland, 1898)

60. John C. Munro, 'Ligation of the ductus arteriosus', *Annals of Surgery* 46, no. 3 (1907), 335–8

61. Russell Brock, 'The development of heart surgery in children', *Archives of Disease in Childhood* 40, no. 210 (1965), 123–7

62. W. Hardy Hendren, 'Robert E. Gross (1905–1988) and patent ductus arteriosus', in *Children's Surgery: A Worldwide History* (ed. John G. Raffensperger; London: McFarland & Co, 2012), 130–39

63. Robert E. Gross, 'Surgical management of the patent ductus arteriosus: with summary of four surgically treated cases', *Annals of Surgery* 110, no. 3 (1939), 321–56

64. Hardy Hendren, op. cit.

65. Frances Hess, 'The fire and explosive hazards involved in the use of cyclopropane as an anesthetic', *Bulletin of the National Association of Nurse Anesthetists* 5, no. 3 (1937), 359–63

66. Boston Children's Hospital Archives Oral History Project, 'Interview with Betty Lank OH' (1999)

67. Robert E. Gross and Luther A. Longino, 'The patent ductus arteriosus: observations from 412 surgically treated cases', *Circulation* 3, no. 1 (1951), 125–37

68. Robert E. Gross and John P. Hubbard, 'Surgical ligation of a patent ductus arteriosus: report of first successful case', *JAMA* 112, no. 8 (1939), 729–31

69. Boston Children's Hospital Archives Oral History Project, 'Interview with Lorraine Sweeney Nicoli' (2011)

70. 'Interview with Judson G. Randolph', in Stoney (ed.), op. cit.

71. Boston Children's Hospital Archives Oral History Project, 'Interview with Dr Hardy Hendren' (2000)

72. Robert Gross, 'Surgical management of the patent ductus arteriosus …', op. cit.

73. Alfred Blalock, 'Recent advances in surgery', *New England Journal of Medicine* 231 (1944), 261; 293

74. Gross and Longino, op. cit.

75. Helen B. Taussig, 'The surgery of congenital heart disease', *British Heart Journal* 10, no. 2 (1948), 65–79

76. Maurice Campbell, 'Natural history of coarctation of the aorta', *British Heart Journal* 32, no. 5 (1970), 633–40

77. M. J. Shapiro, 'Coarctation of the aorta: ten years' observation of a patient still living', *JAMA* 100, no. 9 (1933), 640–42

78. Paul D. White, *Heart Disease* (3rd ed.; New York: Macmillan, 1944), 307

79. Taussig, 'The surgery of congenital heart disease', op. cit.

80. John-Peder E. Kvitting and Christian L. Olin, 'Clarence Crafoord: a giant in cardiothoracic surgery, the first to repair aortic coarctation', *Annals of Thoracic Surgery* 87, no. 1 (2009), 342–6

81. Clarence Crafoord and G. Nylin, 'Congenital coarctation of the aorta and its surgical treatment', *Journal of Thoracic Surgery* 14 (1945), 347–61

82. Hardy Hendren, op. cit.

83. 'Interview with Viking Bjork', in Stoney (ed.), op. cit.

84. Allan Kozinn, 'Samuel Sanders is dead at 62; accompanied noted performers', *New York Times*, 12 July 1999

85. 'Pioneers in Cardiac Surgery – Clarence Crafoord': www.youtube.com/watch?v=mz4w-oHDp-E

86. Willis J. Potts, Sidney Smith and Stanley Gibson, 'Anastomosis of the aorta to a pulmonary artery: certain types in congenital heart disease', *JAMA* 132, no. 11 (1946), 627–31

87. Russell Brock, 'In memoriam: Alfred Blalock', *Annals of the Royal College of Surgeons of England* 36, no. 1 (1965), 62–5

3. 'A SENSIBLE HISSING'

1. Giovanni B. Morgagni, *The Seats and Causes of Diseases Investigated by Anatomy* (abridged and elucidated with notes by W. Cooke, 1822), 1: 431–2

2. ibid.

3. René T. H. Laennec and John Forbes, *A Treatise of the Diseases of the Chest* (Philadelphia: J. Webster, 1823), 276

4. William Hunter, 'The history of an aneurysm of the aorta, with some remarks on aneurysms in general', *Medical Observations and Inquiries* 1 (1757), 323–57

5. Henry Mason, *Lectures upon the Heart, Lungs, Pericardium, Pleura, Aspera Arteria, Membrana Intersepiens, or Mediastinum* (Reading, 1765), 37

6. Denton A. Cooley and Michael E. DeBakey, 'Surgical considerations of intrathoracic aneurysms of the aorta and great vessels', *Annals of Surgery* 135, no. 5 (1952), 660

7. Michael E. DeBakey and Denton A. Cooley, 'Successful resection of aneurysm of thoracic aorta and replacement by graft', *JAMA* 152, no. 8 (1953), 673–6

8. William Osler, *Bibliotheca Osleriana* (Oxford: Clarendon Press, 1929), 40

9. P. Prioreschi, *A History of Medicine: Roman Medicine* (Edwin Mellen Press, 1998), 164–5

10. Charles Harris, *The Heart and the Vascular System in Ancient Greek Medicine: From Alcmaeon to Galen* (Oxford: Clarendon Press, 1973), 449–51

11. W. E. Stehbens, 'History of aneurysms', *Medical History* 2, no. 4 (1958), 274

12. Ambroise Paré and Thomas Johnson, *The Workes of that Famous Chirurgien Ambrose Parey* (London: T. Cotes and R. Young, 1634), 224–5

13. Lloyd A. Wells, 'The William Osler Medal essay: Aneurysm and physiological surgery', *Bulletin of the History of Medicine* 44, no. 5 (1970), 411–24

14. John Hunter and James F. Palmer, *The Works of John Hunter, FRS* (London: Longman, 1835–1837), 3: 594–611

15. Wells, op. cit.

16. Astley P. Cooper and Frederick Tyrrell, *The Lectures of Sir Astley Cooper, Bart., FRS, on the Principles and Practice of Surgery* (London: Thomas & George Underwood, 1824–27), 3: 50

17. ibid., 67–71

18. Alexander Monro, *Observations on Aneurism of the Abdominal Aorta* (Edinburgh: P. Neill, 1827), 24–9

19. Charles H. Moore and Charles Murchison, 'On a new method of procuring the consolidation of fibrin in certain incurable aneurisms: With the report of a case in which an aneurism of the ascending aorta was treated by the insertion of wire', *Medico-Chirurgical Transactions* 47 (1864), 129–49

20. ibid.

21. Timothy Holmes and John G. Westmacott, *A Treatise on Surgery: Its Principles and Practice* (2nd ed.; London: Smith, Elder, 1878)

22. Rudolph Matas, 'Surgery of the vascular system', in *Surgery: Its Principles and Practice* (ed. William W. Keen; 7 vols 5; Philadelphia: W. B. Saunders Co, 1909), 17–350

23. Arthur H. Blakemore and Barry G. King, 'Electrothermic coagulation of aortic aneurysms', *JAMA* 111, no. 20 (1938), 1821–7

24. Holmes and Westmacott, op. cit.

25. 'Reports of societies', *BMJ* 1, no. 1155 (1883), 311–17

26. 'Reports of societies,' *BMJ* 1, no. 1055 (1881), 431–5

27. Henry Goodridge, 'On the treatment of paroxysmal dyspnoea occurring in aneurysm of the arch of the aorta', *BMJ*, no. 1 (1887), 1207

28. National Library of Medicine, 'Oral history interview of Michael DeBakey by Donald A. Schanche', tape 3, cited 27 July 2015: https://profiles.nlm.nih.gov/ps/access/FJBBTG.pdf

29. Rudolph Matas, 'Traumatic aneurysm of the left brachial artery', *Medical News* 53, no. 17 (1888), 462–6

30. Rudolph Matas, 'I. An operation for the radical cure of aneurism based upon arteriorrhaphy', *Annals of Surgery* 37, no. 2 (1903), 161–96

31. Rudolph Matas, 'Aneurysm of the abdominal aorta at its bifurcation into the common iliac arteries', *Annals of Surgery* 112, no. 5 (1940), 909

32. J. R. Cohen and L. M. Graver, 'The ruptured abdominal aortic aneurysm of Albert Einstein', *Surgery, Gynecology & Obstetrics* 170, no. 5 (1990), 455–8

33. Théodore Tuffier, 'Intervention chirurgicale directe pour un aneurysme de la crosse de l'aorte. Ligature du sac', *Presse Medicale*, no. 23 (1902), 267–71

34. I. A. Bigger, 'The surgical treatment of aneurysm of the abdominal aorta', *Annals of Surgery* 112, no. 5 (1940), 879

35. Harris B. Shumacker Jr, 'Coarctation and aneurysm of the aorta: report of a case treated by excision and end-to-end suture of aorta', *Annals of Surgery* 127, no. 4 (1948), 655

36. Denton A. Cooley, *100,000 Hearts: A Surgeon's Memoir* (Austin, TX: Dolph Briscoe Center for American History, University of Texas at Austin, 2012), 73–4

37. Denton A. Cooley, 'Early development of surgical treatment for aortic aneurysms: personal recollections', *Texas Heart Institute Journal* 28, no. 3 (2001), 197–9

38. Cooley, *100,000 Hearts*, op. cit., 34–5

39. 'The Texas tornado', *Time* 85, no. 22 (1965), 54

40. Cooley, *100,000 Hearts*, op. cit., 90–91

41. National Library of Medicine, 'Oral history interview of Michael DeBakey by Donald A. Schanche', tape 13, cited 28 July 2015: https://profiles.nlm.nih.gov/ps/access/FJBBTS.pdf

42. Cooley and DeBakey, 'Surgical considerations of intrathoracic aneurysms of the aorta and great vessels', op. cit.

43. ibid.

44. DeBakey and Cooley, 'Successful resection of aneurysm of thoracic aorta and replacement by graft', op. cit.

45. Stephen Westaby and Cecil Bosher, *Landmarks in Cardiac Surgery* (Oxford: ISIS Medical Media, 1997), 234

46. Henry Swan et al., 'Arterial homografts: II. Resection of thoracic aortic aneurysm using a stored human arterial transplant', *Archives of Surgery* 61, no. 4 (1950), 732–7

47. National Library of Medicine, 'Oral history interview of Michael DeBakey by Donald A. Schanche', tape 7, cited 27 July 2015: https://profiles.nlm.nih.gov/ps/access/FJBBTL.pdf

48. National Library of Medicine, "Oral history interview of Michael DeBakey … ' op. cit., tape 13

49. W. S. Edwards, *Alexis Carrel: Visionary Surgeon* (Springfield, Illinois: Thomas, 1974), 13

50. Theodore I. Malinin, *Surgery and Life: The Extraordinary Career of Alexis Carrel* (1st ed.; New York: Harcourt Brace Jovanovich, 1979), 4

51. Steven G. Friedman, *A History of Vascular Surgery* (2nd ed.; Malden, Mass., Oxford: Blackwell Futura, 2005), 21

52. A. Carrel, 'The surgery of blood vessels', *Johns Hopkins Hospital Bulletin* 18 (1907), 18–28

53. Robert Dalbey, 'An English surgeon in America', *Littell's Living Age* 332 (1927), 9

54. Alexis Carrel, 'Results of the transplantation of blood vessels, organs and limbs', *JAMA* 51, no. 20 (1908), 1662–7

55. Alexis Carrel, 'VIII. On the experimental surgery of the thoracic aorta and heart', *Annals of Surgery* 52, no. 1 (1910), 83

56. A. Carrel, 'The transplantation of organs: a preliminary communication', *JAMA* 45, no. 22 (1905), 1645–6

57. Alexis Carrel, 'Permanent intubation of the thoracic aorta', *Journal of Experimental Medicine* 16, no. 1 (1912), 17–24

58. Friedman, op. cit., 121–3

59. Arthur B. Voorhees Jr., Alfred Jaretzki III, Arthur H. Blakemore, 'The use of tubes constructed from Vinyon "N" cloth in bridging arterial defects: a preliminary report', *Annals of Surgery* 135, no. 3 (1952), 332

60. National Library of Medicine, 'Oral history interview of Michael DeBakey by Donald A. Schanche', tape 1, cited 17 July 2015: https://profiles.nlm.nih.gov/ps/access/FJBBTD.pdf

61. Michael E. DeBakey and Antonio M. Gotto, *The New Living Heart* (Holbrook, MA: Adams Media Corp, 1997), 216

62. J. Harold Harrison, 'Synthetic materials as vascular prostheses: II. A comparative study of nylon, dacron, orlon, ivalon sponge and teflon in large blood vessels with tensile strength studies', *American Journal of Surgery* 95, no. 1 (1958), 16–24

63. H. I. Rustad, R. O. Gregg and J. T. Prior, 'The effect of hypercholesterolemia upon aortic homografts and teflon-nylon prostheses in the rabbit; absence of arteriosclerosis in prostheses', *Surgery* 44, no. 4 (1958), 726–34

64. National Library of Medicine, 'Oral history interview of Michael DeBakey … ', op. cit., tape 1

65. National Library of Medicine, 'Oral history interview of Michael DeBakey … ', op. cit., tape 7

66. R. A. Deterling Jr and S. B. Bhonslay, 'An evaluation of synthetic materials and fabrics suitable for blood vessel replacement', *Surgery* 38, no. 1 (1955), 71–91

67. Michael E. DeBakey et al., 'Clinical application of a new flexible knitted Dacron arterial substitute', *Archives of Surgery* 77, no. 5 (1958), 713–24

68. Ricky Harminder Bhogal and Richard Downing, 'The evolution of aortic aneurysm repair: past lessons and future directions', in *Aneurysmal Disease of the Thoracic and Abdominal Aorta* (ed. Marvin D. Atkins and Ruth L. Bush; INTECH, 2011), 21–54

69. Ralph S. Brown and Wilmarth S. Lewis, *Horace Walpole's Correspondence with George Montagu* (48 vols; New Haven: Yale University Press, 1941), 9: 311

70. F. Nicholls, 'Observations concerning the body of his late Majesty, October 26, 1760, by Frank Nicholls, MD, FRS, Physician to his late Majesty', *Philosophical Transactions* 52 (1761), 265–75

71. Michael E. DeBakey, Denton A. Cooley and Oscar Creech Jr, 'Surgical considerations of dissecting aneurysm of the aorta', *Annals of Surgery* 142, no. 4 (1955), 586

72. Michael DeBakey et al., 'Surgical treatment of dissecting aneurysm of the aorta. Analysis of seventy-two cases', *Circulation* 24, no. 2 (1961), 290–303

73. Walter S. Henly and Baylor College of Medicine, 'Interview with Dr Walter S. Henly, MD', cited 16 July 2015: http://profiles.nlm.nih.gov/ps/retrieve/ResourceMetadata/FJBBQS

4. ICE BATHS AND MONKEY LUNGS

1. Samuel A. Levine, *Clinical Heart Disease* (Philadelphia, London: W. B. Saunders Co, 1936), 313

2. Gordon Murray, 'Closure of defects in cardiac septa', *Annals of Surgery* 128, no. 4 (1948), 843–52

3. F. R. Edwards et al., 'Surgical treatment of atrial septal defects', *BMJ* 2, no. 4954 (1955), 1463–9

4. Robert E. Gross et al., 'A method for surgical closure of interauricular septal defects', *Surgery, Gynecology & Obstetrics* 96, no. 1 (1953), 1–24

5. J. H. Gibbon, 'Application of a mechanical heart and lung apparatus to cardiac surgery', *Minnesota Medicine* 37, no. 3 (1954), 171–85

6. J. H. Gibbon, 'Successful suture of a penetrating wound of the heart', *JAMA* 46, no. 6 (1906), 431

7. Ada Romaine-Davis, *John Gibbon and his Heart-Lung Machine* (Philadelphia: University of Pennsylvania Press, 1991), 4

8. J. H. Gibbon, 'The development of the heart-lung apparatus', *Review of Surgery* 27, no. 4 (1970), 231–44

9. P. S. Hasleton, 'The internal surface area of the adult human lung', *Journal of Anatomy* 112, Part 3 (1972), 391–400

10. Robert Hooke, 'An account of an experiment made by Mr Hooke, of preserving animals alive by blowing through their lungs with bellows', *Philosophical Transactions* 2, 23–32 (1666), 539–40

11. Richard Lower and Kenneth Franklin, *A Facsimile Edition of Tractatus de Corde* (Oxford, 1932)

12. J. J. C. Legallois, N. C. Nancrede and J. G. Nancrede, *Experiments on the Principle of Life: And Particularly on the Principle of the Motion of the Heart and on the Seat of this Principle / Translated by N. C. and J. G. Nancrede* (Philadelphia: M. Thomas, 1813), 130–31

13. J. Prevost, 'Examen du sang et de son action dans les divers phénomènes de la vie', *Annales de Chimie et de Physique* 18 (1821), 280–96

14. Michael J. Aminoff, *Brown-Séquard: An Improbable Genius who Transformed Medicine* (Oxford, New York: Oxford University Press, 2011), 276–7

15. Charles E. Brown-Séquard, *Experimental Researches Applied to Physiology and Pathology* (New York: H. Bailliere, 1853), 88–94

16. C. Ludwig and A. Schmidt, 'Das Verhalten der Gase, Welche mit dem Blut durch die reizbaren Säugethiermuskelz strömen', *Leipzig Berichte*, no. 20 (1868), 12–72

17. T. Lauder Brunton, 'On the use of artificial respiration and transfusion as a means of preserving life', *BMJ*, no. 1 (1873), 555

18. W. von Schroder, 'Uber die Bildungstatte des Harnstoffs', *Archiv Fur Experimentelle Pathologie und Pharmakologie*, no. 15 (1882), 364–402

19. M. von Frey and M. Gruber, 'Untersuchungen über den Stoffwechsel isolierter Organe. Ein Respirations-Apparat für isolierte Organe', *Virchov's Archiv fur Physiologie* 9 (1885), 519–32

20. J. W. Hurst, W. B. Fye and Heinz-Gerd Zimmer, 'The heart-lung machine was invented twice – the first time by Max von Frey', *Clinical Cardiology* 26, no. 9 (2003), 443–5

21. Robert L. Hewitt and Oscar Creech, 'History of the pump oxygenator', *Archives of Surgery* 93, no. 4 (1966), 680–96

22. Nikolai Krementsov, 'Off with your heads: isolated organs in early Soviet science and fiction', *Studies in History and Philosophy of Biological and Biomedical Sciences* 40, no. 2 (2009), 87

23. 'George Bernard Shaw tempted to have head cut off when he is told of scientist's feat', Associated Press, 17 March 1929

24. Igor E. Konstantinov and Vladimir V. Alexi-Meskishvili, 'Sergei S. Brukhonenko: the development of the first heart-lung machine for total body perfusion', *Annals of Thoracic Surgery* 69, no. 3 (2000), 962–6

25. Jay McLean, 'The discovery of heparin', *Circulation* 19, no. 1 (1959), 75–8

26. ibid.

27. W. G. Bigelow, *Mysterious Heparin: The Key to Open Heart Surgery* (Toronto: McGraw-Hill Ryerson, 1990), 10–15

28. W. H. Howell and Emmett Holt, 'Two new factors in blood coagulation – Heparin and Pro-antithrombin', *American Journal of Physiology* 47, no. 3 (1918), 328–41

29. D. W. G. Murray et al., 'Heparin and vascular occlusion', *Canadian Medical Association Journal* 35, no. 6 (1936), 621–2

30. Bigelow, op. cit., 36–40

31. Murray et al., op. cit.

32. Charles H. Best, 'Preparation of heparin and its use in the first clinical cases', *Circulation* 19, no. 1 (1959), 79–86

33. Bigelow, op. cit., 42

34. Gibbon, 'The development of the heart-lung apparatus', op. cit.

35. J. H. Gibbon, 'The gestation and birth of an idea', *Philadelphia Medicine* 13 (1963), 913–16

36. Romaine-Davis, op. cit., 56–7

37. Harris B. Shumacker, *A Dream of the Heart: The Life of John H. Gibbon, Jr, Father of the Heart-Lung Machine* (Santa Barbara, CA: Fithian Press, 1999), 126

38. J. H. Gibbon, 'Artificial maintenance of circulation during experimental occlusion of pulmonary artery', *Archives of Surgery* 34, no. 6 (1937), 1105–31

39. J. H. Gibbon, 'The maintenance of life during experimental occlusion of the pulmonary artery followed by survival', *Surgery, Gynecology & Obstetrics* 69 (1939), 602–14

40. Shumacker, op. cit., 128

41. Gibbon, 'The development of the heart-lung apparatus', op. cit.

42. 'The last field', *Time* 54, no. 13 (1949), 40

43. Bernard J. Miller, John H. Gibbon, Jr, Mary H. Gibbon, 'Recent advances in the development of a mechanical heart and lung apparatus', *Annals of Surgery* 134, no. 4 (1951), 694

44. Shumacker, op. cit., 156

45. Romaine-Davis, op. cit., 93–7

46. Michael E. DeBakey and Charles E. Schmidt, 'Surgical pump', US Patent no. 2018998, 1935

47. National Library of Medicine, 'Oral history interview of Michael DeBakey by Donald A. Schanche', tape 3, cited 27 July 2015: https://profiles.nlm.nih.gov/ps/access/FJBBTG.pdf

48. Denton A. Cooley, 'Development of the roller pump for use in the cardiopulmonary bypass circuit', *Texas Heart Institute Journal* 14, no. 2 (1987), 112

49. Clarence Dennis, Dwight S. Spreng Jr, George E. Nelson, Karl E. Karlson, Russell M. Nelson, John V. Thomas, Walter Phillip Eder, Richard L. Varco, 'Development of a pump-oxygenator to replace the heart and lungs: an apparatus applicable to human patients and application to one case', *Annals of Surgery* 134, no. 4 (1951), 709

50. Shumacker, op. cit., 158–9

51. Gibbon, 'Application of a mechanical heart …', op. cit.

52. Kelly D. Hedlund, 'A tribute to Frank F. Allbritten, Jr: origin of the left ventricular vent during the early years of open-heart surgery with the Gibbon heart-lung machine', *Texas Heart Institute Journal* 28, no. 4 (2001), 292–6

53. Gibbon, 'The development of the heart-lung apparatus', op. cit.

54. Romaine-Davis, op. cit., 98

55. Joeann G. T. Fraser, 'Retrospective on Dr Gibbon and his heart-lung machine', *Annals of Thoracic Surgery* 76, no. 6 (2003), S2197–8

56. Romaine-Davis, op. cit., 118–22

57. Gibbon, 'The development of the heart-lung apparatus', op. cit.

58. ibid.

59. Gibbon, 'Application of a mechanical heart …', op. cit.

60. Romaine-Davis, op. cit., 130–31

61. 'Historic operation', *Time* 61, no. 20 (1953), 33

62. F. J. Lewis, Richard L. Varco and Mansur Taufic, 'Repair of atrial septal defects in man under direct vision with the aid of hypothermia', *Surgery* 36, no. 3 (1954), 538–56

63. W. G. Bigelow, *Cold Hearts: The Story of Hypothermia and the Pacemaker in Heart Surgery* (Toronto: McClelland and Stewart, 1984), 40

64. Lawrence W. Smith and Temple Fay, 'Temperature factors in cancer and embryonal cell growth', *JAMA* 113, no. 8 (1939), 653–60

65. Bigelow, *Cold Hearts*, op. cit., 45–7

66. W. G. Bigelow, W. K. Lindsay and W. F. Greenwood, 'Hypothermia; its possible role in cardiac surgery: an investigation of factors governing survival in dogs at low body temperatures', *Annals of Surgery* 132, no. 5 (1950), 849–66

67. Bigelow, *Cold Hearts*, op. cit., 50–51

68. Bigelow, *Cold Hearts*, op. cit., 55–6

69. H. Swan et al., 'Surgery by direct vision in the open heart during hypothermia', *JAMA* 153, no. 12 (1953), 1081–5

70. ibid.

71. H. Swan, 'Hypothermia for general and cardiac surgery; with techniques of some open intracardiac procedures under hypothermia,' *The Surgical Clinics of North America* (1956), 1009–24

72. Bigelow, *Cold Hearts*, op. cit., 61

73. Stephen Westaby and Cecil Bosher, *Landmarks in Cardiac Surgery* (Oxford: ISIS Medical Media, 1997), 56

74. Swan et al., 'Surgery by direct vision ...', op. cit.

75. 'Discussion on the application of hypothermia to surgical procedures', *Proceedings of the Royal Society of Medicine* 49, no. 6 (1956), 345

76. I. Boerema et al., 'High atmospheric pressure as an aid to cardiac surgery', *Archivum Chirurgicum Neerlandicum* 8, no. 3 (1956), 193–211

77. I. Boerema, 'An operating room with high atmospheric pressure', *Bulletin de la Société Internationale de Chirurgie* 21 (1962), 170–76

78. 'Interview with C. Walton Lillehei', in *Pioneers of Cardiac Surgery* (ed. William S. Stoney; Nashville, TN: Vanderbilt University Press, 2008), 83–99

79. A. T. Andreasen and F. Watson, 'Experimental cardiovascular surgery: discussion of results so far obtained and report on experiments concerning a donor circulation', *British Journal of Surgery* 41, no. 166 (1953), 195–206

80. 'Interview with Richard A. DeWall', in Stoney (ed.), op. cit., 100–111

81. James Kay-Shuttleworth, *The Physiology, Pathology, and Treatment of Asphyxia, etc* (London: Longman, 1834)

82. L. Blum and S. J. Megibow, 'Exclusion of the dog heart by parabiosis', *Journal of the Mount Sinai Hospital, New York* 17, no. 1 (1950), 38–43

83. 'Interview with Lillehei', in Stoney (ed.), op. cit., 89–90

84. H. E. Warden et al., 'Controlled cross circulation for open intracardiac surgery: physiologic studies and results of creation and closure of ventricular septal defects', *Journal of Thoracic Surgery* 28, no. 3 (1954), 331

85. 'Interview with Lillehei', in Stoney (ed.), op. cit., 90–91

86. C. W. Lillehei et al., 'The first open-heart repairs of ventricular septal defect, atrioventricular communis, and tetralogy of Fallot using extracorporeal circulation by cross-circulation: a 30-year follow-up', *Annals of Thoracic Surgery* 41, no. 1 (1986), 4–21

87. Warden et al., op. cit.

88. 'Interview with DeWall', in Stoney (ed.), op. cit., 104

89. 'Discussion on the application of hypothermia to surgical procedures', op. cit.

90. Romaine-Davis, op. cit., 143

91. Lillehei et al., 'The first open-heart repairs ...', op. cit.

92. G. S. Campbell, N. W. Crisp, and E. B. Brown, 'Total cardiac by-pass in humans utilizing a pump and heterologous lung oxygenator (dog lungs)', *Surgery* 40, no. 2 (1956), 364–71

93. 'Medicine: answer in a dog's lung', *Time* 65, no. 14 (1955), 27

94. W. T. Mustard and J. A. Thomson, 'Clinical experience with the artificial heart lung preparation', *Canadian Medical Association Journal* 76, no. 4 (1957), 265

95. W. T. Mustard et al., 'A surgical approach to transposition of the great vessels with extracorporeal circuit', *Surgery* 36, no. 1 (1954), 31–51

96. Mustard and Thomson, op. cit.

97. Hewitt and Creech, op. cit.

98. J. W. Kirklin et al., 'Studies in extracorporeal circulation. I. Applicability of Gibbon-type pump-oxygenator to human intracardiac surgery: 40 cases', *Annals of Surgery* 144, no. 1 (1956), 2

99. 'Interview with Lillehei', in Stoney (ed.), op. cit., 91

100. Richard A. DeWall, 'The evolution of the helical reservoir pump-oxygenator system at the University of Minnesota', *Annals of Thoracic Surgery* 76, no. 6 (2003), S2210–15

101. 'Interview with Lillehei', in Stoney (ed.), op. cit., 92

102. Stanton P. Nolan, Richard Zacour and J. F. Dammann, 'Reflections on the evolution of cardiopulmonary bypass', *Annals of Thoracic Surgery* 64, no. 5 (1997), 1540–43

103. R. A. DeWall et al., 'A simple, expendable, artificial oxygenator for open heart surgery', *Surgical Clinics of North America* (1956), 1025–34

104. Vincent L. Gott et al., 'A self-contained, disposable oxygenator of plastic sheet for intracardiac surgery: experimental development and clinical application', *Thorax* 12, no. 1 (1957), 1

105. D. B. Effler et al., 'Disposable membrane oxygenator (heart-lung machine) and its use in experimental surgery', *Journal of Thoracic Surgery* 32, no. 5 (1956), 620–29

106. J. G. Allen (ed.), *Extracorporeal Circulation* (Springfield, IL: Thomas, 1958)

107. Russell C. Brock, 'The present position of cardiac surgery: Bradshaw Lecture delivered at the Royal College of Surgeons of England on 11th December 1957', *Annals of the Royal College of Surgeons of England* 23, no. 4 (1958), 213

108. A. M. Dogliotti and E. Ciocatto, 'Personal experiences in physiopathological bases of hypothermia and possibilities of association between hypothermia and extracorporal circulation', *Schweizerische Medizinische Wochenschrift* 83, no. 31 (1953), 707–10

109. Will C. Sealy, Ivan W. Brown Jr, W. Glenn Young Jr et al., 'A report on the use of both extracorporeal circulation and hypothermia for open heart surgery', *Annals of Surgery* 147, no. 5 (1958), 603

110. N. E. Shumway, R. R. Lower and R. C. Stofer, 'Selective hypothermia of the heart in anoxic cardiac arrest', *Surgery, Gynecology & Obstetrics* 109 (1959), 750–54

111. James Wardrop, *On the Nature and Treatment of the Diseases of the Heart* (London: J. Churchill, 1851), 318

112. D. G. Melrose et al., 'Elective cardiac arrest', *The Lancet* 269, no. 6879 (1955), 21–2

113. ibid.

114. Westaby and Bosher, op. cit., 66–7

115. A. R. Cordell, 'Milestones in the development of cardioplegia', *Annals of Thoracic Surgery* 60, no. 3 (1995), 793–6

116. D. J. Hearse, D. A. Stewart and M. V. Braimbridge, 'Cellular protection during myocardial ischemia: the development and characterization of a procedure for the induction of reversible ischemic arrest', *Circulation* 54, no. 2 (1976), 193–202

117. D. J. Hearse, 'Cardioplegia: the protection of the myocardium during open heart surgery: a review', *Journal de Physiologie* 76, no. 7 (1980), 751–68

118. S. Westaby, 'Complement and the damaging effects of cardiopulmonary bypass', *Thorax* 38, no. 5 (1983), 321

5. RUBBER BALLS AND PIG VALVES

1. 'Heart valve replaced by rubber ball', *Register-Guard* (Eugene, Oregon), 13 October 1960

2. Ann Sullivan, 'Engineer applies pump experience to create artificial heart valve', *Oregonian*, 3 December 1963

3. Bilal Ayub et al., 'Durability, reliability, viability: 48-year-survival of a Starr–Edwards mitral valve', *Heart, Lung & Circulation* 23, no. 1 (2014), 96–7

4. H. Milton, 'Mediastinal surgery', *The Lancet* 149, no. 3839 (1897), 872–5

5. Peter C. English, *Rheumatic Fever in America and Britain: A Biological, Epidemiological, and Medical History* (New Brunswick, NJ: Rutgers University Press, 1999), 1

6. Michael D. Seckeler and Tracey R. Hoke, 'The worldwide epidemiology of acute rheumatic fever and rheumatic heart disease', *Clinical Epidemiology* 3 (2011), 67–84

7. William C. Wells, 'On rheumatism of the heart', *Transactions of the Society for the Improvement of Medical and Chirurgical Knowledge* 3 (1812), 373–424

8. William C. Wells, *An Essay on Dew; and Several Appearances Connected with it* (London: Printed for Taylor and Hessey, 1814)

9. William C. Wells, *Two Essays* (London: Longman, Hurst, Rees, Orme and Brown, 1818)

10. Wells, 'On rheumatism of the heart', op. cit.

11. Norman Moore, *Lumleian Lectures on Rheumatic Fever and Valvular Disease* (London: reprinted from *The Lancet*, 1909), 10–11

12. D. W. Samways, 'Cardiac peristalsis: its nature and effects', *The Lancet* 151, no. 3892 (1898), 927

13. Lauder Brunton, 'Preliminary note on the possibility of treating mitral stenosis by surgical methods', *The Lancet* 159, no. 4093 (1902), 352

14. Editorial, *The Lancet* 159, no. 4094 (1902), 460–62

15. Lauder Brunton et al., 'Surgical operation for mitral stenosis', *The Lancet* 159, no. 4095 (1902), 547–8

16. Rudolph Matas, 'Surgery of the vascular system', in *Surgery: Its Principles and Practice* (7 vols, vol. 5 ed. William W. Keen; Philadelphia: W. B. Saunders Co., 1909), 17–350

17. B. M. Ricketts, *Surgery of the Thorax and its Viscera, Symptoms, Diagnosis, Indications and Treatment* (Cincinnati, 1918), 26

18. Théodore Tuffier, 'La chirurgie du coeur', in *Cinquieme Congrès de la Société Internationale de Chirurgie: Paris, 19–23 juillet 1920: rapports, procès-verbaux et discussions* (Brussels: Hayez, 1921), 66–75

19. E. Doyen, 'Chirurgie des malformations congénitales ou acquises du coeur', *Presse Medicale* 21 (1913), 860–75

20. Duff S. Allen and Evarts A. Graham, 'Intracardiac surgery – a new method: preliminary report', *JAMA* 79, no. 13 (1922), 1028–30

21. Lawrence H. Cohn, 'The first successful surgical treatment of mitral stenosis: the 70th anniversary of Elliott Cutler's mitral commissurotomy', *Annals of Thoracic Surgery* 56, no. 5 (1993), 1187–90

22. Claude S. Beck and Elliott C. Cutler, 'A cardiovalvulotome', *Journal of Experimental Medicine* 40, no. 3 (1924), 375–9

23. Elliott C. Cutler and S. A. Levine, 'Cardiotomy and valvulotomy for mitral stenosis; experimental observations and clinical notes concerning an operated case with recovery', *Boston Medical and Surgical Journal* 188, no. 26 (1923), 1023–7

24. ibid.

25. Cohn, op. cit.

26. Elliott C. Cutler and Claude S. Beck, 'The present status of the surgical procedures in chronic valvular disease of the heart: final report of all surgical cases', *Archives of Surgery* 18 (1929), 403–16

27. H. S. Souttar, 'The surgical treatment of mitral stenosis', *BMJ* 2, no. 3379 (1925), 603–06

28. Brian Blades, 'Intrathoracic surgery, 1905–1955', in *Fifty Years of Surgical Progress, 1905–1955* (ed. Loyal Davis; Chicago: Franklin H. Martin Memorial Foundation, 1955)

29. Souttar, op. cit.

30. Blades, op. cit., 172

31. ibid.

32. Fred A. Crawford, 'Horace Smithy: pioneer heart surgeon', *Annals of Thoracic Surgery* 89, no. 6 (2010), 2067–71

33. H. G. Smithy and E. F. Parker, 'Experimental aortic valvulotomy; a preliminary report', *Surgery, Gynecology & Obstetrics* 84, 4–A (1947), 625–8

34. 'Operation saves girl', *News-Journal*, (Mansfield, OH), 16 February 1948

35. H. G. Smithy, J. A. Boone and J. M. Stallworth, 'Surgical treatment of constrictive valvular disease of the heart', *Surgery, Gynecology & Obstetrics* 90, no. 2 (1950), 175

36. Crawford, op. cit.

37. 'Surgeon dies, too weak for own cure', *Salt Lake Tribune*, 29 October 1948

38. Allen B. Weisse, *Conversations in Medicine: The Story of Twentieth-Century American Medicine in the Words of Those who Created it* (New York: New York University Press, 1984), 136–7

39. Stephen Westaby and Cecil Bosher, *Landmarks in Cardiac Surgery* (Oxford: ISIS Medical Media, 1997)

40. Weisse, op. cit., 139–40

41. ibid., 142

42. ibid., 138–9

43. Charles P. Bailey, 'The surgical treatment of mitral stenosis (mitral commissurotomy): discussion', *Chest* 15, no. 4 (1949), 393–7

44. ibid.

45. Dwight E. Harken et al., 'The surgical treatment of mitral stenosis', *New England Journal of Medicine* 239, no. 22 (1948), 801–09

46. T. Treasure and A. Hollman, 'The surgery of mitral stenosis 1898–1948: why did it take 50 years to establish mitral valvotomy?', *Annals of the Royal College of Surgeons of England* 77, no. 2 (1995), 145–51

47. Charles Baker, R. C. Brock and Maurice Campbell, 'Valvulotomy for mitral stenosis', *BMJ* 1, no. 4665 (1950), 1283–93

48. Weisse, op. cit., 141

49. Dwight E. Harken et al., 'The surgery of mitral stenosis: III. Finger-fracture valvulo-plasty', *Annals of Surgery* 134, no. 4 (1951), 722–41

50. Claude S. Beck, 'The technique of opening the stenotic mitral valve', *JAMA* 156, no. 15 (1954), 1400–01

51. Charles Baker et al., 'Valvotomy for mitral stenosis', *BMJ* 1, no. 4767 (1952), 1043–55

52. R. C. Brock, 'Valvotomy in pregnancy', *Proceedings of the Royal Society of Medicine* 45, no. 8 (1952), 538–40

53. C. Dubost, 'Presentation d'un nouvel instrument dilatateur pour commissurotomie mitrale', *Presse Medicale* 62 (1954), 253

54. D. E. Harken et al., 'The surgical correction of mitral insufficiency', *Journal of Thoracic Surgery* 28, no. 6 (1954), 604–24

55. C. P. Bailey, H. E. Bolton and H. Perez Redondo-Ramierez, 'Surgery of the mitral valve', *Surgical Clinics of North America* (1952), 1807–48

56. Shelley McKellar, *Surgical Limits: The Life of Gordon Murray* (Toronto, Buffalo, London: University of Toronto Press, 2003), 24

57. Gordon Murray, *Medicine in the Making* (Toronto: The Ryerson Press, 1960), 128

58. Victor W. M. van Hinsbergh, 'Endothelium – role in regulation of coagulation and inflammation', *Seminars in Immunopathology* 34, no. 1 (2012), 93–106

59. Gordon Murray, F. R. Wilkinson and R. MacKenzie, 'Reconstruction of the valves of the heart', *Canadian Medical Association Journal* 38, no. 4 (1938), 317–19

60. Bailey, 'The surgical treatment ...', op. cit.

61. Murray, op. cit., 135

62. John Y. Templeton and John H. Gibbon, 'Experimental reconstruction of cardiac valves by venous and pericardial grafts', *Annals of Surgery* 129, no. 2 (1949), 161–76

63. Gordon Murray, 'The surgical treatment of mitral stenosis', *Canadian Medical Association Journal* 62, no. 5 (1950), 444–7

64. C. A. Hufnagel, 'Permanent intubation of the thoracic aorta', *Archives of Surgery* 54, no. 4 (1947), 382–9

65. J. M. Campbell, 'An artificial aortic valve; preliminary report', *Journal of Thoracic Surgery* 19, no. 2 (1950), 312–18

66. C. A. Hufnagel and W. P. Harvey, 'The surgical correction of aortic regurgitation: pre-liminary report', *Bulletin – Georgetown University Medical Center* 6, no. 3 (1953), 60–61

67. John C. Rose et al., 'The hemodynamic alterations produced by a plastic valvular pros-thesis for severe aortic insufficiency in man', *Journal of Clinical Investigation* 33, no. 6 (1954), 891–900

68. Charles A. Hufnagel and Alberto Villegas, 'Aortic valvular replacement', *ASAIO Journal* 4, no. 1 (1958), 235–9

69. Conwell Carlson, 'Doctors on rare jury', *Kansas City Times*, 15 February 1956

70. Baylor College of Medicine, 'Interview with Dr Walter S. Henly, MD', cited 16 July 2015: http://profiles.nlm.nih.gov/ps/retrieve/ResourceMetadata/FJBBQS

71. Anita F. Norman, 'The first mitral valve replacement', *Annals of Thoracic Surgery* 51, no. 3 (1991), 525–6

72. N. S. Braunwald, 'It will work: the first successful mitral valve replacement', *Annals of Thoracic Surgery* 48, 3 Suppl. (1989), 3

73. Nina S. Braunwald, Theodore Cooper and Andrew G. Morrow, 'Clinical and experimental replacement of the mitral valve: Experience with the use of a flexible polyurethane prosthesis', in *Prosthetic Valves for Cardiac Surgery* (ed. K. A. Merendino; Springfield, IL: Charles C. Thomas, 1961), 307–39

74. Lillehei et al., 'Aortic valve reconstruction and replacement by total valve prosthesis', in Merendino (ed.), op. cit.

75. 'Interview with Albert Starr', in *Pioneers of Cardiac Surgery* (ed. William S. Stoney; Nashville, TN: Vanderbilt University Press, 2008), 271–84

76. Ann Sullivan, 'M. L. Edwards, inventor, dies at 84', *Oregonian*, 9 April 1982

77. Annette Matthews, 'Interview with Miles J. Edwards', Oregon Health and Science University Oral History Collection, 1998: http://digitalcommons.ohsu.edu/hca-oralhist/2

78. 'Interview with Albert Starr', in Stoney (ed.), op. cit., 278–9

79. F. H. Ellis Jr and A. H. Bulbulian, 'Prosthetic replacement of the mitral valve. I. Preliminary experimental observations', *Proceedings of the Staff Meetings: Mayo Clinic* 33, no. 21 (1958), 532

80. J. B. Williams, 'Improved bottle-stopper', US Patent no. 19323A, 1858

81. A. M. Matthews, 'The development of the Starr–Edwards heart valve', *Texas Heart Institute Journal* 25, no. 4 (1998), 282–93

82. Albert Starr, 'How it came about', *Journal of Thoracic and Cardiovascular Surgery* 135, no. 6 (2008), 1198–200

83. Edward A. Lefrak and Albert Starr, *Cardiac Valve Prostheses*, (New York: Appleton-Century-Crofts, 1979), 67–8

84. Matthews, op. cit.

85. Starr, op. cit.

86. Wayne E. Quinton et al., 'An accelerated fatigue pump for testing prosthetic aortic valves', in Merendino (ed.), op. cit., 235–43

87. Albert Starr and M. L. Edwards, 'Mitral replacement: clinical experience with a ball-valve prosthesis', *Annals of Surgery* 154, no. 4 (1961), 726–40

88. Elliott L. Chaikof, 'The development of prosthetic heart valves – lessons in form and function: Interview with Albert Starr on the invention of the first successful artificial heart valve', *New England Journal of Medicine* 357, no. 14 (2007), 1368–71

89. Starr and Edwards, op. cit.

90. ibid.

91. ibid.

92. 'Discussion', *Annals of Surgery* 154, no. 4 (1961), 740

93. William Blot et al., 'Twenty-five-year experience with the Björk–Shiley convexoconcave heart valve. A continuing clinical concern', *Circulation* 111, no. 21 (2005), 2850–57

94. D. Farley, 'Shiley saga leads to improved communication', *FDA Consumer* 28, no. 1 (1994), 12–17

95. M. A. Villafana, '"It will never work!" – the St Jude valve', *Annals of Thoracic Surgery* 48, 3 Suppl (1989), 4

96. G. Murray, 'Homologous aortic-valve-segment transplants as surgical treatment for aortic and mitral insufficiency', *Angiology* 7, no. 5 (1956), 466–71

97. A. J. Kerwin, S. C. Lenkei and D. R. Wilson, 'Aortic-valve homograft in the treatment of aortic insufficiency. Report of nine cases, with one followed for six years', *New England Journal of Medicine* 266 (1962), 852–7

98. D. N. Ross, 'Homograft replacement of the aortic valve', *The Lancet* 280, no. 7254 (1962), 487

99. 'Interview with Donald Ross', in Stoney (ed.), op. cit., 285–96

100. Ross, op. cit.

101. Stoney, op. cit.

102. 'Interview with Alain Carpentier', in Stoney (ed.), op. cit., 322–31

103. J. P. Binet, 'Pioneering in heterografts', *Annals of Thoracic Surgery* 48, 3 Suppl (1989), 2

104. A. Carpentier et al., 'Biological factors affecting long-term results of valvular heterografts', *Journal of Thoracic and Cardiovascular Surgery* 58, no. 4 (1969), 467–83

105. A. Carpentier, 'From valvular xenograft to valvular bioprosthesis: 1965–1970', *Annals of Thoracic Surgery* 48, 3 Suppl (1989), 4

106. A. Senning, 'Fascia lata replacement of aortic valves', *Journal of Thoracic and Cardiovascular Surgery* 54, no. 4 (1967), 465–70

107. Marian I. Ionescu et al., 'Autologous fascia lata for heart valve replacement', *Thorax* 25, no. 1 (1970), 46–56

108. M. I. Ionescu et al., 'Results of aortic valve replacement with frame-supported fascia lata and pericardial grafts', *Journal of Thoracic and Cardiovascular Surgery* 64, no. 3 (1972), 340–53

109. Alain Carpentier, David H. Adams and Farzan Filsoufi, *Carpentier's Reconstructive Valve Surgery* (Philadelphia, PA: Saunders Elsevier, 2010), v

110. A. Carpentier et al., 'A new reconstructive operation for correction of mitral and tricuspid insufficiency', *Journal of Thoracic and Cardiovascular Surgery* 61, no. 1 (1971), 1–13

111. A. Carpentier, 'Cardiac valve surgery – the "French correction"', *Journal of Thoracic and Cardiovascular Surgery* 86, no. 3 (1983), 323–37

112. 'Interview with Alain Carpentier', in Stoney (ed.), op. cit.

6. METRONOMES AND NUCLEAR REACTORS

1. Roger Ebert, 'Peter Sellers dies at 54', *Chicago Sun-Times,* 24 July 1980

2. H. G. Mond and A. Proclemer, 'The 11th world survey of cardiac pacing and implantable cardioverter-defibrillators: calendar year 2009 – a World Society of Arrhythmias project', *Pacing and Clinical Electrophysiology: PACE* 34, no. 8 (2011), 1013–27

3. Dwight Reynolds et al., 'A leadless intracardiac transcatheter pacing system', *New England Journal of Medicine* 374, no. 6 (2016), 533–41

4. Jean Jallabert, *Experiences sur l'Electricité: Avec Quelques Conjectures sur la Cause de ses Effets* (Geneva: Chez Barrillot & Fils, 1748): 75–7

5. John Wesley, *The Desideratum: Or, Electricity Made Plain and Useful. By a Lover of Mankind, and of Common Sense* (London: W. Flexney, 1760), 39

6. ibid., 62

7. Philippe-Nicolas Pia et al., *Détail des succès de l'établissement que la ville de Paris a fait en faveur des personnes noyées et qui a été adopté dans diverses provinces de France. Quatrième partie. Année 1775* (Paris, 1776)

8. H. Bence Jones, 'Remedial action of electricity', *London Journal of Medicine* 1, no. 2 (1849), 125–9

9. Rudolf von Koelliker, 'Nachweis der negativen Schwarlkung des Muskelstroms am natürlich sich kontrahierenden Herzen', *Verhandlungen der Physikalisch-Medizinischen Gesellschaft in Würzburg* 6 (1856), 528–33

10. A. D. Waller, 'A demonstration on man of electromotive changes accompanying the heart's beat', *Journal of Physiology* 8, no. 5 (1887), 229–34

11. W. Einthoven, 'The string galvanometer and the human electrocardiogram', *KNAW, Proceedings* 6 (1903–1904), 107–15

12. 'Science notes', *BMJ* 2, no. 2591 (1910), 558

13. Wilhelm His Jr, 'The activity of the embryonic human heart and its significance for the understanding of the heart movement in the adult', *Journal of the History of Medicine and Allied Sciences* 4, no. 3 (1949), 289–318

14. M. R. Boyett and H. Dobrzynski, 'The sinoatrial node is still setting the pace 100 years after its discovery', *Circulation Research* 100, no. 11 (2007), 1543–5

15. Mark McGrouther, 'World's first black marlin caught on rod and reel – Australian Museum', cited 15 March 2016: http://australianmuseum.net.au/worlds-first-black-marlin-caught-on-rod-and-reel

16. H. G. Mond, J. G. Sloman and R. H. Edwards, 'The first pacemaker', *Pacing and Clinical Electrophysiology: PACE* 5, no. 2 (1982), 278–82

17. Mark C. Lidwill, 'Cardiac disease in relation to anaesthesia', in *Transactions of the Third Session, Sydney: Australasian Medical Congress (British Medical Association), September 2 to 7* (ed. Mervyn Archdall; Sydney, 1930), 160–62

18. D. C. Schechter, 'Background of clinical cardiac electrostimulation. V. Direct electrostimulation of heart without thoracotomy', *New York State Journal of Medicine* 72, no. 5 (1972), 605–19

19. Albert S. Hyman, 'Resuscitation of the stopped heart by intracardiac therapy', *Archives of Internal Medicine* 46, no. 4 (1930), 553–68

20. Albert S. Hyman, 'Resuscitation of the stopped heart by intracardial therapy: II. Experimental use of an artificial pacemaker', *Archives of Internal Medicine* 50, no. 2 (1932), 283–305

21. Howard W. Blakeslee, 'Electricity restores life after heart stops beating', *Salt Lake Tribune*, 1 January 1933

22. 'Heart victims are restored after "death"', *Belvidere Daily Republican*, 13 June 1933

23. 'Heart pacer saves lives', *Evening Review* (East Liverpool, Ohio), 11 June 1934

24. 'Heart victims are restored after "death"', op. cit.

25. Schechter, op. cit.

26. 'Scientist seeks permit to revive gas chamber dead', *Bluefield Daily Telegraph*, 16 October 1934

27. 'New electric needle starts heart, is claim', *Pottstown Mercury*, 11 February 1936

28. Kirk Jeffrey, *Machines in our Hearts: The Cardiac Pacemaker, the Implantable Defibrillator, and American Health Care* (Baltimore: Johns Hopkins University Press, 2001), 33–4

29. Graeme Gooday, *Domesticating Electricity: Technology, Uncertainty and Gender, 1880–1914* (London: Pickering & Chatto, 2008), 66

30. J. L. Prevost and F. Batelli, 'Sur quelques effets des decharges electriques sur le coeur des Mammiferes', *Comptes Rendus des Seances de l'Academie des Sciences* 129 (1899), 1267–8

31. Louise G. Robinovitch, 'Methods of resuscitating electrocuted animals. Different effects of various electric currents according to the method used. Importance of excluding from the circuit the central nervous system', *Journal of Mental Pathology* 8 (1907), 129–36

32. Louise G. Robinovitch, 'Triple interrupter of direct currents for resuscitation. Portable model for ambulance service', *Journal of Mental Pathology* 8 (1907), 195–7

33. Schechter, op. cit., 270–84

34. D. R. Hooker, W. B. Kouwenhoven and O. R. Langworthy, 'The effect of alternating electrical currents on the heart', *American Journal of Physiology* 103, no. 2 (1933), 444–54

35. D. C. Schechter, 'Background of clinical cardiac electrostimulation. III. Electrical regulation of rapid cardiac dysrhythmias', *New York State Journal of Medicine* 72, no. 2 (1972), 270–84

36. Milton B. Dolinger, 'Boy who "died" is alive through prayers', *Sandusky Register*, 12 December 1947

37. C. S. Beck, W. H. Pritchard and H. S. Feil, 'Ventricular fibrillation of long duration abolished by electric shock', *JAMA* 135, no. 15 (1947), 985–6

38. Dolinger, op. cit.

39. W. G. Bigelow, *Cold Hearts: The Story of Hypothermia and the Pacemaker in Heart Surgery* (Toronto: McClelland and Stewart, 1984), 89–90

40. John A. Hopps, 'The development of the pacemaker', *Pacing and Clinical Electrophysiology: PACE* 4, no. 1 (1981), 106–08

41. J. C. Callaghan and W. G. Bigelow, 'An electrical artificial pacemaker for standstill of the heart', *Annals of Surgery* 134 (1951), 8–17

42. Schechter, 'Background of clinical cardiac electrostimulation. V. Direct electrostimulation of heart without thoracotomy', op. cit.

43. Bigelow, op. cit.

44. K. Jeffrey, 'The invention and reinvention of cardiac pacing', *Cardiology Clinics* 10, no. 4 (1992), 561–71

45. Paul M. Zoll, 'Development of electric control of cardiac rhythm', *JAMA* 226, no. 8 (1973), 881–6

46. Paul M. Zoll, 'Resuscitation of the heart in ventricular standstill by external electric stimulation', *New England Journal of Medicine* 247 (1952), 768–71

47. 'Plug failing hearts into AC outlet', *Council Bluffs Nonpareil*, 13 November 1952

48. David Rhees, 'Interview with Earl Bakken and C. Walton Lillehei', 1997: http://collections.mnhs.org/cms/display.php?irn=10445338&return=brand%3Dcms%26q%3DLillehei

49. Seymour Furman, 'Attempted suicide', *Pacing and Clinical Electrophysiology: PACE* 3, no. 2 (1980), 129

50. W. L. Weirich et al., 'The treatment of complete heart block by the combined use of a myocardial electrode and an artificial pacemaker', *Circulation Research* 6 (1958), 410–15

51. 'Interview with C. Walton Lillehei', in *Pioneers of Cardiac Surgery* (ed. William S. Stoney; Nashville, TN: Vanderbilt University Press, 2008), 83–99

52. Earl E. Bakken, *One Man's Full Life* (Minneapolis, MN: Medtronic, Inc, 1999), 36–7

53. Rhees, op. cit.

54. Bakken, op. cit., 38

55. C. W. Lillehei et al., 'Transistor pacemaker for treatment of complete atrioventricular dissociation', *JAMA* 172, no. 18 (1960), 2006–10

56. Steven M. Spencer, 'Making a heartbeat behave', *Saturday Evening Post*, 4 March 1961

57. Rhees, op. cit.

58. 'Conference on artificial pacemakers and cardiac prosthesis: sponsored by the Medical Electronics Center of the Rockefeller Institute, 1958', *Pacing and Clinical Electrophysiology: PACE* 16, 7 Pt 1 (1993), 1445–82

59. Oktay Tutarel and Mechthild Westhoff-Bleck, 'Åke Senning', *Clinical Cardiology* 32, no. 8 (2009), E66–7

60. Åke Senning, 'Cardiac pacing in retrospect', *American Journal of Surgery* 145, no. 6 (1983), 733–9

61. ibid.

62. D. E. Harken, 'Pacemakers, past-makers, and the paced: an informal history from A to Z (Aldini to Zoll)', *Biomedical Instrumentation and Technology* 25, no. 4 (1991), 299–321

63. M. Nicholls, 'Pioneers of cardiology: Rune Elmqvist, MD', *Circulation* 115, no. 22 (2007), 11

64. R. Elmqvist and Å. Senning, 'An implantable pacemaker for the heart', in *Medical Electronics: Proceedings of the Second International Conference on Medical Electronics, Paris, 24–27 June 1959* (ed. C. N. Smyth; London: Iliffe, 1960), 253–4

65. Patrik Hidefjäll, *The Pace of Innovation: Patterns of innovation in the cardiac pacemaker industry* (Linköping: Linköping University, 1997), 160, 87–8

66. B. Larsson et al., 'Lessons from the first patient with an implanted pacemaker: 1958–2001', *Pacing and Clinical Electrophysiology: PACE* 26, 1 Pt 1 (2003), 114–24

67. Hidefjäll, op. cit., 89–90

68. A. H. Siddons and O. Humphries, 'Complete heart block with Stokes–Adams attacks treated by indwelling pacemaker', *Proceedings of the Royal Society of Medicine* 54, no. 3 (1961), 237–8

69. Wilson Greatbatch, *The Making of the Pacemaker: Celebrating a Life-Saving Invention* (Amherst, NY: Prometheus Books, 2000)

70. ibid., 30

71. William M. Chardack, 'Recollections – 1958–1961', *Pacing and Clinical Electrophysiology: PACE* 4, no. 5 (1981), 592–6

72. Greatbatch, op. cit., 32

73. William M. Chardack, Andrew A. Gage and Wilson Greatbatch, 'A transistorized, self-contained, implantable pacemaker for the long-term correction of complete heart block', *Surgery* 48 (1960), 643–54

74. Spencer, op. cit.

75. Chardack, Gage and Greatbatch, op. cit.

76. Bakken, op. cit., 40

77. Rhees, op. cit.

78. Mark A. Wood and Kenneth A. Ellenbogen, 'Cardiac pacemakers from the patient's perspective', *Circulation* 105, no. 18 (2002), 2136–8

79. 'Facts and Statistics, Medtronic', cited 24 March 2016: http://www.medtronic.com/us-en/about-3/medtronic-plc-facts.html?cmpid=mdt_plc_2015_US_about_3_story_panel_featured_company_facts_cta_text_link_learn_more

80. Chardack, Gage and Greatbatch, op. cit.

81. J. S. Butterworth and Charles A. Poindexter, 'Short PR interval associated with a prolonged QRS complex: a clinical and experimental study', *Archives of Internal Medicine* 69, no. 3 (1942), 437–45

82. M. J. Folkman and E. Watkins, 'An artificial conduction system for the management of experimental complete heart block', *Surgical Forum* 8 (1957), 331–4

83. David A. Nathan et al., 'An implantable, synchronous pacemaker for the long-term correction of complete heart block', *Circulation* 27, no. 4 (1963), 682–5

84. Victor Parsonnet et al., 'Clinical use of an implantable standby pacemaker', *JAMA* 196, no. 9 (1966), 784–6

85. Cesar A. Castillo et al., 'Bifocal demand pacing', *Chest* 59, no. 4 (1971), 360–64

86. E. Sowton and J. G. Davies, 'Investigation of failure of artificial pacing', *BMJ* 1, no. 5396 (1964), 1470–74

87. L. D. Abrams and W. A. Hudson, 'The treatment of complete heart block', *Postgraduate Medical Journal* 37, no. 427 (1961), 240–44

88. Greatbatch, op. cit., 126–7

89. Victor Parsonnet et al., 'Thirty-one years of clinical experience with "nuclear-powered" pacemakers', *Pacing and Clinical Electrophysiology: PACE* 29, no. 2 (2006), 195–200

90. 'Nuclear power inside a human body?' *Popular Science* 195, no. 2 (1969), 22

91. Michael Jeffries, 'Atom heart mother named', *Evening Standard,* 16 July 1970

92. Ron Geesin, *The Flaming Cow: The Making of Pink Floyd's Atom Heart Mother* (The History Press, 2013), 80–81

93. V. Parsonnet et al., 'Clinical experience with nuclear pacemakers', *Surgery* 78, no. 6 (1975), 776–86

94. Kenneth Owen, 'Cardiology: contract for nuclear pacemakers', *The Times,* 11 November 1975

95. Parsonnet et al., 'Thirty-one years of clinical experience ...', op. cit.

96. Greatbatch, op. cit., 128–9

97. NRC Preliminary Notification of Event PNO-III-98-027: Accidental incineration of a nuclear powered cardiac pacemaker, 1998

98. P. J. Morrell, 'The exploding body', *Practitioner* 219, no. 1309 (1977), 109

99. C. P. Gale and G. P. Mulley, 'Pacemaker explosions in crematoria: problems and possible solutions', *Journal of the Royal Society of Medicine* 95, no. 7 (2002), 353–5

100. P. M. Zoll et al., 'Termination of ventricular fibrillation in man by externally applied electric countershock', *New England Journal of Medicine* 254, no. 16 (1956), 727–32

101. 'Dwight Harken: pioneer in surgery', *Biomedical Instrumentation and Technology* 25, no. 4 (1991), 263–4

102. B. Lown, R. Amarasingham and J. Neuman, 'New method for terminating cardiac arrhythmias. Use of synchronized capacitor discharge', *JAMA* 182 (1962), 548–55

103. W. B. Kouwenhoven et al., 'Closed-chest cardiac massage', *JAMA* 173 (1960), 1064–7

104. Claude S. Beck and David S. Leighninger, 'Death after a clean bill of health: so-called fatal heart attacks and treatment with resuscitation techniques', *JAMA* 174, no. 2 (1960), 133–5

105. D. G. Julian, 'Treatment of cardiac arrest in acute myocardial ischaemia and infarction', *The Lancet* 2, no. 7207 (1961), 840–44

106. D. G. Julian, 'The history of coronary care units', *British Heart Journal* 57, no. 6 (1987), 497–502

107. J. A. Kastor, 'Michel Mirowski and the automatic implantable defibrillator', *American Journal of Cardiology* 63, no. 13 (1989a), 977–82

108. ibid.

109. M. Mirowski et al., 'Standby automatic defibrillator. An approach to prevention of sudden coronary death', *Archives of Internal Medicine* 126, no. 1 (1970), 158–61

110. Albert I. Mendeloff, 'Michel Mirowski and the Department of Medicine at the Sinai Hospital of Baltimore', *Pacing and Clinical Electrophysiology: PACE* 14, no. 5 (1991), 873–4

111. B. Lown and P. Axelrod, 'Implanted standby defibrillators', *Circulation* 46, no. 4 (1972), 637–9

112. Kastor, op. cit., no. 15 (1989b), 1121–6

113. Morton M. Mower, 'Building the AICD with Michel Mirowski', *Pacing and Clinical Electrophysiology: PACE* 14, no. 5 (1991), 928–34

114. Hidefjäll, op. cit., 260–64

115. M. Mirowski et al., 'A chronically implanted system for automatic defibrillation in active conscious dogs. Experimental model for treatment of sudden death from ventricular fibrillation', *Circulation* 58, no. 1 (1978), 90–94

116. Kastor, op. cit.

117. Mirowski et al., 'A chronically implanted system for automatic debfibrillation … ', op. cit.

118. M. Mirowski et al., 'Termination of malignant ventricular arrhythmias with an implanted automatic defibrillator in human beings', *New England Journal of Medicine* 303, no. 6 (1980), 322–4

119. ibid.

120. M. Mirowski et al., 'The automatic implantable defibrillator. New modality for treatment of life-threatening ventricular arrhythmias', *Pacing and Clinical Electrophysiology: PACE* 5, no. 3 (1982), 384–401

121. M. Mirowski et al., 'Clinical performance of the implantable cardioverter-defibrillator', *Pacing and Clinical Electrophysiology: PACE* 7, 6 Pt 2 (1984), 1345–50

122. M. Mirowski, 'The automatic implantable cardioverter-defibrillator: An overview', *Journal of the American College of Cardiology* 6, no. 2 (1985), 461–6

123. ibid.

124. M. S. Heilman, 'Collaboration with Michel Mirowski on the development of the AICD', *Pacing and Clinical Electrophysiology: PACE* 14, no. 5 (1991), 910–15

125. Mond and Proclemer, 'The 11th world survey of cardiac pacing …', op. cit.

126. David R. Ramsdale and Archana Rao, *Cardiac Pacing and Device Therapy* (London: Springer, 2012), 37–8

127. D. Halperin et al., 'Pacemakers and implantable cardiac defibrillators: software radio attacks and zero-power defenses', in *IEEE World Symposium on Security and Privacy*, IEEE, 2008

128. Richard B. Cheney, Jonathan Reiner and Liz Cheney, *Heart: An American Medical Odyssey* (New York: Scribner, 2013), 220

7. 'STRONG AND PECULIAR SYMPTOMS'

1. John Hunter and Everard Home, *A Treatise on the Blood, Inflammation, and Gunshot Wounds* (London: Thomas Bradford, 1796), lxi

2. Caleb H. Parry, *An Inquiry into the Symptoms and Causes of the Syncope Anginosa, Commonly Called Angina Pectoris; Illustrated by Dissections* (Bath, 1799), 3–5

3. Hunter and Home, op. cit., xlv–xlvi

4. ibid., lxi

5. J. T. Willerson and R. Teaff, 'Egyptian contributions to cardiovascular medicine', *Texas Heart Institute Journal* 23, no. 3 (1996), 191–200

6. Girish Dwivedi and Shridhar Dwivedi, 'Sushruta – the clinician–teacher par excellence', *Indian Journal of Chest Diseases and Allied Sciences* 49, no. 4 (2007), 243–4

7. William Heberden, *Commentaries on the History and Cure of Diseases* (3rd ed.; London: T. Payne, 1806), 364–5

8. ibid., 368–9

9. John Fothergill, 'Farther account of the angina pectoris', *Medical Observations and Inquiries* 5 (1776), 252–8

10. Parry, op. cit.

11. Hunter and Home, op. cit., lxiii

12. John P. Collier and T. Smollett, 'Parry on the Syncope Anginosa', *Critical Review, or, Annals of Literature* 31, January (1801), 79–83

13. Parry, op. cit., 156

14. G.-B Duchenne, *De l'Electrisation Localisée: Et de son Application a la Physiologie, a la Pathologie et a la Thérapeutique* (Paris: Chez J.-B. Baillière, 1855)

15. T. L. Brunton, 'On the use of nitrite of amyl in angina pectoris', *The Lancet* 90, no. 2291 (1867), 97–8

16. James D. Morgan, 'Angina pectoris', *JAMA* 33, no. 1 (1899), 22–4

17. H. W. Verdon, 'The gastric origin of angina pectoris', *BMJ* 1, no. 2620 (1911), 613–14

18. J. Mackenzie, 'An inquiry into the cause of angina pectoris', *BMJ* 2, no. 2336 (1905), 845–7

19. James B. Herrick, 'Clinical features of sudden obstruction of the coronary arteries', *JAMA* 59, no. 23 (1912), 2015–22

20. James H. Means, *The Association of American Physicians: Its First Seventy-five Years* (New York: McGraw-Hill, 1961), 108

21. Herrick, op. cit.

22. T. Jonnesco, 'Angine de poitrine guerie par la resection du sympathique cervico-thoracique', *Bulletin de l'Académie Nationale de Médecine* 84 (1920), 93–102

23. ibid.

24. P. K. Brown and W. B. Coffey, 'Surgical treatment of angina pectoris', *Transactions of the American Climatological and Clinical Association* 40 (1924), 35–42

25. Martin Stritesky et al., 'Endoscopic thoracic sympathectomy – its effect in the treatment of refractory angina pectoris', *Interactive CardioVascular and Thoracic Surgery* 5, no. 4 (2006), 464–8

26. Samuel A. Levine, Elliott C. Cutler and Eugene C. Eppinger, 'Thyroidectomy in the treatment of advanced congestive heart failure and angina pectoris', *New England Journal of Medicine* 209, no. 14 (1933), 667–79

27. ibid.

28. Herrman L. Blumgart, Samuel A. Levine and David D. Berlin, 'Congestive heart failure and angina pectoris: the therapeutic effect on patients without clinical or pathologic evidence of thyroid toxicity', *Archives of Internal Medicine* 51, no. 6 (1933), 866–77

29. Claude S. Beck, 'The development of a new blood supply to the heart by operation', *Annals of Surgery* 102, no. 5 (1935), 801–13

30. A. R. Moritz, C. L. Hudson and E. S. Orgain, 'Augmentation of the extracardiac anastomoses of the coronary arteries through pericardial adhesions', *Journal of Experimental Medicine* 56, no. 6 (1932), 927–31

31. 'Wife watched surgeons operate on husband in angina pectoris cure', *Dunkirk Evening Observer*, 28 February 1935

32. Beck, op. cit.

33. 'Finds "borrowed" time too dear', *Daily Chronicle* (Kalb, IL), 15 February 1937

34. 'Miracles and blunders', *Daily Independent* (Murphysboro, IL), 16 February 1937

35. 'West London Medico-Chirurgical Society', *The Lancet* 230, no. 5963 (1937), 1377–8

36. Laurence O'Shaughnessy, 'An experimental method of providing a collateral circulation to the heart', *British Journal of Surgery* 23, no. 91 (1936), 665–70

37. Daniel Davies et al., 'Surgical treatment of angina pectoris and allied conditions', *The Lancet* 231, no. 5966 (1938), 1–11

38. ibid., no. 5967 (1938), 76–82

39. George Orwell, *Diaries* (ed. Peter Davison; London: Penguin, 2010), 248

40. Claude S. Beck and David S. Leighninger, 'Operations for coronary artery disease', *JAMA* 156, no. 13 (1954), 1226–33

41. Claude S. Beck et al., 'Revascularization of heart by graft of systemic artery into coronary sinus', *JAMA* 137, no. 5 (1948), 436–42

42. Claude S. Beck, 'Coronary artery disease – Physiologic concepts – Surgical operation', *Annals of Surgery* 145, no. 4 (1957), 439–60

43. ibid.

44. Beck and Leighninger, op. cit.

45. J. A. Key et al., 'A method of supplementing the coronary circulation by a jejunal pedicle graft', *Journal of Thoracic Surgery* 28, no. 3 (1954), 320–30

46. A. M. Vineberg, 'Development of an anastomosis between the coronary vessels and a transplanted internal mammary artery', *Canadian Medical Association Journal* 55, no. 2 (1946), 117–19

47. A. Vineberg and G. Miller, 'Treatment of coronary insufficiency', *Canadian Medical Association Journal* 64, no. 3 (1951), 204–10

48. ibid.

49. A. Vineberg, 'Internal mammary artery implant in the treatment of angina pectoris: a three year follow up', *Canadian Medical Association Journal* 70, no. 4 (1954), 367–78

50. A. Vineberg, 'Coronary vascular anastomoses by internal mammary artery implantation', *Canadian Medical Association Journal* 78, no. 11 (1958), 871–9

51. L. A. Cobb et al., 'An evaluation of internal-mammary-artery ligation by a double-blind technic', *New England Journal of Medicine* 260, no. 22 (1959), 1115–18

52. 'Discussion', *Transactions of the American Surgical Association* 83 (1963), 222–4

53. Albert V. Bruschke et al., 'A half century of selective coronary arteriography', *Journal of the American College of Cardiology* 54, no. 23 (2009), 2139–44

54. D. B. Effler et al., 'Increased myocardial perfusion by internal mammary artery implant: Vineberg's operation', *Annals of Surgery* 158, no. 4 (1963), 526–34

55. On Topaz et al., 'The Vineberg procedure revisited: Angiographic evaluation and coronary artery bypass surgery in a patient 21 years following bilateral internal mammary artery implantation', *Catheterization and Cardiovascular Diagnosis* 25, no. 3 (1992), 218–22

56. K. B. Absolon et al., 'Surgical treatment of occlusive coronary artery disease by endarterectomy or anastomotic replacement', *Surgery, Gynecology & Obstetrics* 103, no. 2 (1956), 180–85

57. Charles P. Bailey, Angelo May and William M. Lemmon, 'Survival after coronary endarterectomy in man', *JAMA* 164, no. 6 (1957), 641–6

58. P. N. Sawyer et al., 'Experimental and clinical experience with coronary gas endarterectomy', *Archives of Surgery* 95, no. 5 (1967), 736–42

59. A. Senning, 'Strip grafting in coronary arteries. Report of a case', *Journal of Thoracic and Cardiovascular Surgery* 41 (1961), 542–9

60. 'Interview with René G. Favaloro', in *Pioneers of Cardiac Surgery* (ed. William S. Stoney; Nashville, TN: Vanderbilt University Press, 2008), 357–68

61. R. G. Favaloro et al., 'Double internal mammary artery-myocardial implantation. Clinical evaluation of results in 150 patients', *Circulation* 37, no. 4 (1968), 549–55

62. René G. Favaloro, 'Critical analysis of coronary artery bypass graft surgery: a 30-year journey', *Journal of the American College of Cardiology* 31, 4, Supplement 2 (1998), 1–63

63. René G. Favaloro, 'The present era of myocardial revascularization – some historical landmarks', *International Journal of Cardiology* 4, no. 3 (1983), 331–44

64. Alexis Carrel, 'VIII. On the experimental surgery of the thoracic aorta and heart', *Annals of Surgery* 52, no. 1 (1910), 83

65. I. E. Konstantinov, 'At the cutting edge of the impossible: a tribute to Vladimir P. Demikhov', *Texas Heart Institute Journal* 36, no. 5 (2009), 453–8

66. G. Murray et al., 'Anastomosis of a systemic artery to the coronary', *Canadian Medical Association Journal* 71, no. 6 (1954), 594–7

67. A. Chaikhouni, 'The magnificent century of cardiothoracic surgery', *Heart Views* 11, no. 1 (2010), 31–7

68. David C. Sabiston, *At the Heart of Medicine: Essays on the Practice of Surgery and Surgical Education* (Durham, NC: Carolina Academic Press, 2006), 10

69. H. E. Garrett, E. W. Dennis and M. E. DeBakey, 'Aortocoronary bypass with saphenous vein graft. Seven-year follow-up', *JAMA* 223, no. 7 (1973), 792–4

70. I. E. Konstantinov, 'Vasilii I. Kolesov: a surgeon to remember', *Texas Heart Institute Journal* 31, no. 4 (2004), 349–58

71. Valery M. Sedov and Alexander S. Nemkov, 'Vasilii Ivanovich Kolesov: pioneer of coronary surgery', *European Journal of Cardio-Thoracic Surgery* 45, no. 2 (2014), 220–24

72. V. I. Kolessov, 'Mammary artery-coronary artery anastomosis as method of treatment for angina pectoris', *Journal of Thoracic and Cardiovascular Surgery* 54, no. 4 (1967), 535–44

73. Favaloro, 'The present era of myocardial revascularization ...', op. cit.

74. Jonathan Bor, 'Once radical, now commonplace surgery', *Baltimore Sun*, 22 September 1996

75. G. Captur, 'Memento for René Favaloro', *Texas Heart Institute Journal* 31, no. 1 (2004), 47–60

76. Bor, op. cit.

77. Favaloro, 'Critical analysis of coronary artery bypass ...', op. cit.

78. R. G. Favaloro, 'Direct myocardial revascularization with saphenous vein autograft: clinical experience in 100 cases', *Diseases of the Chest*, 56, no. 4 (1969), 279–83

79. Favaloro, 'Critical analysis of coronary artery bypass ...', op. cit.

80. R. G. Favaloro, 'Landmarks in the development of coronary artery bypass surgery', *Circulation* 98, no. 5 (1998), 466–78

81. George E. Green, Simon H. Stertzer and Edmund H. Reppert, 'Coronary arterial bypass grafts', *Annals of Thoracic Surgery* 5, no. 5 (1968), 443–50

82. Malathy Iyer, 'Man survives 17 blocks in heart', *Times of India*, 23 March 2014

83. Bard Lindeman, 'Dr Christiaan Barnard says: heart transplant "superior to bypass"', *Santa Ana Register*, 10 September 1976

84. D. W. Miller et al., 'Current practice of coronary artery bypass surgery. Results of a national survey', *Journal of Thoracic and Cardiovascular Surgery* 73, no. 1 (1977), 75–83

85. H. D. McIntosh and J. A. Garcia, 'The first decade of aortocoronary bypass grafting, 1967–1977. A review', *Circulation* 57, no. 3 (1978), 405–31

86. 'Consensus development conference on coronary artery bypass surgery: medical and scientific aspects. National Institutes of Health, December 3–5, 1980, Bethesda, Maryland', *Circulation* 65, 7 Pt 2 (1982), 1–129

87. Floyd D. Loop et al., 'Influence of the internal-mammary-artery graft on 10-year survival and other cardiac events', *New England Journal of Medicine* 314, no. 1 (1986), 1–6

88. Enio Buffolo et al., 'Coronary artery bypass grafting without cardiopulmonary bypass', *Annals of Thoracic Surgery* 61, no. 1 (1996), 63–6

89. F. J. Benetti et al., 'Direct myocardial revascularization without extracorporeal circulation. Experience in 700 patients', *Chest* 100, no. 2 (1991), 312–16

90. David Reekie, 'Federico Benetti, champion of beating heart surgery', cited 20 April 2016: http://cxvascular.com/cn-archives/cardiovascular-news-issue-2/federico-benetti-champion-of-beating-heart-surgery

91. Harold L. Lazar, 'Should off-pump coronary artery bypass grafting be abandoned?' *Circulation* 128, no. 4 (2013), 406–13

92. A. C. Deppe et al., 'Current evidence of coronary artery bypass grafting off-pump versus on-pump: a systematic review with meta-analysis of over 16,900 patients investigated in randomized controlled trials', *European Journal of Cardio-Thoracic Surgery* 49, no. 4 (2016), 1031–41

93. 'Interview with René G. Favaloro', in Stoney (ed.), op. cit., 367

94. 'La última carta de Favaloro antes de morir: René Favaloro, Fernando de la Rúa, Cristina Kirchner – Infobae', cited 10 April 2016: http://infobae.com/2013/10/09/1514794-la-ultima-carta-favaloro-antes-morir

8. ONE LIFE, TWO HEARTS

1. D. A. Cooley, 'In memoriam: tribute to Åke Senning, pioneering cardiovascular surgeon', *Texas Heart Institute Journal* 27, no. 3 (2000), 234–5

2. M. Clark, 'The heart: miracle in Cape Town', *Newsweek*, 18 December 1967

3. K. B. Kansupada and J. W. Sassani, 'Sushruta: The father of Indian surgery and ophthalmology', *Documenta Ophthalmologica* 93, 1–2 (1997), 159–67

4. Martha Teach Gnudi, Gaspare Tagliacozzi and Jerome P. Webster, *The Life and Times of Gaspare Tagliacozzi, Surgeon of Bologna, 1545–1599* (New York: Herbert Reichner, 1950), 285

5. Vladimir P. Demikhov, *Experimental Transplantation of Vital Organs* (New York: Consultants Bureau, 1962), 3–4

6. E. Ullmann, 'Tissue and organ transplantation', *Annals of Surgery* 60, no. 2 (1914), 195–219

7. R. T. Morris, 'A case of heteroplastic ovarian grafting, followed by pregnancy, and the delivery of a living child', *Buffalo Medical Journal* 62 (1906), 393–402

8. Roger G. Gosden, 'Ovary and uterus transplantation', *Reproduction* 136, no. 6 (2008), 671–80

9. A. Carrel, 'The surgery of blood vessels, etc', *Bulletin of the Johns Hopkins Hospital* 18 (1907), 18–28

10. Charles C. Guthrie, *Blood-Vessel Surgery and its Applications* (London: Edward Arnold, 1912), 251–2

11. Carrel, op. cit.

12. Simon Flexner, 'Tendencies in pathology', *Science* 27, no. 682 (1908), 128–36

13. 'May transplant the human heart', *New York Times*, 2 January 1908

14. Edgar Jepson, 'The Rejuvenation of Bellamy Grist', *Los Angeles Herald*, 5 July 1908

15. Frank C. Mann et al., 'Transplantation of the intact mammalian heart', *Archives of Surgery* 26, no. 2 (1933), 219–24

16. Ullmann, op. cit.

17. P. B. Medawar, 'The behaviour and fate of skin autografts and skin homografts in rabbits: A report to the War Wounds Committee of the Medical Research Council', *Journal of Anatomy* 78, Pt 5 (1944), 176–99

18. Demikhov, op. cit., 179–86

19. ibid., 162–4

20. ibid., 69

21. ibid., 126–7

22. ibid., 125–6

23. Emanuel Marcus et al., 'Homologous heart grafts: I. Technique of interim parabiotic perfusion; II. Transplantation of the heart in dogs', *Archives of Surgery* 66, no. 2 (1953), 179–91

24. William S. Stoney, 'Interview with Norman E. Shumway', in *Pioneers of Cardiac Surgery* (ed. William S. Stoney; Nashville, TN: Vanderbilt University Press, 2008), 427–39

25. M. H. Cass and R. Brock, 'Heart excision and replacement', *Guy's Hospital Reports* 108 (1959), 285–90

26. R. R. Lower and N. E. Shumway, 'Studies on orthotopic homotransplantation of the canine heart', *Surgical Forum* 11 (1960), 18–19

27. Cass and Brock, op. cit.

28. J. H. Harrison, J. P. Merrill and J. E. Murray, 'Renal homotransplantation in identical twins', *Surgical Forum* 6 (1956), 432–6

29. Norman E. Shumway and Richard R. Lower, 'Special problems in transplantation of the heart', *Annals of the New York Academy of Sciences* 120, no. 1 (1964), 773–7

30. James D. Hardy et al., 'Lung homotransplantation in man: report of the initial case', *JAMA* 186, no. 12 (1963), 1065–74

31. 'Human heart is transplanted', Associated Press, 18 January 1964

32. James D. Hardy et al., 'Heart transplantation in man: developmental studies and report of a case', *JAMA* 188, no. 13 (1964), 1132–40

33. 'Chimp's kidneys keep longshoreman alive', Associated Press, 17 December 1963

34. Keith Reemtsma et al., 'Reversal of early graft rejection after renal heterotransplantation in man', *JAMA* 187, no. 10 (1964), 691–6

35. James D. Hardy, *The World of Surgery, 1945–1985: Memoirs of One Participant* (Philadelphia: University of Pennsylvania Press, 1986), 271

36. James Hardy et al., op. cit.

37. Hardy, *The World of Surgery*, op. cit., 276

38. Hardy et al., op. cit.

39. Hardy, *The World of Surgery*, op. cit., 278–80

40. Stoney, op. cit., 432–3

41. 'Heart transplant dog doing fine', Associated Press, 17 May 1965

42. S. Lansman, M. A. Ergin and R. B. Griepp, 'History of cardiac transplantation', in *Heart and Heart-Lung Transplantation* (ed. John Wallwork; Philadelphia, London: W. B. Saunders, 1989), 3–19

43. Y. Kondo, F. Grädel and A. Kantrowitz, 'Homotransplantation of the heart in puppies under profound hypothermia: long survival without immunosuppressive treatment', *Annals of Surgery* 162, no. 5 (1965), 837–48

44. A. Kantrowitz, 'America's first human heart transplantation: the concept, the planning, and the furor', *ASAIO Journal* 44, no. 4 (1998), 244–52

45. J. H. Louw and C. N. Barnard, 'Congenital intestinal atresia: observations on its origin', *The Lancet* 266, no. 6899 (1955), 1065–7

46. David Cooper, *Chris Barnard: By Those Who Know Him* (Vlaeberg, South Africa: Vlaeberg Publishers, 1992), 232–3

47. 'Interview with Christiaan Barnard', in Stoney (ed.), op. cit., 440–45

48. V. Schrire, W. Beck and C. N. Barnard, 'An analysis of cardiac surgery at Groote Schuur Hospital and Red Cross War Memorial Children's Hospitals, Cape Town, for the 14 years April 1951–April 1965', *South African Medical Journal* 40, no. 20 (1966), 461–7

49. Marius Barnard and Simon Norval, *Defining Moments: An Autobiography* (Cape Town: Zebra Press, 2011)

50. D. J. Rowe, 'Dr Christiaan Barnard: renowned surgeon, egoist but an old-fashioned family doctor at heart. Interview by Robert MacNeil', *Canadian Medical Association Journal* 120, no. 1 (1979), 98–9

51. Christiaan Barnard and Curtis B. Pepper, *Christiaan Barnard: One Life* (Cape Town: Howard Timmins, 1969), 327–8

52. ibid., 314–15

53. Barnard and Norval, op. cit.

54. V. Schrire and W. Beck, 'Human heart transplantation – the pre-operative assessment', *South African Medical Journal* 41, no. 48 (1967), 1263–5

55. Barnard and Pepper, op. cit., 260

56. J. Ozinsky, 'Cardiac transplantation–the anaesthetist's view: a case report', *South African Medical Journal* 41, no. 48 (1967), 1268–70

57. C. N. Barnard, 'The operation. A human cardiac transplant: an interim report of a successful operation performed at Groote Schuur Hospital, Cape Town', *South African Medical Journal* 41, no. 48 (1967), 1271–4

58. Barnard and Norval, op. cit.

59. Barnard, 'The operation … ', op. cit.

60. Barnard and Norval, op. cit.

61. Barnard and Pepper, op. cit., 357

62. C. N. Barnard, 'Human cardiac transplantation. An evaluation of the first two operations performed at the Groote Schuur Hospital, Cape Town', *American Journal of Cardiology* 22, no. 4 (1968), 584–96

63. J. G. Thomson, 'Heart transplantation in man – necropsy findings', *BMJ* 2, no. 5604 (1968), 511–17

64. Kantrowitz, op. cit.

65. Adrian Kantrowitz et al., 'Transplantation of the heart in an infant and an adult', *American Journal of Cardiology* 22, no. 6 (1968), 782–90

66. Jordan D. Haller and Marcial M. Cerruti, 'Heart transplantation in man: compilation of cases', *American Journal of Cardiology* 22, no. 6 (1968), 840–43

67. Edward B. Stinson et al., 'Initial clinical experience with heart transplantation', *American Journal of Cardiology* 22, no. 6 (1968), 791–803

68. 'Barnard faces his critics', *Tomorrow's World*, BBC1, 2 February 1968

69. Introduction, *American Journal of Cardiology* 22, no. 6 (1968), 761

70. Haller and Cerruti, op. cit.

71. Lyman A. Brewer, 'Cardiac transplantation: an appraisal', *JAMA* 205, no. 10 (1968), 691–2

72. Denton A. Cooley, *100,000 Hearts: A Surgeon's Memoir* (Austin, TX: Dolph Briscoe Center for American History, University of Texas at Austin, 2012), 124–5

73. Denton A. Cooley et al., 'Transplantation of the human heart: report of four cases', *JAMA* 205, no. 7 (1968), 479–86

74. Thomas Thompson, 'The year they changed hearts', *Life,* 17 September 1971

75. D. A. Cooley et al., 'Cardiac transplantation: general considerations and results', *Annals of Surgery* 169, no. 6 (1969), 892–905

76. Haller and Cerruti, op. cit.

77. Philip Blaiberg, *Looking at My Heart* (London: Heinemann, 1969), 118–19

78. K. Simpson, 'The moment of death – a new medico-legal problem', *South African Medical Journal* 41, no. 46 (1967), 1188–91

79. 'British heart transplant may be too early', *The Times,* 4 May 1968

80. 'Heart operation held in secrecy', *Guardian,* 4 May 1968

81. Donald Ross, 'Report of a heart transplant operation', *American Journal of Cardiology* 22, no. 6 (1968), 838–9

82. E. M. Tansey and L. A. Reynolds (eds), *Early Heart Transplant Surgery in the UK* (Wellcome Witnesses to Twentieth Century Medicine 3; London, 1999), 33

83. 'News and notes', *BMJ* 2, no. 5604 (1968), 567–70

84. 'Doctor criticises heart transplant "vultures"', *The Times,* 11 September 1968

85. S. S. Gilder, 'Twenty-second World Medical Assembly', *BMJ* 3, no. 5616 (1968), 493–4

86. 'A definition of irreversible coma. Report of the Ad Hoc Committee of the Harvard Medical School to Examine the Definition of Brain Death', *JAMA* 205, no. 6 (1968), 337–40

87. Robert J. Joynt, 'A new look at death', *JAMA* 252, no. 5 (1984), 680–82

88. Japan Organ Transplant Network, 'Japan Organ Transplant Network: the history of transplanting', cited 11 May 2016: http://www.jotnw.or.jp/english/01.html

89. Maria-Keiko Yasuoka, *Organ Donation in Japan: A Medical Anthropological Study* (Lanham, MD: Lexington Books, 2015), 9

90. Asako Saegusa, 'Japan's transplant law "is too stringent"', *Nature* 398, no. 6723 (1999), 95

91. Thompson, op. cit.

92. Tansey and Reynolds, op. cit., 35

93. David K. Cooper, 'Christiaan Barnard and his contributions to heart transplantation', *Journal of Heart and Lung Transplantation* 20, no. 6 (2001), 599–610

94. ibid.

95. J. Hassoulas and C. N. Barnard, 'Heterotopic cardiac transplantation. A 7-year experience at Groote Schuur Hospital, Cape Town', *South African Medical Journal* 65, no. 17 (1984), 675–82

96. Cooley et al., 'Cardiac transplantation: general considerations and results', op. cit.

97. Tansey and Reynolds, op. cit., 29–30

98. C. N. Barnard, A. Wolpowitz and J. G. Losman, 'Heterotopic cardiac transplantation with a xenograft for assistance of the left heart in cardiogenic shock after cardiopulmonary bypass', *South African Medical Journal* 52, no. 26 (1977), 1035–8

99. Barnard and Norval, op. cit.

100. Barnard, Wolpowitz and Losman, op. cit.

101. L. L. Bailey et al., 'Baboon-to-human cardiac xenotransplantation in a neonate', *JAMA* 254, no. 23 (1985), 3321–9

102. 'Baby Fae critical, but stable', Press Association, 29 October 1984

103. Bailey et al., op. cit.

104. Olga Jonasson and Mark A. Hardy, 'The case of Baby Fae', *JAMA* 254, no. 23 (1985), 3358–9

105. Heidi Evans, 'Talk about a guy with a lot of heart', *New York Daily News,* 13 April 2003

106. D. A. Clark et al., 'Cardiac transplantation in man. Review of first three years' experience', *American Journal of Medicine* 54, no. 5 (1973), 563–76

107. 'Interview with Norman E. Shumway', in Stoney (ed.), op. cit., 435

108. P. K. Caves et al., 'Diagnosis of human cardiac allograft rejection by serial cardiac biopsy', *Journal of Thoracic and Cardiovascular Surgery* 66, no. 3 (1973), 461–6

109. A. F. Graham et al., 'Acute rejection in the long-term cardiac transplant survivor. Clinical diagnosis, treatment and significance', *Circulation* 49, no. 2 (1974), 361–6

110. 'Interview with Norman E. Shumway', in Stoney (ed.), op. cit., 435

111. Author's interview with Terence English, 29 October 2015

112. ibid.

113. ibid.

114. J. F. Borel, Z. L. Kis and T. Beveridge, 'The history of the discovery and development of cyclosporine (Sandimmune®)', in *The Search for Anti-Inflammatory Drugs: Case Histories from Concept to Clinic* (ed. Vincent J. Merluzzi and Julian Adams; Boston: Birkhäuser, 1995), 27–63

115. C. J. Green and A. C. Allison, 'Extensive prolongation of rabbit kidney allograft survival after short-term cyclosporin – a treatment', *The Lancet* 1, no. 8075 (1978), 1182–3

116. R. Y. Calne et al., 'Prolonged survival of pig orthotopic heart grafts treated with cyclosporin A', *The Lancet* 1, no. 8075 (1978), 1183–5

117. Author's interview with Terence English, 29 October 2015

118. D. M. Canafax and N. L. Ascher, 'Cyclosporine immunosuppression', *Clinical Pharmacy* 2, no. 6 (1983), 515–24

119. The International Society for Heart and Lung Transplantation, 'Heart/Lung Transplant Registry', cited 8 July 2016: https://www.ishlt.org/registries/slides.asp?slides=heartLungRegistry

120. 'Interview with Norman E. Shumway', in Stoney (ed.), op. cit.

121. C. N. Barnard and D. K. Cooper, 'Clinical transplantation of the heart: a review of 13 years' personal experience', *Journal of the Royal Society of Medicine* 74, no. 9 (1981), 670–74

122. Alan Richman, 'Christiaan Barnard endorses cosmetics and the famous heart surgeon gets creamed', *People,* 14 April 1986

123. David Charter, Michael Theodoulou and Michael Dynes, 'Farewell to Barnard, the playboy king of hearts', *The Times,* 3 September 2001

9. CLINICAL TRIAL BY MEDIA

1. Ronald Ross, 'The Vivisector Vivisected', in *Horror Stories: Classic Tales from Hoffmann to Hodgson* (ed. Darryl Jones; Oxford: Oxford University Press, 2014), 176–89
2. 'Artificial hearts seen becoming major industry', United Press International, 17 August 1968
3. H. H. Dale and E. H. Schuster, 'A double perfusion-pump', *Journal of Physiology* 64, no. 4 (1928), 356–64
4. Richard J. Bing, 'Recollections of an eyewitness', Perspectives in Biology and Medicine 39, no.2 (1996), 227–38
5. C. A. Lindbergh, 'An apparatus for the culture of whole organs', *Journal of Experimental Medicine* 62, no. 3 (1935), 409–31
6. Alexis Carrel and Charles A. Lindbergh, *The Culture of Organs* (New York: P. B. Hoeber Inc., 1938), 219
7. *The Walking Dead* (director, Michael Curtiz), Warner Bros, 1936
8. V. P. Demikhov, *Experimental Transplantation of Vital Organs* (New York: Consultants Bureau, 1962), 212–13
9. W. H. Sewell Jr and W. W. Glenn, 'Experimental cardiac surgery. I. Observation on the action of a pump designed to shunt the venous blood past the right heart directly into the pulmonary artery', *Surgery* 28, no. 3 (1950), 474–94
10. W. J. Kolff et al., 'The artificial kidney: a dialyser with a great area', *Journal of Internal Medicine* 117, no. 2 (1944), 121–34
11. Peter F. Salisbury, 'History – The American Society for Artificial Internal Organs', *Transactions – American Society for Artificial Internal Organs* 6, no. 1 (1960), ii–vi
12. Peter F. Salisbury, 'Implantation of physiological machines into the mammalian organism. Identification of problems connected with the implantation of artificial hearts and of artificial kidneys. Experimental results to date', *Transactions – American Society for Artificial Internal Organs* 3, no. 1 (1957), 37–42
13. T. Akutsu and Willem J. Kolff, 'Permanent substitutes for valves and hearts', *Transactions – American Society for Artificial Internal Organs* 4, no. 1 (1958), 230–34
14. Kazuhiko Atsumi et al., 'Artificial heart incorporated in the chest', *Transactions – American Society for Artificial Internal Organs* 9, no. 1 (1963), 292–8
15. D. Liotta et al., 'Artificial heart in the chest: preliminary report', *Transactions – American Society for Artificial Internal Organs* 7 (1961), 318–22
16. Paul Winchell, 'Artificial heart', US patent no. 3097366A, 1963
17. Don B. Olsen, *True Valor: Barney Clark and the Utah Artificial Heart* (Salt Lake City: The University of Utah Press, 2015), 398
18. B. K. Kusserow, 'A permanently indwelling intracorporeal blood pump to substitute for cardiac function', *Transactions – American Society for Artificial Internal Organs* 4, no. 1 (1958), 227–9
19. Yukihiko Nosé, Martin Schamaun and Adrian Kantrowitz, 'Experimental use of an electronically controlled prosthesis as an auxiliary left ventricle', *Transactions – American Society for Artificial Internal Organs* 9, no. 1 (1963), 269–74

20. C. W. Hall et al., 'Development of artificial intrathoracic circulatory pumps', *American Journal of Surgery* 108 (1964), 685–92

21. Domingo Liotta et al., 'Prolonged assisted circulation during and after cardiac or aortic surgery', *American Journal of Cardiology* 12, no. 3 (1963), 399–405

22. Edwin Chen, 'Artificial heart – a case of pushing science "too fast"', *Los Angeles Times*, 12 January 1990

23. Hall et al., op. cit.

24. National Library of Medicine, 'Oral history interview of Michael DeBakey by Donald A. Schanche', tape 16, cited 19 July 2016: https://profiles.nlm.nih.gov/ps/retrieve/ResourceMetadata/FJBBTW

25. ibid.

26. Michael E. DeBakey, 'Left ventricular bypass pump for cardiac assistance', *American Journal of Cardiology* 27, no. 1 (1971), 3–11

27. 'Brooklyn doctor did such surgery 2½ months ago', United Press International, 22 April 1966

28. Adrian Kantrowitz et al., 'A clinical experience with an implanted mechanical auxiliary ventricle', *JAMA* 197, no. 7 (1966), 525–9

29. A. Kantrowitz, 'Moments in history. Introduction of left ventricular assistance', *Transactions – American Society for Artificial Internal Organs* 33, no. 1 (1987), 39–48

30. Adrian Kantrowitz and Arthur Kantrowitz, 'Experimental augmentation of coronary flow by retardation of the arterial pressure pulse', *Surgery* 34, no. 4 (1953), 678–87

31. John A. Jacobey et al., 'A new therapeutic approach to acute coronary occlusion', *American Journal of Cardiology* 11, no. 2 (1963), 218–27

32. R. H. Clauss et al., 'Assisted circulation by counter-pulsation with an intra-aortic balloon. Methods and effects', in *Digest of the 1962 15th Annual Conference on Engineering in Medicine and Biology, Chicago, Illinois, November 5–7, 1962* (ed. Hans U. Wessel; Chicago, 1962), 44

33. Spyridon D. Moulopoulos, Stephen Topaz and Willem J. Kolff, 'Diastolic balloon pumping (with carbon dioxide) in the aorta – A mechanical assistance to the failing circulation', *American Heart Journal* 63, no. 5 (1962), 669–75

34. Wladimir Schilt et al., 'Temporary non-surgical intraarterial cardiac assistance', *Transactions – American Society for Artificial Internal Organs* 13, no. 1 (1967), 322–7

35. Adrian Kantrowitz et al., 'Initial clinical experience with intraaortic balloon pumping in cardiogenic shock', *JAMA* 203, no. 2 (1968), 113–18

36. DeBakey, op. cit.

37. M. E. DeBakey et al., 'Orthotopic cardiac prosthesis: preliminary experiments in animals with biventricular artificial heart', *Cardiovascular Research Center Bulletin* 7, no. 4 (1969), 127–42

38. National Library of Medicine, 'Oral history interview of Michael DeBakey … ', tape 12, cited 2 August 2016: https://profiles.nlm.nih.gov/ps/retrieve/ResourceMetadata/FJBBTR

39. D. A. Cooley et al., 'Orthotopic cardiac prosthesis for two-staged cardiac replacement', *American Journal of Cardiology* 24, no. 5 (1969), 723–30

40. United States Court of Appeals, Fifth Circuit, Karp v Cooley and Liotta, 493, 1974

41. Cooley et al., op. cit.

42. 'Karp's wife pleads for donor of heart', Associated Press, 5 April 1969

43. Denton A. Cooley, *100,000 Hearts: A Surgeon's Memoir* (Austin, TX: Dolph Briscoe Center for American History, University of Texas at Austin, 2012), 142–3

44. Cooley et al., op. cit.

45. 'Ready for probe, says Dr Cooley', Associated Press, 11 April 1969

46. National Library of Medicine, 'Oral history interview of Michael DeBakey … ', tape 11, cited 2 August 2016: https://profiles.nlm.nih.gov/ps/retrieve/ResourceMetadata/FJBBTQ

47. ibid.

48. 'Surgeon draws censure letter', Associated Press, 10 December 1969

49. United States Court of Appeals, Fifth Circuit, Karp v Cooley and Liotta, 493, 1974

50. National Library of Medicine, 'Oral history interview of Michael DeBakey … ', tape 17, cited 19 July 2016: https://profiles.nlm.nih.gov/ps/retrieve/ResourceMetadata/FJBBTX

51. Thomas Thompson, 'The Texas Tornado v Dr Wonderful', *Life* 68, no. 13 (1970), 62–74

52. Max Lerner, 'Ethics of transplants', *New York Post*, 16 April 1969

53. Cooley et al., op. cit.

54. William E. Mott, 'Nuclear power for the artificial heart', *Biomaterials, Medical Devices, and Artificial Organs* 3, no. 2 (1975), 181–91

55. D. W. Cole, W. S. Holman and W. E. Mott, 'Status of the USAEC's nuclear-powered artificial heart', *Transactions – American Society for Artificial Internal Organs* 19 (1973), 537–41

56. National Heart and Lung Institute, Artificial Heart Assessment Panel, *The Totally Implantable Artificial Heart; Economic, Ethical, Legal, Medical, Psychiatric [and] Social Implications; a Report* (Bethesda: National Institutes of Health, 1973), 113–16

57. ibid., 107–09

58. A. R. Jonsen, 'The artificial heart's threat to others', *Hastings Center Report* 16, no. 1 (1986), 9–11

59. C. S. Kwan-Gett et al., 'Total replacement artificial heart and driving system with inherent regulation of cardiac output', *Transactions – American Society for Artificial Internal Organs* 15 (1969), 245–66

60. Yoshitsugu Kito et al., 'Recent results in total artificial heart', *Transactions – American Society for Artificial Internal Organs* 19, no. 1 (1973), 573–7

61. H. Oster et al., 'Survival for 18 days with a Jarvik-type artificial heart', *Surgery* 77, no. 1 (1975), 113–17

62. Arthur S. Freese, 'The pump that works like a heart', *Popular Mechanics* 134, no. 35 (1970), 128–201

63. Renée C. Fox and Judith P. Swazey, *Spare Parts: Organ Replacement in American Society* (New York, Oxford: Oxford University Press, 1992), 106

64. W. L. Hastings et al., 'A retrospective study of nine calves surviving five months on the pneumatic total artificial heart', *Transactions – American Society for Artificial Internal Organs* 27 (1981), 71–6

65. 'Interview with William C. DeVries', in Stoney (ed.), op. cit., 476

66. O. H. Frazier, T. Akutsu and D. A. Cooley, 'Total artificial heart (TAH) utilization in man', *Transactions – American Society for Artificial Internal Organs* 28 (1982), 534–8

67. Archives West: Barney B. Clark papers, 1910–1984, cited 24 July 2016: http://archiveswest.orbiscascade.org/ark:/80444/xv15817#historicalID

68. Willem Kolff Interview, Academy of Achievement, p. 6/9, cited 2 August 2016: http://www.achievement.org/autodoc/page/kol0int-6

69. Preface, *After Barney Clark: Reflections on the Utah Artificial Heart Program* (ed. Margery W. Shaw; Austin: University of Texas Press, 1984), ix–xi

70. William C. DeVries et al., 'Clinical use of the total artificial heart', *New England Journal of Medicine* 310, no. 5 (1984), 273–8

71. W. C. DeVries, 'Surgical technique for implantation of the Jarvik-7-100 total artificial heart', *JAMA* 259, no. 6 (1988), 875–80

72. Clyde Haberman, 'Artificial hearts ticking along decades after Jarvik-7 debate', *New York Times,* 20 March 2016, cited 26 August 2016: http://www.nytimes.com/2016/03/21/us/artificial-hearts-ticking-along-decades-after-jarvik-7-debate.html?_r=0

73. William C. DeVries, 'The physician, the media, and the "spectacular" case', *JAMA* 259, no. 6 (1988), 886–90

74. DeVries et al., 'Clinical use of the total artificial heart', op. cit.

75. Denton A. Cooley, 'Total artificial heart implantation', in *Reflections and Observations: Essays of Denton A. Cooley* (ed. Marianne Kneipp; Austin, TX: Eakin Press, 1984), 139–41

76. 'Interview with William C. DeVries', in Stoney (ed.), op. cit., 481–2

77. Fox and Swazey, op. cit., 116–17

78. Jonsen, op. cit.

79. 'Interview with William C. DeVries', in Stoney (ed.), op. cit., 480–81

80. Laurence Gonzales, 'The rock 'n' roll heart of Robert Jarvik; creator of artificial heart', *Playboy* 33, no. 4 (1986)

81. W. C. DeVries, 'The permanent artificial heart. Four case reports', *JAMA* 259, no. 6 (1988), 849–59

82. ibid.

83. K. E. Johnson et al., 'Registry report. Use of total artificial hearts: summary of world experience, 1969–1991', *Transactions – American Society for Artificial Internal Organs* 38, no. 3 (1992), M486–92

84. V. A. Starnes et al., 'Isolated left ventricular assist as bridge to cardiac transplantation', *Journal of Thoracic and Cardiovascular Surgery* 96, no. 1 (1988), 62–71

85. 'St Laurent dies 20 years after heart transplant', cited 26 August 2016: http://news.stanford.edu/news/2004/december8/med-stlaurent-1208.html

86. H. Wilkens, W. Regelson and F. S. Hoffmeister, 'The physiologic importance of pulsatile blood flow', *New England Journal of Medicine* 267 (1962), 443–6

87. Sigmund A. Wesolowski, 'The role of the pulse in maintenance of the systemic circulation during heart-lung bypass', *Transactions – American Society for Artificial Internal Organs* 1 (1955), 84–6

88. L. R. Golding et al., 'Chronic nonpulsatile blood flow', *Transactions – American Society for Artificial Internal Organs* 28 (1982), 81–5

89. O. H. Frazier et al., 'Clinical experience with the Hemopump', *Transactions – American Society for Artificial Internal Organs* 35, no. 3 (1989), 604–06

90. M. E. DeBakey, 'Development of a ventricular assist device', *Artificial Organs* 21, no. 11 (1997), 1149–53

91. G. M. Wieselthaler et al., 'First clinical experience with the DeBakey VAD continuous-axial-flow pump for bridge to transplantation', *Circulation* 101, no. 4 (2000), 356–9

92. Eric A. Rose et al., 'Long-term use of a left ventricular assist device for end-stage heart failure', *New England Journal of Medicine* 345, no. 20 (2001), 1435–43

93. NICE, 'Implantation of a left ventricular assist device for destination therapy in people ineligible for heart transplantation; 1-recommendations; Guidance and guidelines', cited 30 August 2016: https://www.nice.org.uk/guidance/IPG516/chapter/1-Recommendations

94. G. Gerosa et al., 'Successful heart transplant after 1374 days living with a total artificial heart', *European Journal of Cardiothoracic Surgery* 49, no. 4 (2016), e88–9

95. Denton A. Cooley and Joseph S. Coselli, 'Feuds: social and medical', *Texas Heart Institute Journal* 37, no. 6 (2010), 649–51

96. Lawrence Altman, 'The feud', *New York Times*, 27 November 2007

10. FANTASTIC VOYAGE

1. Charles T. Dotter, *Transluminal Angioplasty*, training film, 1965

2. Claude Bernard, *Leçons de Physiologie Opératoire* (Paris: Librarie J-B Bailliere et Fils, 1879), 277–9

3. Auguste Chauveau and Étienne-Jules Marey, 'Appareils et expériences cardiographiques: Démonstration nouvelle de mécanisme des mouvements du coeur par l'emploi des instruments enregistreurs a indications continues', *Mémoires de l'Académie Impériale de Médecine* 26 (1863), 268–319

4. Werner Forssmann, *Experiments on Myself: Memoirs of a Surgeon in Germany* (New York: St Martin's Press, 1974), 81–2

5. ibid., 83

6. ibid., 85–6

7. Werner Forssmann, 'Catheterization of the right heart', in *Classics of Cardiology* (ed. John A. Callahan, Thomas E. Keys and Jack D. Key; 4 vols; Krieger, 1983), 3: 252–5

8. 'Medical contact with the heart', *Brooklyn Daily Eagle*, 6 November 1929

9. Forssmann, *Experiments on Myself*, op. cit., 99

10. Werner Forssmann, 'Über Kontrastdarstellung der Höhlen des lebenden rechten Herzens und der Lungenschlagader', *Munchener Medizinische Wochenschrift* 78 (1931), 490–92

11. Forssmann, *Experiments on Myself*, op. cit., 128–9

12. Pierre Ameuille, 'Remarques sur quelques cas d'artériographie pulmonaire chez l'homme vivant', *Bulletins et Mémoires de la Société Médicale des Hôpitaux* 52 (1936), 729–39

13. Allen B. Weisse, *Heart to Heart: The Twentieth Century Battle Against Cardiac Disease: an Oral History* (New Brunswick, NJ: Rutgers University Press, 2002), 33

14. A. J. Dunning, 'Interview with André Cournand at Leiden, November 1979', in *History and Perspectives of Cardiology: Catherization, Angiography, Surgery, and Concepts of Circular Control* (ed. H. A. Snellen, A. J. Dunning and Alexander C. Arntzenius; The Hague, Boston, Hingham, MA: Leiden University Press, 1981), 33–7

15. A. Cournand, 'Cardiac catheterization; development of the technique, its contributions to experimental medicine, and its initial applications in man', *Acta Medica Scandinavica. Supplementum* 579 (1975), 3–32

16. André Cournand and Hilmert A. Ranges, 'Catheterization of the right auricle in man', *Experimental Biology and Medicine* 46, no. 3 (1941), 462–6

17. Eleanor Baldwin, Lucille V. Moore and Robert P. Noble, 'The demonstration of ventricular septal defect by means of right heart catheterization', *American Heart Journal* 32, no. 2 (1946), 152–62

18. Emmett S. Brannon, H. S. Weens and James V. Warren, 'Atrial septal defect: study of hemodynamics by the technique of right heart catheterization', *American Journal of the Medical Sciences* 210, no. 4 (1945), 480–90

19. S. Howarth, J. McMichael and E. P. Sharpey-Schafer, 'Cardiac catheterization in cases of patent interauricular septum, primary pulmonary hypertension, Fallot's tetralogy, and pulmonary stenosis', *British Heart Journal* 9, no. 4 (1947), 292–303

20. A. J. Benatt, 'Cardiac catheterization; a historical note', *The Lancet* 1, no. 6557 (1949), 746

21. The Nobel Prize in Physiology or Medicine 1956, cited 16 September 2016: http://www. nobelprize.org/nobel_prizes/medicine/laureates/1956/

22. Forssmann, *Experiments on Myself*, op. cit., 284

23. P. L. Fariñas, 'A new technique for the arteriographic examination of the abdominal aorta and its branches', *American Journal of Roentgenology* 46 (1941), 641–5

24. Henry A. Zimmerman, Roy W. Scott and Norman O. Becker, 'Catheterization of the left side of the heart in man', *Circulation* 1, no. 3 (1950), 357–9

25. J. Willis Hurst, 'History of cardiac catheterization', in *Coronary Arteriography and Angioplasty* (ed. Spencer B. King and John S. Douglas; New York, London: McGraw-Hill, 1985), 1–9

26. John Ross Jr, 'Transseptal left heart catheterization: a 50-year odyssey', *Journal of the American College of Cardiology* 51, no. 22 (2008), 2107–15

27. Gunnar Jönsson, 'Selective visualization in angiocardiography', *Journal of the Faculty of Radiologists* 3, no. 2 (1951), 125–9

28. C. T. Dotter, 'Cardiac catheterization and angiographic technics of the future. Background and current status of clinical catheter angiography', *Ceskoslovenska Radiologie* 19, no. 4 (1965), 217–36

29. Josef Rösch, Frederick S. Keller and John A. Kaufman, 'The birth, early years, and future of interventional radiology', *Journal of Vascular and Interventional Radiology* 14, no. 7 (2003), 841–53

30. T. J. Fogarty et al., 'A method for extraction of arterial emboli and thrombi', *Surgery, Gynecology & Obstetrics* 116 (1963), 241–4

31. Richard Mullins, 'Interview with Albert Starr, MD', 2006: http://digitalcommons.ohsu. edu/cgi/viewcontent.cgi?article=1080&context=hca-oralhist

32. M. M. Payne, 'Charles Theodore Dotter: The father of intervention', *Texas Heart Institute Journal* 28, no. 1 (2001), 28–38

33. Charles T. Dotter and Melvin P. Judkins, 'Transluminal treatment of arteriosclerotic obstruction', *Circulation* 30, no. 5 (1964), 654–70

34. 'Portraits in radiology: Charles T. Dotter, MD', *Applied Radiology* 10 (1981), 116

35. T. J. Fogarty et al., 'Intraoperative transluminal angioplasty', in *Haimovici's Vascular Surgery* (ed. Henry Haimovici; 4th ed.; Cambridge, MA, Oxford: Blackwell Science, 1996), 257–66

36. Josef Rösch and Frederick S. Keller, 'Historical account: cardiovascular interventional radiology', in *Catheter-Based Cardiovascular Interventions: A Knowledge-Based Approach* (ed. P. Lanzer; Heidelberg, New York: Springer, 2013), 15–26

37. P. Jerie, 'Thirty years of the balloon catheter – A. Grüntzig and percutaneous balloon angioplasty', *Casopis Lekaru Ceskych* 143, no. 12 (2004), 866–71

38. M. Barton et al., 'Balloon angioplasty – the legacy of Andreas Grüntzig, MD (1939–1985)', *Frontiers in Cardiovascular Medicine* 1 (2014), 15

39. ibid.

40. Jerie, op. cit.

41. Spencer B. King, 'The development of interventional cardiology', *Journal of the American College of Cardiology* 31, No. 4, Supplement 2 (1998), 64B–88B

42. M. Schlumpf, '30 Jahre Ballonkatheter: Andreas Grüntzig, ein Pionier in Zürich', *Schweizerische Ärztezeitung* 85, no. 7 (2004), 346–51

43. Barton et al., op. cit.

44. ibid.

45. Bernhard Meier, Dölf Bachmann and Thomas F. Lüscher, '25 years of coronary angioplasty: almost a fairy tale', *The Lancet* 361, no. 9356 (2003), 527

46. J. W. Hurst, 'The first coronary angioplasty as described by Andreas Gruentzig', *American Journal of Cardiology* 57, no. 1 (1986), 185–6

47. Barton et al., op. cit.

48. H. J. Swan, 'Coronary stents – Introduction', in *Coronary Stents* (ed. Ulrich Sigwart and George I. Frank; Berlin, Heidelberg: Springer Berlin Heidelberg, 1992), 1–3

49. Kenneth M. Kent et al., 'Long-term efficacy of percutaneous transluminal coronary angioplasty (PTCA): Report from the National Heart, Lung, and Blood Institute PTCA Registry', *American Journal of Cardiology* 53, no. 12 (1984), C27–31

50. K. P. Rentrop et al., 'Initial experience with transluminal recanalization of the recently occluded infarct-related coronary artery in acute myocardial infarction – Comparison with conventionally treated patients', *Clinical Cardiology* 2, no. 2 (1979), 92–105

51. Geoffrey O. Hartzler, Barry D. Rutherford and David R. McConahay, 'Percutaneous transluminal coronary angioplasty: application for acute myocardial infarction', *American Journal of Cardiology* 53, no. 12 (1984), C117–121

52. Jerie, op. cit.

53. 'Andreas Gruentzig dies in air crash', UPI, 28 October 1985

54. W. Rutsch, 'Transluminale koronare Angioplastie: 20 Jahre Follow-up der ersten 6 Patienten aus Zürich und Frankfurt', *Zeitschrift für Kardiologie* 87, no. 15 (1998), s1–7

55. Bernhard Meier, 'The world's longest follow-up after percutaneous coronary intervention, 37 years and still going strong', *European Heart Journal* 36, no. 19 (2015), 1154

56. Ariel Roguin, 'Stent: the man and word behind the coronary metal prosthesis', *Circulation: Cardiovascular Interventions* 4, no. 2 (2011), 206–09

57. Dotter and Judkins, op. cit.

58. C. T. Dotter, 'Transluminally-placed coilspring endarterial tube grafts. Long-term patency in canine popliteal artery', *Investigative Radiology* 4, no. 5 (1969), 329–32

59. Author's interview with Ulrich Sigwart, 22 September 2016

60. Ulrich Sigwart, 'Living history of medicine: vascular scaffolding, from dream to reality', *European Heart Journal*, 2016: http://eurheartj.oxfordjournals.org/content/early/2016/01/19/eurheartj.ehv656.long

61. Aaron S. Kesselheim, Shuai Xu and Jerry Avorn, 'Clinicians' contributions to the development of coronary artery stents: a qualitative study of transformative device innovation', *Plos One* 9, no. 2 (2014), e88664

62. Sigwart, op. cit.

63. Kesselheim, Xu and Avorn, op. cit.

64. Sigwart, op. cit.

65. Author's interview with Ulrich Sigwart

66. U. Sigwart et al., 'Intravascular stents to prevent occlusion and restenosis after transluminal angioplasty', *New England Journal of Medicine* 316, no. 12 (1987), 701–06

67. Author's interview with Tony Gershlick, 15 December 2015

68. D. L. Fischman et al., 'A randomized comparison of coronary-stent placement and balloon angioplasty in the treatment of coronary artery disease. Stent Restenosis Study Investigators', *New England Journal of Medicine* 331, no. 8 (1994), 496–501

69. Nadim M. Zacca et al., 'Treatment of symptomatic peripheral atherosclerotic disease with a rotational atherectomy device', *American Journal of Cardiology* 63, no. 1 (1989), 77–80

70. Patrick W. Serruys et al., 'Angiographic follow-up after placement of a self-expanding coronary-artery stent', *New England Journal of Medicine* 324, no. 1 (1991), 13–17

71. A. M. Lincoff, E. J. Topol and S. G. Ellis, 'Local drug delivery for the prevention of restenosis. Fact, fancy, and future', *Circulation* 90, no. 4 (1994), 2070–84

72. Claude Vézina, Alicia Kudelski and S. N. Sehgal, 'Rapamycin (AY-22, 989), a new antifungal antibiotic', *Journal of Antibiotics* 28, no. 10 (1975), 721–6

73. Marie-Claude Morice et al., 'A randomized comparison of a sirolimus-eluting stent with a standard stent for coronary revascularization', *New England Journal of Medicine* 346, no. 23 (2002), 1773–80

74. Joanna J. Wykrzykowska, Yoshinobu Onuma and Patrick W. Serruys, 'Vascular restoration therapy: the fourth revolution in interventional cardiology and the ultimate "Rosy" prophecy', *EuroIntervention* 5, F (2009), F7–8

75. John A. Ormiston et al., 'A bioabsorbable everolimus-eluting coronary stent system for patients with single de-novo coronary artery lesions (ABSORB): A prospective open-label trial', *The Lancet* 371, no. 9616 (2008), 899–907

76. Eurostat, 'Cardiovascular diseases statistics', cited 28 September 2016: http://ec.europa.eu/eurostat/statistics-explained/index.php/Cardiovascular_diseases_statistics

77. Healthcare Quality Improvement Partnership, *National Audit of Percutaneous Coronary Interventions – Annual Report*, 2016

78. W. J. Rashkind, 'Transcatheter treatment of congenital heart disease', *Circulation* 67, no. 4 (1983), 711–16

79. W. J. Rashkind and W. W. Miller, 'Creation of an atrial septal defect without thoracotomy. A palliative approach to complete transposition of the great arteries', *JAMA* 196, no. 11 (1966), 991–2

80. 'Balloon to save a baby', *Time* 60, no. 21 (1966), 65–6

81. S. C. Park et al., 'Clinical use of blade atrial septostomy', *Circulation* 58, no. 4 (1978), 600–06

82. Michael DeVault, 'King of hearts', cited 29 September 2016: http://www.bayoulifemag.com/king-of-hearts/

83. N. L. Mills and T. D. King, 'Nonoperative closure of left-to-right shunts', *Journal of Thoracic and Cardiovascular Surgery* 72, no. 3 (1976), 371–8

84. J. S. Kan et al., 'Percutaneous balloon valvuloplasty: a new method for treating congenital pulmonary-valve stenosis', *New England Journal of Medicine* 307, no. 9 (1982), 540–42

85. Colin K. Phoon, 'Jean S. Kan, MD: A conversation with Colin K.L. Phoon, MPhil, MD', *American Journal of Cardiology* 101, no. 1 (2008), 129–38

86. J. E. Lock et al., 'Percutaneous catheter commissurotomy in rheumatic mitral stenosis', *New England Journal of Medicine* 313, no. 24 (1985), 1515–18

87. Patrick Wintour and Sarah Boseley, 'Tony Blair in heart scare', *Guardian*, 20 October 2003

88. Hasan Goran, 'Professor Hein J. J. Wellens: 33 years of cardiology and arrhythmology', *Circulation* 104, no. 12 (2001), e64

89. D. Durrer et al., 'The role of premature beats in the initiation and the termination of supraventricular tachycardia in the Wolff–Parkinson–White syndrome', *Circulation* 36, no. 5 (1967), 644–62

90. F. R. Cobb et al., 'Successful surgical interruption of the bundle of Kent in a Patient with Wolff–Parkinson–White syndrome', *Circulation* 38, no. 6 (1968), 1018–29

91. R. Gonzalez et al., 'Closed-chest electrode-catheter technique for His bundle ablation in dogs', *American Journal of Physiology* 241, no. 2 (1981), H283–7

92. W. M. Jackman et al., 'Catheter ablation of accessory atrioventricular pathways (Wolff–Parkinson–White syndrome) by radiofrequency current', *New England Journal of Medicine* 324, no. 23 (1991), 1605–11

93. Harvey W. Cushing, 'Electro-surgery as an aid to the removal of intracranial tumors. With a preliminary note on a new surgical-current generator by W. T. Bovie', *Surgery, Gynecology & Obstetrics* 47 (1928), 751–84

94. 'Electric knife is used to restore lost sanity', *Popular Mechanics* 48, no. 4 (1927), 604–05

95. T. Budde et al., 'Initial experiences with high-frequency electric ablation of the AV conduction system in the human', *Zeitschrift für Kardiologie* 76, no. 4 (1987), 204–10

96. Jackman et al., op. cit.

97. Author's interview with Andrew Grace, 1 December 2015

11. I, ROBOT (SURGEON)

1. Bridget Cherry and Nikolaus Pevsner, *The Buildings of England: London 2: South* (London: Yale University Press, 2002), 94

2. Jochen Reinöhl et al., 'Effect of availability of transcatheter aortic-valve replacement on clinical practice', *New England Journal of Medicine* 373, no. 25 (2015), 2438–47

3. Hywel Davies, 'Catheter-mounted valve for temporary relief of aortic insufficiency', *The Lancet* 285, no. 7379 (1965), 250

4. Aarhus University, 'The Andersen Patent', cited 7 November 2016: http://www.au.dk/en/about/profile/publications/ordogbilleder/2003/chapter12/

5. H. R. Andersen, L. L. Knudsen and J. M. Hasenkam, 'Transluminal implantation of artificial heart valves. Description of a new expandable aortic valve and initial results with implantation by catheter technique in closed chest pigs', *European Heart Journal* 13, no. 5 (1992), 704–08

6. P. Bonhoeffer et al., 'Percutaneous replacement of pulmonary valve in a right-ventricle to pulmonary-artery prosthetic conduit with valve dysfunction', *The Lancet* 356, no. 9239 (2000), 1403–05

7. Alain Cribier, 'Development of transcatheter aortic valve implantation (TAVI): a 20-year odyssey', *Archives of Cardiovascular Diseases* 105, no. 3 (2012), 146–52

8. Alain Cribier et al., 'Percutaneous transcatheter implantation of an aortic valve prosthesis for calcific aortic stenosis: First human case description', *Circulation* 106, no. 24 (2002), 3006–08

9. ibid.

10. Cribier, 'Development of transcatheter aortic valve …', op. cit.

11. M. B. Leon et al., 'Transcatheter aortic-valve implantation for aortic stenosis in patients who cannot undergo surgery', *New England Journal of Medicine* 363, no. 17 (2010), 1597–607

12. C. R. Smith et al., 'Transcatheter versus surgical aortic-valve replacement in high-risk patients', *New England Journal of Medicine* 364, no. 23 (2011), 2187–98

13. Lars Søndergaard et al., 'First-in-human case of transfemoral CardiAQ mitral valve implantation', *Circulation: Cardiovascular Interventions* 8, no. 7 (2015), e002135

14. S. L. Goldberg and T. Feldman, 'Percutaneous mitral valve interventions: overview of new approaches', *Current Cardiology Reports* 12, no. 5 (2010), 404–12

15. J. G. Webb et al., 'Percutaneous transvenous mitral annuloplasty: initial human experience with device implantation in the coronary sinus', *Circulation* 113, no. 6 (2006), 851–5

16. Lindsey D. Allan, Lisa K. Hornberger and G. K. Sharland, *Textbook of Fetal Cardiology* (London: Greenwich Medical Media, 2000)

17. L. D. Allan et al., 'Echocardiographic and anatomical correlates in the fetus', *Heart* 44, no. 4 (1980), 444–51

18. L. D. Allan et al., 'Identification of congenital cardiac malformations by echocardiography in midtrimester fetus', *British Heart Journal* 46, no. 4 (1981), 358–62

19. D. Maxwell, L. Allan and M. J. Tynan, 'Balloon dilatation of the aortic valve in the fetus: a report of two cases', *British Heart Journal* 65, no. 5 (1991), 256–8

20. J. I. Hoffman and S. Kaplan, 'The incidence of congenital heart disease', *Journal of the American College of Cardiology* 39, no. 12 (2002), 1890–900

21. Doff B. McElhinney, Wayne Tworetzky and James E. Lock, 'Current status of fetal cardiac intervention', *Circulation* 121, no. 10 (2010), 1256–63

22. Author's interview with Jay VanDerwerken, 1 November 2016

23. A. C. Marshall et al., 'Results of in utero atrial septoplasty in fetuses with hypoplastic left heart syndrome', *Prenatal Diagnosis* 28, no. 11 (2008), 1023–8

24. A. Carpentier, 'Cardiac valve surgery – the "French correction"', *Journal of Thoracic and Cardiovascular Surgery* 86, no. 3 (1983), 323–37

25. G. Kelling, 'Die Tamponade der Bauchhöhle mit Luft zur Stillung lebensgefährlicher Intestinalblutungen', *Munchener Medizinische Wochenschrift* 48 (1901), 1480–83

26. José L. Navia and Delos M. Cosgrove, 'Minimally invasive mitral valve operations', *Annals of Thoracic Surgery* 62, no. 5 (1996), 1542–4

27. R. A. Felder et al., 'Robotics in the medical laboratory', *Clinical Chemistry* 36, no. 9 (1990), 1534–43

28. A. Carpentier et al., 'Computer assisted open heart surgery. First case operated on with success', *Comptes Rendus de l'Academie des Sciences. Serie III, Sciences de la Vie* 321, no. 5 (1998), 437–42

29. V. Falk et al., 'Robot-assisted minimally invasive solo mitral valve operation', *Journal of Thoracic and Cardiovascular Surgery* 115, no. 2 (1998), 470–71

30. Friedrich W. Mohr et al., 'Computer-enhanced "robotic" cardiac surgery: Experience in 148 patients', *Journal of Thoracic and Cardiovascular Surgery* 121, no. 5 (2001), 842–53

31. Didier Loulmet et al., 'Endoscopic coronary artery bypass grafting with the aid of robotic assisted instruments', *Journal of Thoracic and Cardiovascular Surgery* 118, no. 1 (1999), 4–10

32. N. J. Verberkmoes et al., 'Distal anastomotic patency of the Cardica C-PORT(R) xA system versus the hand-sewn technique: a prospective randomized controlled study in patients undergoing coronary artery bypass grafting', *European Journal of Cardio-Thoracic Surgery* 44, no. 3 (2013), 512–18

33. E. Soylu et al., 'A systematic review of the safety and efficacy of distal coronary artery anastomotic devices in MIDCAB and TECAB surgery', *Perfusion* 31, no. 7 (2016), 537–43

34. Rakesh M. Suri et al., 'Mitral valve repair using robotic technology: Safe, effective, and durable', *Journal of Thoracic and Cardiovascular Surgery* 151, no. 6 (2016), 1450–54

35. Murali Chakravarthy et al., 'Conscious cardiac surgery with cardiopulmonary bypass using thoracic epidural anesthesia without endotracheal general anesthesia', *Journal of Cardiothoracic and Vascular Anesthesia* 19, no. 3 (2005), 300–05

36. NHS Blood and Transplant, *Annual Report on Cardiothoracic Transplantation 2013/2014* (2016)

37. Author's interview with André Simon, 24 November 2015

38. Saez D. Garcia et al., 'Evaluation of the Organ Care System in heart transplantation with an adverse donor/recipient profile', *Annals of Thoracic Surgery* 98, no. 6 (2014), 2099–2105

39. A. Ali et al., 'Cardiac recovery in a human non-heart-beating donor after extracorporeal perfusion: source for human heart donation?' *Journal of Heart and Lung Transplantation* 28, no. 3 (2009), 290–93

40. Kumud K. Dhital et al., 'Adult heart transplantation with distant procurement and ex-vivo preservation of donor hearts after circulatory death: A case series', *The Lancet* 385, no. 9987 (2015), 2585–91

41. S. Messer and S. Large, 'Resuscitating heart transplantation: the donation after circulatory determined death donor', *European Journal of Cardio-Thoracic Surgery* 49, no. 1 (2016), 1–4

42. Author's interview with Stephen Large, 1 December 2015

43. T. Noterdaeme et al., 'What is the potential increase in the heart graft pool by cardiac donation after circulatory death?' *Transplant International* 26, no. 1 (2013), 61–6

44. Author's interview with André Simon, 24 November 2015

45. Corbin E. Goerlich, O. H. Frazier and William E. Cohn, 'Previous challenges and current progress – the use of total artificial hearts in patients with end-stage heart failure', *Expert Review of Cardiovascular Therapy* 14, no. 10 (2016), 1095–8

46. A. Carpentier et al., 'First clinical use of a bioprosthetic total artificial heart: report of two cases', *The Lancet* 386, no. 10003 (2015), 1556–63

47. Carmat press release, 'Information regarding the feasibility study of the CARMAT bioprosthetic artificial heart', 21 January 2016. Online: http://www.carmatsa.com/en/media-gb/press-releases/item/download/485_3000d273837bd1dd6337628cf466c668

48. Roy Calne, 'Xenografting – the future of transplantation, and always will be?' *Xenotransplantation* 12, no. 1 (2005), 5–6

49. Author's interview with David Cooper, 25 May 2016

50. A. M. Rosengard et al., 'Tissue expression of human complement inhibitor, decay-accelerating factor, in transgenic pigs. A potential approach for preventing xenograft rejection', *Transplantation* 59, no. 9 (1995), 1325–33

51. Nuala Moran, 'Pig-to-human heart transplant slated to begin in 1996', *Nature Medicine* 1, no. 10 (1995), 987

52. C. Patience, Y. Takeuchi and R. A. Weiss, 'Infection of human cells by an endogenous retrovirus of pigs', *Nature Medicine* 3, no. 3 (1997), 282–6

53. C. J. Phelps et al., 'Production of alpha 1,3-galactosyltransferase-deficient pigs', *Science* 299, no. 5605 (2003), 411–14

54. K. Kuwaki et al., 'Heart transplantation in baboons using α1,3-galactosyltransferase gene-knockout pigs as donors: initial experience', *Nature Medicine* 11, no. 1 (2005), 29–31

55. Author's interview with David Cooper, 25 May 2016

56. B. Petersen et al., 'Pigs transgenic for human thrombomodulin have elevated production of activated protein C', *Xenotransplantation* 16, no. 6 (2009), 486–95

57. M. M. Mohiuddin et al., 'One-year heterotopic cardiac xenograft survival in a pig to baboon model', *American Journal of Transplantation* 14, no. 2 (2014), 488–9

58. Raghav Murthy et al., 'Heart xenotransplantation: historical background, experimental progress, and clinical prospects', *Annals of Thoracic Surgery* 101, no. 4 (2016), 1605–13

59. Author's interview with David Cooper, 25 May 2016

60. Calne, op. cit.

61. Wayne Paris et al., 'Psychosocial challenges of xenotransplantation: the need for a multidisciplinary, religious, and cultural dialogue', *Xenotransplantation* 23, no. 5 (2016), 335–7

62. Ernest W. Goodpasture, *Leo Loeb, 1869–1959: A Biographical Memoir* (New York: National Academy of Sciences, 1961), 209–10

63. C. A. Vacanti, 'The history of tissue engineering', *Journal of Cellular and Molecular Medicine* 10, no. 3 (2006), 569–76

64. R. Langer and J. Vacanti, 'Tissue engineering', *Science* 260, no. 5110 (1993), 920–26

65. Toshiharu Shin'oka, Yasuharu Imai and Yoshito Ikada, 'Transplantation of a tissue-engineered pulmonary artery', *New England Journal of Medicine* 344, no. 7 (2001), 532–3

66. J. A. Thomson et al., 'Embryonic stem cell lines derived from human blastocysts', *Science* 282, no. 5391 (1998), 1145–7

67. K. Takahashi et al., 'Induction of pluripotent stem cells from adult human fibroblasts by defined factors', *Cell* 131, no. 5 (2007), 861–72

68. Author's interview with Sanjay Sinha, 25 October 2016

69. D. Kehl, B. Weber and S. P. Hoerstrup, 'Bioengineered living cardiac and venous valve replacements: current status and future prospects', *Cardiovascular Pathology* 25, no. 4 (2016), 300–05

70. B. Schmitt et al., 'Percutaneous pulmonary valve replacement using completely tissue-engineered off-the-shelf heart valves: six-month in vivo functionality and matrix remodelling in sheep', *EuroIntervention* 12, no. 1 (2016), 62–70

71. Rachael W. Quinn et al., 'Performance of allogeneic bioengineered replacement pulmonary valves in rapidly growing young lambs', *Journal of Thoracic and Cardiovascular Surgery* 152, no. 4 (2016), 1156–65.e4

72. H. C. Ott et al., 'Perfusion-decellularized matrix: using nature's platform to engineer a bioartificial heart', *Nature Medicine* 14, no. 2 (2008), 213–21

73. A. Weymann et al., 'Bioartificial heart: a human-sized porcine model – the way ahead', *Plos One* 9, no. 11 (2014)

74. L. A. Hockaday et al., 'Rapid 3D printing of anatomically accurate and mechanically heterogeneous aortic valve hydrogel scaffolds', *Biofabrication* 4, no. 3 (2012), 35005

75. Thomas J. Hinton et al., 'Three-dimensional printing of complex biological structures by freeform reversible embedding of suspended hydrogels', *Science Advances* 1, no. 9 (2015), e1500758

76. Carnegie Mellon University, 'Carnegie Mellon researchers hack off-the-shelf 3D printer toward rebuilding the heart', cited 5 December 2016: https://engineering.cmu.edu/media/feature/2015/10_23_feinberg_paper.html

77. H. M. Sherman, 'The future of heart surgery', *California State Journal of Medicine* 8, no. 7 (1910), 227–32

78. Judith Mackay et al., *The Atlas of Heart Disease and Stroke* (Geneva: World Health Organization, 2004), 75

79. Harry M. Sherman, 'Suture of heart wounds: oration on surgery, delivered before the fifty-third annual meeting of the American Medical Association at Saratoga Springs, NY, June 10–13, 1902', *JAMA* 38, no. 24 (1902), 1560–68

INDEX